Dengue: Prevention, Diagnosis and Treatment

Dengue: Prevention, Diagnosis and Treatment

Edited by Marcel Soto

AMERICAN
MEDICAL PUBLISHERS
www.americanmedicalpublishers.com

American Medical Publishers,
41 Flatbush Avenue,
1st Floor, New York,
NY 11217, USA

Visit us on the World Wide Web at:
www.americanmedicalpublishers.com

ISBN: 978-1-63927-221-1

Cataloging-in-Publication Data

Dengue : prevention, diagnosis and treatment / edited by Marcel Soto.
p. cm.
Includes bibliographical references and index.
ISBN 978-1-63927-221-1
1. Dengue. 2. Dengue--Prevention. 3. Dengue--Diagnosis. 4. Dengue--Treatment.
5. Hemorrhagic fever. 6. Dengue viruses. I. Soto, Marcel.
RC137 .D46 2022
616.918 52--dc23

Table of Contents

Preface

Dengue fever is a tropical disease that is caused by the dengue virus. It is spread by various species of female Aedes type mosquitoes. The symptoms of dengue appear after three to fourteen days of infection. The most common symptoms include headache, fever, vomiting, muscle and joint pains and skin rashes. It can be life-threatening in some cases. It can also affect other body systems. A few of the neurological disorders can also occur in dengue such as transverse myelitis and Guillain-barre syndrome. It can cause miscarriage, low birth rate and premature birth in a pregnant woman. Dengue can develop into dengue hemorrhagic fever that causes bleeding, low levels of blood platelets and blood plasma leakage. The diagnosis of dengue is based on physical examination and symptoms. The book presents researches and studies performed by experts across the globe. It contains some path-breaking studies about dengue. It will serve as a valuable source of reference for graduate and post graduate students.

After months of intensive research and writing, this book is the end result of all who devoted their time and efforts in the initiation and progress of this book. It will surely be a source of reference in enhancing the required knowledge of the new developments in the area. During the course of developing this book, certain measures such as accuracy, authenticity and research focused analytical studies were given preference in order to produce a comprehensive book in the area of study.

This book would not have been possible without the efforts of the authors and the publisher. I extend my sincere thanks to them. Secondly, I express my gratitude to my family and well-wishers. And most importantly, I thank my students for constantly expressing their willingness and curiosity in enhancing their knowledge in the field, which encourages me to take up further research projects for the advancement of the area.

Editor

1

Accuracy of clinical criteria and an immunochromatographic strip test for dengue diagnosis in a DENV-4 epidemic

Sibelle Nogueira Buonora[1*], Sonia Regina Lambert Passos[1], Cleber Nascimento do Carmo[2], Fernanda Moisés Quintela[1], Diana Neves Rodrigues de Oliveira[1], Flavia Barreto dos Santos[4], Yara Hahr Marques Hökerberg[1], Rita Maria Ribeiro Nogueira[4] and Regina Paiva Daumas[3]

Abstract

Background: Early diagnosis of dengue infection is important for decision-making and timely implementation of therapeutic measures. Although rapid NS1 assays have been used for dengue diagnosis since 2008, their performance in DENV-4 cases has not yet been fully assessed.

Methods: We evaluated the accuracy of NS1 Bioeasy™ immunochromatographic strip test and of three clinical criteria for dengue diagnosis. Patients presenting at an emergency care center within 72 h of an acute febrile illness during the 2013 DENV-4 epidemic in Rio de Janeiro were consecutively enrolled for clinical and laboratory evaluation. We classified patients as suspected dengue or not according to three clinical criteria: WHO 2009, WHO 1997, and INI-FIOCRUZ. Dengue diagnosis was defined by RNA detection using RT-PCR and the negative cases were negative for all dengue serotypes and also Platelia™ NS1 ELISA. We obtained accuracy indices for NS1 Bioeasy™ alone and in combination with the clinical criteria.

Results: RT-PCR for DENV-4 was positive in 148 out of 325 patients. Positive likelihood ratio, sensitivity, and specificity of NS1 Bioeasy™ with WHO 2009, WHO 1997, and INI-FIOCRUZ criteria were 22.6 (95 % CI 7.2–70.6), 40.6 % (95 % CI 32.3–49.3), and 98.2 % (95 % CI 94.9–99.6); 18.3 (95 % CI 6.8–49.2), 44.2 (95 % CI 35.8–52.9), 97.6 (95 % CI 94.0–99.3); 26.2 (95 % CI 6.5–106.5), 29.7 (95 % CI 22.4–37.8), 98.9 (95 % CI 96.0–99.9), respectively. WHO 1997 clinical criteria presented high sensitivity to rule out disease, but extremely low specificity. INI-FIOCRUZ had moderate sensitivity and specificity, and could target a group to a more specific test.

Conclusions: Although the large rates of false negative results using NS1 Bioeasy™ rapid test advise against its use for triaging (rule out) purposes in DENV-4 epidemics, it could be used as a confirmatory tool in a bedside algorithm.

Keywords: Dengue, Accuracy, Sensitivity, Specificity, Diagnosis, Point-of-care systems, NS1

Background

Dengue is an acute viral febrile disease mainly transmitted by the *Aedes aegypti* mosquito. Dengue virus has four serotypes (DENV 1-4) defined by phylogenetic and antigenic characteristics. The immunity resulting from infection is serotype-specific and does not protect the individual against other serotypes [1].

* Correspondence: sibellebuonora@gmail.com
[1]Laboratory of Clinical Epidemiology, Evandro Chagas National Institute of Infectious Diseases, Oswaldo Cruz Foundation, Rio de Janeiro, Brazil
Full list of author information is available at the end of the article

A recent study estimated that about 390 million cases of dengue occurred in 2010, which is more than three times the World Health Organization (WHO) estimates for that same period [2]. However, only 96 million were symptomatic. Brazil has the highest dengue reporting rates worldwide and between 2000 and 2007, over three million cases were reported in the country, corresponding to approximately 60 % of cases in the Americas [3].

In Brazil, dengue outbreaks have occurred yearly since 1986 and during epidemic seasons the entire health care system is overwhelmed by a three to four-fold increase in patient visits. In the state of Rio de Janeiro, epidemics occurred in 1986 [4], 1990 [5], 2000 [6], and 2008 [7] by DENV-1, DENV-2, DENV-3, and by the reemergence of DENV-2, respectively, usually followed by dissemination to other regions of the country. DENV-4 was first identified in this Brazilian state in 2011 [8] and accounted for 218,000 reported cases in the 2013 epidemic.

Early diagnosis is critical because some patients may progress from a mild to a severe disease in a short period of time [9, 10]. Repeated monitoring of platelet count and hematocrit is recommended, as an abrupt decrease in platelet count is a warning sign and a significant hematocrit increase is an indirect sign of plasma leakage [7]. In 1997, WHO proposed as a dengue clinical case a patient that presented with fever and two or more of the following: headache, retro-orbital pain, myalgia, arthralgia, rash, hemorrhagic manifestations, and leukopenia [11]. However, due to the low specificity (36 %) of these criteria [12], a new set was proposed in 2009 that grouped myalgia and arthralgia in body aches, included nausea and vomiting, and added some warning signs and symptoms [1]. The 80 % sensitivity and 57 % specificity of the newly proposed WHO criteria [12], supports the importance of laboratory confirmation.

A previous study carried out at the Evandro Chagas National Institute of Infectious Diseases, Oswaldo Cruz Foundation (INI-FIOCRUZ) in Rio de Janeiro analyzed clinical and hematological data in ambulatory febrile patients and derived another diagnostic set of clinical criteria for dengue diagnosis [13]. In this study population the prediction rule, based on the presence of conjunctival hyperemia and leukocyte count, shown 81 % sensitivity and 71 % specificity [13].

Dengue laboratory diagnosis can be performed directly, by identifying the virus or its components, or indirectly, through serological tests detecting antibodies produced against the virus. The sensitivity of each method relies on disease duration at the moment of the clinical specimen collection [14]. The indirect methods are the more commonly used but have limited usefulness in the acute dengue diagnosis. IgM peaks occur around the third to fourth day of disease onset, and therefore a second clinical specimen collection is needed around day 14 to confirm the IgM rise and conclusively diagnose the disease [15]. However, in scenarios where the prevalence of secondary dengue is high, such as in Rio de Janeiro State, the duration and magnitude of the IgM response is reduced possibly impairing the accuracy of this serologic parameter [16]. Furthermore, pairing IgM are usually not point-of-care techniques, limiting their usefulness in epidemic scenarios.

During the febrile phase, detection of viral RNA or nonstructural protein-1 (NS1) are the main methods for the disease diagnosis. However, detection of viral RNA by reverse transcriptase-polymerase chain reaction (RT-PCR) is relatively complex and expensive, and is therefore not feasible in a number of health care settings, particularly in epidemic situations. For this reason, the identification of NS1 has been suggested as an alternative because it is present in the virus membrane, is highly stable and is secreted in the human serum during the early phase of dengue infection [15]. The sensitivity of the NS1 ELISA is reported to be greater than 90 % in primary infections and varies from 60 to 80 % in secondary infections [17, 18].

The rapid detection of dengue NS1 by immunochromatographic methods represents a potential breakthrough for laboratory case confirmation at early stages of disease in settings with limited infrastructure because they require minimal laboratory expertise and provide results within 15 to 30 min of specimen reception [4, 15, 19]. This laboratory technique, first described in 2000 and widely used since 2008, has now been tested in all dengue scenarios, especially in DENV-1 and DENV-3 scenarios [12, 15]. However, DENV-4 samples are still underrepresented [15, 18, 20, 21].

Ferraz, et al. [22], when evaluating mainly Brazilian DENV-1 samples by three different immunochromatographic assays, identified the NS1 Bioeasy™ as the one with higher sensitivity (63 %) despite the high specificity presented by all three (100 %). Another Brazilian study evaluating accuracy parameters of 4 immunochromatographic tests in a panel of acute DENV-1 to DENV-3 concluded that NS1 Bioeasy™ presented an overall 68 % specificity and a 90 % sensitivity which could reach 95 % in a DENV-1 setting [23].

A simple and accurate test to diagnose acute dengue cases in outpatient healthcare settings is still required. Considering this issue, we evaluated the diagnostic accuracy of three clinical dengue diagnostic criteria (WHO 1997, WHO 2009, INI-FIOCRUZ) and NS1 Bioeasy™ immunochromatographic test in an urgent care center during a DENV-4 epidemic in the city of Rio de Janeiro, Brazil.

Methods

Ethical statement

This prospective cross-sectional diagnostic accuracy study is reported according to the Standards for Reporting of Diagnostic Accuracy Study (STARD) Guideline [24] and was approved by the Research Ethics Committee of the Evandro Chagas National Institute of Infectious Diseases-FIOCRUZ, CAAE 0066.0.009.000-11, on March 23, 2012.

Enrollment, data, and specimen collection

We conducted the study in the city of Rio de Janeiro, Rio de Janeiro, Brazil, from March to April 2013, during an ongoing dengue epidemic. Adult patients (age >18 years) attending a public urgent care center (Unidade de Pronto Atendimento-UPA 24H) within 72 h of onset of an acute febrile illness without an evident focus of infection were eligible for the study.

A trained nurse obtained informed consent and prospectively enrolled the patients during business hours 5 days a week. An infectious disease physician collected data on demographic characteristics, symptoms and physical signs using a summarized version of a previously published and tested semi-structured questionnaire [25]. The tourniquet test was not performed and only spontaneous hemorrhagic manifestations were recorded.

We evaluated all patients according to WHO 1997, WHO 2009, and INI-FIOCRUZ clinical criteria defined elsewhere [1, 11, 13, 26].

Blood samples were collected for complete blood count and specific dengue tests including NS1 Bioeasy™, RT-PCR, Panbio® dengue IgM capture ELISA and dengue IgG ELISA, and Platelia™ Dengue NS1 Ag-ELISA. Acute dengue-4 cases were confirmed by RT-PCR. Serum samples were sent to the Flavivirus Laboratory, a regional reference laboratory for dengue and yellow fever at the Oswaldo Cruz Foundation (FIOCRUZ) where they were frozen at −70 °C until using for dengue specific laboratorial tests.

Index tests

NS1 strip test

All febrile cases were tested by the NS1 Bioeasy™ immunochromatographic strip test (Bioeasy™, Standard Diagnostics INC, Korea). This rapid test was chosen because it has already been used in the state of Rio de Janeiro and in other Brazilian states during dengue outbreaks. However, its performance had not been previously assessed. According to the manufacturer's instruction, the test can be stored at room temperature and can adequately detect the NS1 within 15 min using three drops of whole blood, plasma or serum.

In the immunochromatographic strip test, the NS1 antigen present in the sample will complex with the gold colloidal particles coated with anti-NS1 antibodies. After migration, the complexes will be captured by anti-NS1 antibodies at the test line where a line will appear. The presence of two lines in the cassette's window means a positive result, whereas the absence of the second line means a negative result with an adequate control line, which ensures the test is working properly.

Clinical criteria

Patients were classified as suspected dengue cases according to three sets of clinical criteria described as follows:

WHO 1997: fever with two or more of the following: headache, retro-orbital pain, myalgia, arthralgia, rash, hemorrhagic manifestations, and leukopenia [11]; *WHO 2009*: fever with two or more of the following: nausea/vomiting, rash, pain, leukopenia, and any of the following warning signs: abdominal pain, persistent vomiting, edema, mucosal bleeding, lethargy, hepatomegaly or hemoconcentration associated with a sudden drop in platelet count [1]; and *INI-FIOCRUZ*: presence of conjunctival redness with leukocytes less than 7500/mm^3 or less than 3760 leukocytes/mm^3 independently of other signs or symptoms [13].

Hemoconcentration in a single sample was defined by a hematocrit >53 % in males or 48 % in females [27]. Leukopenia was defined as a total leucocyte count ≤4500 cells/mm^3 [27].

Reference tests

Dengue viral RNA

In order to identify dengue viral RNA and specifically dengue 4 serotype, we performed RT-PCR according to the protocol described by Lanciotti et al. [28]. This highly specific protocol suggested by WHO [1] was considered the "gold standard" method for dengue-4 case confirmation in this study. Briefly, consensus primers (D1-5′-TCAATATGCTGAAACGCGGAGAAACCG-3′) and D2 (5′-TTGCACCAACAGTCAATGTCTTCAGGTTC-3′) were annealed to any of the four dengue serotypes to amplify a 511-bp product in a reverse transcriptase-polymerase reaction. After a second round of amplification (nested PCR) with type-specific primers (TS1 [5′- CGTCTCAGTGATCCGGGGG- 3′], TS2 [5′-CGCCACAAGGGCCATGAACAG-3′], TS3 [5′-TAACATCATCATGAGACAGAGC-3′] and TS4 [5′-CTCTGTTGTCTTAAACAAGAGA-3′]), DNA products specific for each dengue virus serotype were generated.

NS1 antigen detection by ELISA

The Platelia™ Dengue NS1 Ag-ELISA (BioRad Laboratories, France) was used for NS1 antigen capture according to the instructions by the manufacturer.

Immunologic markers

We performed the Panbio® dengue IgM Capture ELISA (Alere™, Minas Gerais, Brasil) and Dengue Virus IgG DxSelect™ ELISA (Focus Diagnostics, California, USA) according to the manufacturers' instructions for the qualitative detection of anti-DENV IgM and anti-DENV IgG antibodies, respectively.

Case definition

Since we aimed to describe only dengue 4 cases, a dengue (D4) case was defined as a patient confirmed with DENV-4 by RT-PCR. Furthermore, acute DENV-4 cases were classified as primary or secondary infections according to the absence or presence of anti-dengue IgG.

A non dengue (ND) case was defined as a patient with negative results for all dengue biomarkers (viral genome from any serotype, anti-dengue IgM and NS1).

Patients with negative RT-PCR and Platelia™ Dengue NS1 Ag-ELISA and/or dengue IgM positive results were considered indeterminate [29]. Indeterminate cases and patients with dengue infection by serotypes other than DENV-4 were excluded.

Laboratory personnel performing one test were blinded to the results of other tests.

Data processing and analysis

All clinical and laboratory data were collected and recorded in a database using the EpiData© 3.1 software [30]. Exploratory analysis was performed using the SPSS© v 17.0 software (SPSS Inc., Chicago, Illinois). MedCalc© 14.8.1 program was used to calculate 95 % confidence intervals (CI) for sensitivity, specificity, positive predictive value (PPV), negative predictive value (NPV), and likelihood ratios of NS1 Bioeasy™ and dengue clinical criteria.

A sample size of 137 positive dengue patients was determined as necessary to estimate, with 95 % confidence level, a sensitivity of 85 % with an absolute error of 6 %. Considering a prevalence of 40 % among febrile patients, 342 febrile subjects should be evaluated.

Role of funding source

The Brazilian National Council of Scientific and Technological Development (CNPq) funded this study (PROEP 402068/2012, REBRATS 401366/2013-8 and Grant level 2 CNPq 311414/2013-3); however, the funder was not involved in the design, sample handling, analysis, data interpretation, conclusions or decision to publish.

Results

In this study, we evaluated a total of 375 acutely febrile patients. Of those, 38 (10.1 %) were excluded, for reasons shown in Fig. 1. For this reason, 12 patients in the RT-PCR negative group were excluded for presenting positive or indeterminate results for specific dengue IgM or Platelia™ Dengue NS1 Ag-ELISA (Fig. 1).

From the 325 patients included in the study, 148 (45.5 %) had confirmed DENV-4 infection. No significant differences in age and gender distributions were observed

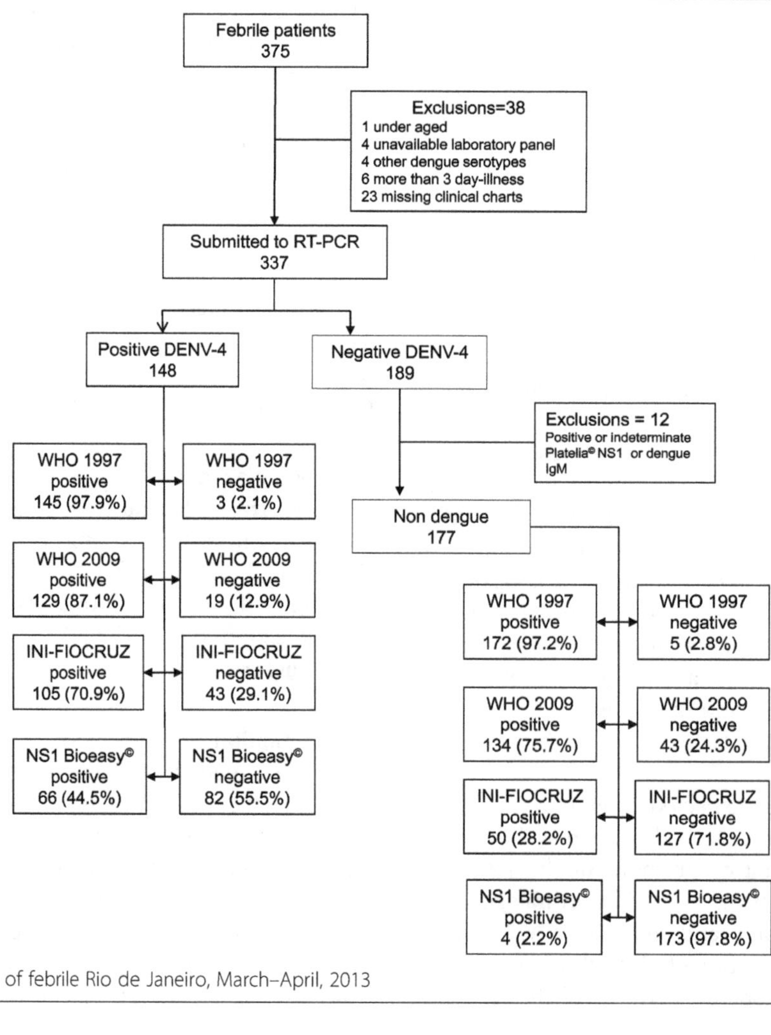

Fig. 1 STARD flow diagram of febrile Rio de Janeiro, March–April, 2013

between D4 and ND groups. The hematocrits were similar in both groups, but the platelet and leukocyte counts were lower among D4 patients (Table 1). The median time from onset of symptoms and medical care was 2 days in both groups.

The secondary infections, defined by anti-dengue IgG detection in the D4 group, were characterized in 124/148 (83.7 %) patients, and the NS1 strip test sensitivity was lower (42 %) in secondary (52/124) than in primary dengue cases (62.5 %; 15/24), $p = 0.05$.

We also tested the agreement between the NS1 Bioeasy™ test and the Platelia™ Dengue NS1 Ag-ELISA. The overall agreement, positive and negative concordances between the tests were 84.1, 83.5 and 84.7 %, respectively.

Clinical and laboratory features of eligible patients are shown in Table 2. No sign or symptom alone was able to predict dengue, although leukopenia and thrombocytopenia were more frequent in D4 cases. Leukocyte counts below 4500/mm^3 were almost eight times more likely to be present in D4 cases. In our study population, we did not find warning signs such as nuchal rigidity, altered consciousness, and ascites.

Using the WHO 1997 diagnostic criteria, a total of 145 (97.8 %) D4 and 172 (97.2 %) ND were clinically classified as dengue suspected cases, with a sensitivity of 97.8 % and specificity of 2.8 %. The WHO 2009 criteria clinically classified as dengue 129 (87.1 %) D4 and 134 (75.7 %) ND with 87.1 % sensitivity and 24.3 % specificity. The INI-FIOCRUZ clinical prediction rule classified as dengue suspected 105 (70.9 %) D4 patients but also 50 (28.2 %) ND, with a sensitivity of 70.9 % and specificity of 71.8 % (Table 3).

The NS1 Bioeasy™ immunochromatographic strip test alone was more accurate than the clinical criteria (OR = 34.4) and showed high specificity (97.8 %). However, the test sensitivity was lower (44.5 %). The test incorrectly classified as ND more than half of dengue patients (55.2 %). With these results almost a third of the patients with a negative NS1 Bioeasy™ test in our setting were in fact confirmed dengue cases (PPV = 68.3 %).

Combining the NS1 test with any clinical criteria did not improve the sensitivity or alter the high false negative rates, which remained similar to those obtained by the test alone. But all the evaluated clinical criteria could be complemented by this test resulting in an almost perfect specificity in a clinical setting.

Discussion

This is the first study we are aware of that assesses the combined accuracy of dengue clinical criteria and a NS1 point-of-care immunoassay for early diagnosis in outpatients during a DENV-4 epidemic. The WHO 1997 criteria was better to rule out the disease. When the INI-FIOCRUZ clinical criteria was positive, then the NS1 rapid test should be done. Patients with a positive strip test should be treated as dengue cases; however, negative results should be monitored for dengue or other acute febrile illnesses. As the clinical diagnosis lacks specificity, a definitive dengue case may need laboratory confirmation.

According to Lima, et al. [17], RT-PCR used in the present research showed 90 % sensitivity and more than 95 % specificity on the second day after the onset of disease, the same median time obtained in our sample. It is reasonable to consider this as a good diagnostic tool to confirm dengue fever. However, considering false negative results, we excluded 12 patients with negative RT-PCR and a positive or indeterminate IgM or Platelia™ NS1 results in which we could not identify the serotype.

At the time the study population was evaluated, there were no reports of any other Flavivirus circulating simultaneously in the city of Rio de Janeiro that could interfere in dengue laboratory results. We believe that we obtained a true non-dengue set of patients.

We also evaluated the ability of hematological parameters and individual signs and symptoms to discriminate dengue from non-dengue. We found that leukopenia was more frequent in D4 than in ND, although the overlapping range between the two groups prevented an adequate discrimination between them. The relevance of leukopenia as a discriminant feature of dengue infection has been previously documented, although the cutoff values may vary [13, 31–34].

The platelet counts were lower in the D4 group, although true thrombocytopenia was infrequent in both groups. Similar to findings in other studies [22, 35], there was no significant difference in hematocrit between groups. This may be because both hemoconcentration and platelet drop are usually not seen in the first days of disease [34].

Table 1 Epidemiological characteristics of 325 febrile patients, Rio de Janeiro, March–April, 2013

	Median (IQR)		
	Dengue 4 (*N* = 148)	Non dengue (*N* = 177)	*p*-value
Age in years	36.6 (23.1–50.1)	36.5 (23.0–50.0)	0.99
Hematocrit (%)	42.6 (40.3–45.0)	42.2 (40.0–44.0)	0.45
Leucocyte counts (cells/mm^3)	4251 (3400–4667)	7518 (5467–7900)	<0.05
Platelet counts (cells/ mm^3)	217.812 (187,667–236,667)	256,4945 (221,000–284,667)	<0.05

IQR interquartile range

Table 2 Clinical and laboratory features of 325 febrile patients, Rio de Janeiro, March–April, 2013

	Dengue 4 (*N* = 148)		Non dengue (*N* = 177)		OR (95 % CI)
	N	%	*N*	%	
Clinical					
Exanthema	28	18.9	21	11.8	1.7 (0.9–3.2)
Conjunctival hyperemia	75	50.6	72	40.6	1.5 (1–2.3)
Lethargy[a]	142	95.9	168	94.9	1.3 (0.4–3.6)
Joint pain	110	74.3	128	72.3	1.1 (0.7–1.8)
Pain	143	96.6	171	96.6	1.0 (0.3–3.4)
Retro-orbital pain	105	70.9	124	70.0	1.0 (0.6–1.7)
Nausea/vomiting	99	66.9	120	67.7	1.0 (0.6–1.5)
Edema[a]	3	2.0	4	2.2	0.9 (0.2–4.0)
Liver enlargement[a]	4	2.7	6	3.3	0.8 (0.2–2.9)
Persistent vomiting[a]	35	23.6	48	27.1	0.8 (0.5–1.4)
Myalgia	134	90.5	161	90.9	0.9 (0.4–1.9)
Abdominal tenderness[a]	47	31.7	68	38.4	0.7 (0.5–1.2)
Bleeding[a]	12	8.1	25	14.1	0.5 (0.3–1.1)
Headache	133	89.8	169	95.4	0.4 (0.2–1. 0)
Laboratory					
Leukopenia	95	64.1	33	18.6	7.8 (4.7–13.0)[b]
Thrombocytopenia	17	11.4	8	4.5	2.7 (1.1–6.5)[b]
Anti-dengue IgG	123	83.1	161	90.9	0.5 (0.3–1.0)

OR odds ratio, *CI* confidence interval
[a]warning signs; Leukopenia = leucocyte count <4,500cells/mm^3; thrombocytopenia = platelet count <150,000 cells/mm^3
[b]significant odds ratio

Repeated monitoring of the platelet count and hematocrit is recommended, as an abrupt fall in platelet count is proposed as a warning sign, and a significant hematocrit increase is an indirect sign of plasma leakage [10, 34].

Gan, et al. [36] studied 256 adults in Singapore and reported 87.1 % sensitivity and 26 % specificity for the WHO 2009 criteria, similar to the present research. However, the 20 % sensitivity using the WHO 1997 criteria was far different from those obtained in our study.

Due to its lower sensitivity (70.9 %), the INI-FIOCRUZ clinical criteria does not seem very promising as an exclusive screening alternative. However, it was much more specific than both WHO criteria and showed the best clinical performance for classifying suspected dengue cases. It could be proposed (and tested in a different population) as a screening tool to further confirm using more expensive and time consuming specific laboratory tests.

Among the signs and symptoms in the three sets of clinical criteria, none was significantly more frequent among D4 patients. However, conjunctival hyperemia, a sign used in the INI-FIOCRUZ criteria, had a performance similar to classic signs, such as exanthema. Although not sufficiently accurate to be used as a discriminant feature alone, this was an important finding

Table 3 Accuracy parameters for DENV-4 in 325 febrile patients, Rio de Janeiro, March–April, 2013

	Sensitivity % (95 % CI)	Specificity % (95 % CI)	LR+ (95 % CI)	LR− (95 % CI)	PPV (95 % CI)	NPV (95 % CI)	OR (95 % CI)
WHO 1997	97.8 (93.8–99.6)	2.8 (1.0–6.9)	1.0 (1.0–1.1)	0.7 (0.2–3.0)	45.6 (39.9–51.5)	62.5 (24.5–91.5)	1.4 (0.3–6.0)
WHO 2009	87.1 (80.3–92.1)	24.3 (18.1–31.6)	1.1 (1.0–1.3)	0.5 (0.3–0.9)	48.8 (42.4–55.2)	69.5 (56.1–80.8)	2.2 (1.2–4.0)
INI-FIOCRUZ	70.9 (63.2–78.6)	71.8 (64.5–78.4)	2.5 (2.0–3.3)	0.4 (0.3–0.5)	67.6 (59.5–74.9)	75.3 (68.0–81.7)	6.4 (3.9–10.4)
NS1	44.5 (36.4–53.3)	97.8 (94.2–99.4)	19.5 (7.3–52.2)	0.6 (0.5–0.7)	94.1 (85.6–98.4)	68.3 (62.1–74.0)	34.4 (12.1–97.9)
WHO 1997 and NS1	44.2 (35.8–52.9)	97.6 (94.0–99.3)	18.3 (6.8–49.2)	0.6 (0.5–0.7)	93.9 (85.0–98.3)	67.8 (61.4–73.7)	32.1 (11.3–91.4)
WHO 2009 and NS1	40.6 (32.3–49.3)	98.2 (94.9–99.6)	22.6 (7.2–70.6)	0.6 (0.5–0.7)	94.9 (85.9–98.9)	66.7 (60.4–72.5)	37.3 (11.3–122.9)
INI-FIOCRUZ and NS1	29.7 (22.4–37.8)	98.9 (96.0–99.9)	26.2 (6.5–106.5)	0.7 (0.6–0.8)	95.6 (84.9–99.5)	63.2 (57.2–68.9)	36.9 (8.7–155.5)

LR+ positive likelihood ratio, *LR−* negative likelihood ratio, *PPV* positive predictive value, *NPV* negative predictive value, *OR* odds ratio, *CI* confidence interval because this clinical sign is not included in the WHO criteria. At least three other studies have reported similar results, both in febrile outpatients in early disease stages [13, 35, 37].

As described by Leo, et al. [38] and Paranavitane, et al. [39] our study targeted early dengue disease in outpatient setting, therefore we could not assess warning signs such as nuchal rigidity, altered consciousness, and ascites, abrupt platelet count fall or hemoconcentration, that occur later during the disease.

The WHO 2009 dengue criteria improved rates of correct identification of severe dengue cases, aiding therapeutics and avoiding unnecessary deaths [30]. However, it did not prove to be much more accurate (sensitive) for screening or clinically diagnosing dengue 4 than the WHO 1997 version. INI-FIOCRUZ criteria showed the best-balanced performance and could enhance specificity being used previously to the NS1 rapid test in selecting a group of patients for this more specific test.

The NS1 Bioeasy™ showed excellent specificity (97.8 %) in the study population, which agrees with previous reported results in different countries [15, 40]. However, we found a substantially lower sensitivity (44.5 %) of Bioeasy™ NS1 immunoassay in our DENV-4 patients compared to the 61.3 and 90 % sensitivity described respectively by Ferraz, et al. [22], and Silva, et al. [23] in DENV-1 and DENV-3 scenarios. Lower sensitivity to DENV-4 compared to the other serotypes has also been documented by Pal, et al. [15], varying from 42 to 58 % depending on the test used.

Differing performances according to serotype were also recently described in a meta-analysis evaluating two NS1 ELISA tests for early dengue detection [18]. The study concluded that Platelia™ NS1 and NS1 Panbio® tests showed lower pooled sensitivity for DENV-4 (58 and 37 %, respectively) [18]. The interpretation given by some authors includes the NS1 gene polymorphism associated with immunological epitopes, a low NS1 concentration in DENV-4 cases [20, 41], or low overall viremia [21]. Nevertheless, this latter hypothesis was not confirmed by Allonso, et al. [20] in a recent Brazilian study.

As reported in other studies on NS1 detection using conventional ELISA or rapid tests, we observed lower NS1 Bioeasy™ sensitivity in secondary (42 %) compared to primary (62.5 %) dengue cases [9, 12, 15, 20]. As most of the cases (83.7 %) were secondary infections, this might have contributed to the poor performance of the test in our population. This low performance probably occurred due to a rapid clearance in secondary cases [15] and/or as a result of antigen-antibody complexes that disrupt the test targets impeding the ability of the test to detect free NS1 antigen [42, 43]. Efforts to dissociate immune complexes by acid or heat treatment can probably enhance the assays sensitivities [44].

The high PPV (94.1 %) obtained in this 45.5 % dengue prevalence scenario, similar to that obtained by Pal, et al. [15], indicates that individuals testing positive on NS1 do not require another confirmatory test. The performance on specificity qualifies this test, as a confirmatory one, to streamline the decision to treat the correctly identified dengue patients in the clinical setting. It should be used just after the onset of symptoms in order to avoid complications and deaths and to organize the flow of care at the facility. This rapid test might also be useful for virologic surveillance purposes to select serum samples for RNA detection by PCR.

However, although highly specific, the NS1 rapid test yields high false negative rates (55.5 %) among confirmed DENV-4 patients, and its low sensitivity argues against its incorporation as a screening diagnostic tool in clinical practice. Recently, the Rio de Janeiro State Health Department decided not to include the test for dengue screening in outpatient settings. Its use has been restricted to evaluate critically ill hospitalized patients.

Our study has some limitations: a small sample of primary dengue patients and the absence of the tourniquet test, a WHO sign criteria, considered a painful and lengthy procedure with poor patient compliance. We were also not able to reevaluate the patients in the convalescent period due to the pragmatic diagnostic study outline and the dynamics of the Rio de Janeiro city's health care system. Although the gold standard for dengue diagnosis would be pairing specific dengue IgM in acute and convalescent period, as proposed by WHO [11], recent studies have also exclusively used PCR as the reference test to evaluate early phase dengue [45], to evaluate clinical algorithms [46] or ELISA and NS1 tests [15].

Conclusions

The development of more sensitive point-of-care tests for dengue diagnosis to act as a screening tool remains a challenge, especially for endemic countries, where the prevalence of secondary cases is high. In summary, we proposed a clinical-laboratory algorithm which combines the INI-FIOCRUZ and the WHO 1997 clinical criteria, in order to select ambulatory suspected early dengue cases (within 3 days of onset of disease) eligible for NS1 strip testing. The patients that test positive should be immediately treated for dengue, and the patients that test negative would still require subsequent diagnostic investigation. We recommend external validation in different settings.

Abbreviations

CI: confidence interval; CNPq: Brazilian National Council of Scientific and Technological Development; D4: dengue 4; DENV-1: dengue virus serotype 1; DENV-2: dengue virus serotype 2; DENV-3: dengue virus serotype 3; DENV-4: dengue virus serotype 4; DNA: deoxyribonucleic acid; ELISA: enzyme-linked immunosorbent assay; FIOCRUZ: Oswaldo Cruz Foundation;

IgG: immunoglobulin G; IgM: immunoglobulin M; INI-FIOCRUZ: Evandro Chagas National Institute of Infectious Diseases, Oswaldo Cruz Foundation; IQR: interquartile range; LR+: positive likelihood ratio; LR–: negative likelihood ratio; ND: non-dengue; NPV: negative predictive value; NS1: nonstructural protein-1; OR: odds ratio; PPV: positive predictive value; RNA: ribonucleic acid; RT-PCR: reverse transcriptase-polymerase chain reaction.; STARD: Standards for Reporting of Diagnostic Accuracy Study; UPA 24H: Unidade de Pronto Atendimento; WHO: World Health Organization.

Competing interests
The authors declare that they have no competing interests.

Authors' contributions
SNB, SRLP and RPD conceived of the study, participated in its design and coordination and helped to draft the manuscript. DNRO and FMQ participated in its design, data collection and recording. YHMH participated in the study design, data analysis and interpretation and helped to draft the manuscript. RMRN and FBS carried out the immunoassays, rapid immunochromatographic test, viral characterization and writing the manuscript. CNC participated in the design of the study and performed the statistical analysis. All authors read and approved the final manuscript.

Acknowledgements
We thank Dr Maria Angélica Borges dos Santos for her helpful discussions reviewing this manuscript, Dr Monique da Rocha Queiroz Lima for executing all the specific laboratory assays, Allan and Kate Crean for the careful English editing.

Author details
[1]Laboratory of Clinical Epidemiology, Evandro Chagas National Institute of Infectious Diseases, Oswaldo Cruz Foundation, Rio de Janeiro, Brazil. [2]National School of Public Health, Oswaldo Cruz Foundation, Rio de Janeiro, Brazil. [3]Germano Sinval Faria Teaching Primary Care Center, National School of Public Health, Oswaldo Cruz Foundation, Rio de Janeiro, Brazil. [4]Flavivirus Laboratory, Oswaldo Cruz Institute, Oswaldo Cruz Foundation, Rio de Janeiro, Brazil.

References
1. World Health Organization. Dengue: diagnosis, treatment, prevention and control. Geneva: WHO; 2009. http://www.who.int/neglected_diseases/en/. Accessed in 15 Jan 2015.
2. Bhatt S, Gething PW, Brady OJ, Messina JP, Farlow AW, Moyes CL, et al. The global distribution and burden of dengue. Nature. 2013;496(7446):504–7.
3. San Martin JL, Brathwaite O, Zambrano B, Solorzano JO, Bouckenooghe A, Dayan GH, et al. The epidemiology of dengue in the Americas over the last three decades: a worrisome reality. Am J Trop Med Hyg. 2010;82(1):128–35.
4. Dietz VJ, Gubler DJ, Rigau-Perez JG, Pinheiro F, Schatzmayr HG, Bailey R, et al. Epidemic dengue 1 in Brazil, 1986: evaluation of a clinically based dengue surveillance system. Am J Epidemiol. 1990;131(4):693–701.
5. Nogueira RM, Miagostovich MP, Lampe E, Schatzmayr HG. Isolation of dengue virus type 2 in Rio de Janeiro. Mem Inst Oswaldo Cruz. 1990;85(2):253.
6. Nogueira RM, Schatzmayr HG, de Filippis AM, dos Santos FB, da Cunha RV, Coelho JO, et al. Dengue virus type 3, Brazil, 2002. Emerg Infect Dis. 2005; 11(9):1376–81.
7. Teixeira MG, Costa Mda C, Barreto F, Barreto ML. Dengue: twenty-five years since reemergence in Brazil. Cad Saude Publica. 2009;25 Suppl 1:S7–18.
8. Nogueira RM, Eppinghaus AL. Dengue virus type 4 arrives in the state of Rio de Janeiro: a challenge for epidemiological surveillance and control. Mem Inst Oswaldo Cruz. 2011;106(3):255–6.
9. Hang VT, Nguyet NM, Trung DT, Tricou V, Yoksan S, Dung NM, et al. Diagnostic accuracy of NS1 ELISA and lateral flow rapid tests for dengue sensitivity, specificity and relationship to viraemia and antibody responses. PLoS Negl Trop Dis. 2009;3(1), e360.
10. Brasil. Ministério da Saúde. Secretaria de Vigilância em Saúde. Diretoria Técnica de Gestão. Dengue : diagnóstico e manejo clínico – adulto e criança / Ministério da Saúde, Secretaria de Vigilância em Saúde, Diretoria Técnica de Gestão. – 4. ed. – Brasília : Ministério da Saúde, 2011.
11. World Health Organization. Dengue haemorrhagic fever: diagnosis, treatment, prevention and control. Genebra: WHO; 1997. http://www.who.int/neglected_diseases/en/. Accessed in 15 Nov 2014.
12. Chaterji S, Allen Jr JC, Chow A, Leo YS, Ooi EE. Evaluation of the NS1 rapid test and the WHO dengue classification schemes for use as bedside diagnosis of acute dengue fever in adults. Am J Trop Med Hyg. 2011;84(2):224–8.
13. Daumas RP, Passos SR, Oliveira RV, Nogueira RM, Georg I, Marzochi KB, et al. Clinical and laboratory features that discriminate dengue from other febrile illnesses: a diagnostic accuracy study in Rio de Janeiro, Brazil. BMC Infect Dis. 2013;13:77.
14. Lima MRQ, Nogueira RM, Santos FB. Dengue diagnosis: commercially available kits and laboratory support. In: Clinical insights: dengue: transmission, diagnosis & surveillance. 1st ed. London: Future Medicine Ltd; 2014. p. 27–47.
15. Pal S, Dauner AL, Mitra I, Forshey BM, Garcia P, Morrison AC, et al. Evaluation of dengue NS1 antigen rapid tests and ELISA kits using clinical samples. PLoS One. 2014;9(11), e113411.
16. Domingo C, Alves MJ, de Ory F, Teichmann A, Schmitz H, Muller R, et al. International external quality control assessment for the serological diagnosis of dengue infections. BMC Infect Dis. 2015;15:167.
17. Lima MR, Nogueira RM, Schatzmayr HG, dos Santos FB. Comparison of three commercially available dengue NS1 antigen capture assays for acute diagnosis of dengue in Brazil. PLoS Negl Trop Dis. 2010;4(7), e738.
18. da Costa VG, Marques-Silva AC, Moreli ML. A meta-analysis of the diagnostic accuracy of two commercial NS1 antigen ELISA tests for early dengue virus detection. PLoS One. 2014;9(4), e94655.
19. Fry SR, Meyer M, Semple MG, Simmons CP, Sekaran SD, Huang JX, et al. The diagnostic sensitivity of dengue rapid test assays is significantly enhanced by using a combined antigen and antibody testing approach. PLoS Negl Trop Dis. 2011;5(6), e1199.
20. Allonso D, Meneses MD, Fernandes CA, Ferreira DF, Mohana-Borges R. Assessing positivity and circulating levels of NS1 in samples from a 2012 dengue outbreak in Rio de Janeiro, Brazil. PLoS One. 2014;9(11), e113634.
21. Sea VR, Cruz AC, Gurgel RQ, Nunes BT, Silva EV, Dolabella SS, et al. Underreporting of Dengue-4 in Brazil due to low sensitivity of the NS1 Ag test in routine control programs. PLoS One. 2013;8(5), e64056.
22. Ferraz FO, Bomfim MR, Totola AH, Avila TV, Cisalpino D, Pessanha JE, et al. Evaluation of laboratory tests for dengue diagnosis in clinical specimens from consecutive patients with suspected dengue in Belo Horizonte, Brazil. J Clin Virol. 2013;58(1):41–6.
23. Silva FG, Silva SJS, Rocco IM, Silveira VR, Suzuki A, Katz G, et al. Evaluation of commercial kits for detecting the antigen NS1-dengue- São Paulo. Bepa. 2011;8(9):14–26.
24. Bossuyt PM, Reitsma JB, Bruns DE, Gatsonis CA, Glasziou PP, Irwig LM, et al. Toward complete and accurate reporting of studies of diagnostic accuracy. The STARD initiative. Am J Clin Pathol. 2003;119(1):18–22.
25. Daumas RP, Brasil P, Bressan CS, Oliveira RV, Carvalho BB, Carneiro DV, et al. Interobserver agreement on signs and symptoms of patients with acute febrile illness. Infection. 2011;39(2):135–40.
26. Gutierrez G, Gresh L, Perez MA, Elizondo D, Aviles W, Kuan G, et al. Evaluation of the diagnostic utility of the traditional and revised WHO dengue case definitions. PLoS Negl Trop Dis. 2013;7(8), e2385.
27. Failace R. Hemograma: manual de interpretação. 5th ed. Artmed: Porto Alegre; 2009.
28. Lanciotti RS, Calisher CH, Gubler DJ, Chang GJ, Vorndam AV. Rapid detection and typing of dengue viruses from clinical samples by using reverse transcriptase-polymerase chain reaction. J Clin Microbiol. 1992;30(3):545–51.
29. Setiati TE, Mairuhu AT, Koraka P, Supriatna M, Mac Gillavry MR, Brandjes DP, et al. Dengue disease severity in Indonesian children: an evaluation of the World Health Organization classification system. BMC Infect Dis. 2007;7:22.
30. Lauritsen JM, Bruus M. EpiData 3ed. A comprehensive tool for validated entry and documentation of data. Odense, Denmark: The EpiData Association; 2003.
31. Gregory CJ, Lorenzi OD, Colon L, Garcia AS, Santiago LM, Rivera RC, et al. Utility of the tourniquet test and the white blood cell count to differentiate dengue among acute febrile illnesses in the emergency room. PLoS Negl Trop Dis. 2011;5(12), e1400.
32. Macedo GA, Gonin ML, Pone SM, Cruz OG, Nobre FF, Brasil P. Sensitivity and specificity of the World Health Organization dengue classification schemes for severe dengue assessment in children in Rio de Janeiro. PLoS One. 2014;9(4), e96314.

33. Horstick O, Jaenisch T, Martinez E, Kroeger A, See LL, Farrar J, et al. Comparing the usefulness of the 1997 and 2009 WHO dengue case classification: a systematic literature review. Am J Trop Med Hyg. 2014;91(3):621–34.
34. Huang SY, Lee IK, Wang L, Liu JW, Hung SC, Chen CC, et al. Use of simple clinical and laboratory predictors to differentiate influenza from dengue and other febrile illnesses in the emergency room. BMC Infect Dis. 2014;14:623.
35. Low JG, Ooi EE, Tolfvenstam T, Leo YS, Hibberd ML, Ng LC, et al. Early Dengue infection and outcome study (EDEN) - study design and preliminary findings. Ann Acad Med Singapore. 2006;35(11):783–9.
36. Gan VC, Lye DC, Thein TL, Dimatatac F, Tan AS, Leo YS. Implications of discordance in world health organization 1997 and 2009 dengue classifications in adult dengue. PLoS One. 2013;8(4), e60946.
37. Conroy AL, Gelvez M, Hawkes M, Rajwans N, Liles WC, Villar-Centeno LA, et al. Host biomarkers distinguish dengue from leptospirosis in Colombia: a case-control study. BMC Infect Dis. 2014;14:35.
38. Leo YS, Gan VC, Ng EL, Hao Y, Ng LC, Pok KY, et al. Utility of warning signs in guiding admission and predicting severe disease in adult dengue. BMC Infect Dis. 2013;13:498.
39. Paranavitane SA, Gomes L, Kamaladasa A, Adikari TN, Wickramasinghe N, Jeewandara C, et al. Dengue NS1 antigen as a marker of severe clinical disease. BMC Infect Dis. 2014;14:570.
40. Tan LK, Lye DC, Pok KY, Mok SQ, Chua RC, et al. Diagnosing dengue at the point-of-care: utility of a rapid combined diagnostic kit in Singapore. PLoS One. 2014;9(3), e90037.
41. Colombo TE, Vedovello D, Araki CS, Cogo-Moreira H, dos Santos IN, Reis AF, et al. Dengue-4 false negative results by Panbio®Dengue Early ELISA assay in Brazil. J Clin Virol. 2013;58(4):710–2.
42. Peeling RW, Artsob H, Pelegrino JL, Buchy P, Cardosa MJ, Devi S, et al. Evaluation of diagnostic tests: dengue. Nat Rev Microbiol. 2010;8(12 Suppl):S30–8.
43. Blacksell SD. Commercial dengue rapid diagnostic tests for point-of-care application: recent evaluations and future needs? J Biomed Biotechnol. 2012;2012:151967.
44. Lima MR, Nogueira RM, Filippis AM, Nunes PC, Sousa CS, Silva MH, et al. A simple heat dissociation method increases significantly the ELISA detection sensitivity of the nonstructural-1 glycoprotein in patients infected with DENV type-4. J Virol Methods. 2014;204:105–8.
45. Nujum ZT, Thomas A, Vijayakumar K, Nair RR, Pillai MR, Indu PS, et al. Comparative performance of the probable case definitions of dengue by WHO (2009) and the WHO-SEAR expert group (2011). Pathog Glob Health. 2014;108(2):103–10.
46. Cecilia D, Kakade M, Alagarasu K, Patil J, Salunke A, Parashar D, et al. Development of a multiplex real-time RT-PCR assay for simultaneous detection of dengue and chikungunya viruses. Arch Virol. 2015;160(1):323–7.

2

Thromboelastometry analysis of thrombocytopenic dengue patients

Felipe Maia de Toledo Piza[1*], Thiago Domingos Corrêa[1], Alexandre Rodrigues Marra[1], João Carlos Campos Guerra[1], Roseny dos Reis Rodrigues[1,2], Andrea Aparecida Rocco Villarinho[1], Valdir Fernandes de Aranda[1], Sandra Christina Pereira Lima Shiramizo[1], Maria Roza de Jesus de Lima[1], Esper Georges Kallas[2] and Alexandre Biasi Cavalcanti[2]

Abstract

Background: Dengue virus infection (DVI) is a prevalent and potentially fatal viral disease associated with coagulopathy. So far, the coagulation profile of DVI patients with thrombocytopenia has not been assessed through a viscoelastic test such as rotational thromboelastometry. We aimed to describe the prevalence and characteristics of coagulation abnormalities in dengue fever outpatients with thrombocytopenia, addressed by both rotational thromboelastometry and conventional coagulation tests.

Methods: This was a cross-sectional study conducted between April 6th and May 5th 2015 in São Paulo, Brazil during a dengue outbreak. Thromboelastometry (ROTEM®) and the conventional coagulation tests prothrombin time (PT), international normalized ratio (INR), activated partial thromboplastin time (aPTT), thrombin time (TT), platelet count and fibrinogen levels were performed in 53 patients with DVI and thrombocytopenia.

Results: Despite a median interquartile range (IQR) platelet count of 77 (63–88) x 10^9/L in DVI patients, conventional coagulation tests and plasma fibrinogen levels were within the normal range. Subjects demonstrated hypocoagulability in 71.7% (38/53) in INTEM and 54.7% (29/53) in EXTEM DVI patients. FIBTEM analyses detected only 5.7% (3/53) with hypocoagulability among this population. The median (IQR) clotting time (CT), clot formation time (CFT) and maximum clot firmness (MCF) on INTEM were, respectively, 177 (160–207) sec, 144 (108–178) sec and 48 (42–52) mm. On EXTEM, median (IQR) CT, CFT and MCF were, respectively, 69 (65–78) sec, 148 (126–198) sec and 49 (44–55) mm. Median (IQR) MCF on FIBTEM was 15 (13–18) mm.

Conclusion: Thromboelastometry impairment is highly prevalent in DVI patients with thrombocytopenia, particularly in INTEM and EXTEM analyses, while standard coagulation tests are normal in this setting. Clinical implications remain to be established.

Background

Dengue is by far the most incident human arbovirus disease [1], with over 2.5 billion people living in high-risk transmission areas [2]. The World Health Organization (WHO) estimates 50–100 million of dengue virus infections (DVI) per year, resulting in 500,000 hospitalizations and 20,000 deaths worldwide [1, 2].

Dengue hemorrhagic fever (DHF) represents a severe clinical presentation of DVI and is characterized by the presence of varying degrees of hemostatic disorders [3, 4]. Intense and amplified cytokine release, along with the complement activation, result in endothelial dysfunction, platelet destruction and consumption of coagulation factors, which may lead to a life threatening disseminate intravascular coagulation (DIC) [5, 6]. Indeed, blood coagulation disorders are commonly observed in patients with DHF and dengue shock syndrome [6, 7].

* Correspondence: felipe.piza@einstein.br
[1]Department of Intensive Care Medicine, Hospital Israelita Albert Einstein, Av. Albert Einstein, 627/701, 5° andar, São Paulo CEP: 05651-901, Brazil
Full list of author information is available at the end of the article

Many studies have assessed the coagulation system in DVI through conventional coagulation tests such as the prothrombin time (PT), international normalized ratio (INR), thrombin time (TT), and activated partial thromboplastin time (aPTT) [3, 6, 8, 9]. Nevertheless, conventional coagulation tests were validated to monitor vitamin K antagonists and heparin therapy [10, 11]. Although conventional coagulation tests have not been validated to predict and/or to guide therapy in acute (acquired) hemorrhage, they have been widely used for this purpose [10]. Conventional coagulation tests results may take a few hours to be completed and reported, they track the complexity of hemostatic impairment poorly, and most frequently, they reflect late coagulopathy disorders [10–13].

Rotational thromboelastometry (ROTEM®) is a point of care test that promptly provides (5–30 min) information about the dynamics of clot formation, stabilization and dissolution, reflecting the in vivo hemostasis at the bedside [12]. ROTEM provides more clinically useful and reliable information than the conventional coagulation tests in critically ill patients [13, 14], yielding a graphical presentation of fibrin polymerization process, involving fibrinogen and platelet function, and fibrinolysis [13].

To our knowledge, no study has evaluated the coagulation profile of patients with DVI with rotational thromboelastometry. Therefore, we aimed at describing the prevalence of coagulation abnormalities addressed by both thromboelastometry and conventional coagulation tests in cases of dengue fever outpatients with thrombocytopenia. Additionally, we evaluated the correlation between conventional coagulation tests and thromboelastometry in this population of patients.

Methods

Study design and setting

This was a cross-sectional study conducted during a DVI outbreak in São Paulo, Brazil between April 6th and May 5th 2015. This study was approved by the University of São Paulo Institutional Review Board [*Comissão de Ética para Análise de Projetos e Pesquisas* (CAPPesq), approval number: 0652/09]. All patients provided informed consent prior inclusion in this study.

Participants

Patients were screened at an outpatient clinic established in a neighborhood in the city of São Paulo with high incidence of DVI. Patients with at least 24 h of fever (axillary temperature >37.8 °C), in addition to a positive dengue virus (DV) specific immunoglobulin IgM/IgG or non-structural protein-1 (NS1) antigen rapid test (DENGUE DUO Bioeasy®, Kyonggi-Do, South Korea) and platelet count <100 x 10^9/L were consecutively included in this study (Fig. 1).

Exclusion criteria included pregnancy, presence of oncologic or hematologic disorders, solid or bone marrow transplantation, secondary thrombocytopenia, previous known coagulopathy, chronic hepatitis B or C, chronic renal failure and use of anti-platelet therapy or vitamin K antagonists.

Dengue virus infections triage, support and blood sampling

All patients who visited the outpatient clinic had their clinical history taken to obtain information on length of time, type and severity of symptoms and vital signs analysis (arterial blood pressure, axillary temperature and heart rate) (Fig. 2). Demographic data, comorbidities, clinical presentation, vital signs and the need for hospital admission were recorded.

Once DVI was suspected, blood samples were collected and tested for detection of DV-specific IgM/IgG and NS1 antigen (Fig. 2). Additionally, hemoglobin, hematocrit, white blood cell and platelets count were performed (XS-1000i™; Sysmex Roche®, Kobe, Japan).

Patients with confirmed DVI and arterial hypotension [systolic blood pressure (SBP) <90 mmHg], fever (temperature >37.8 °C), tachycardia [heart rate (HR) >100 bpm) and/or hemoconcentration (hematocrit >50% for men or >48% for women) were admitted for intravenous (I.V.) fluid administration and/or symptomatic support (Fig. 2). In 53 patients with confirmed DVI and

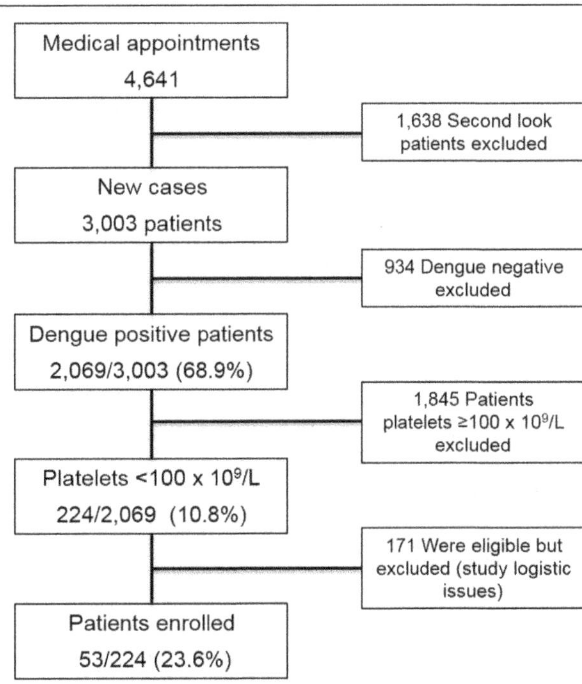

Fig. 1 Patients' flow diagram

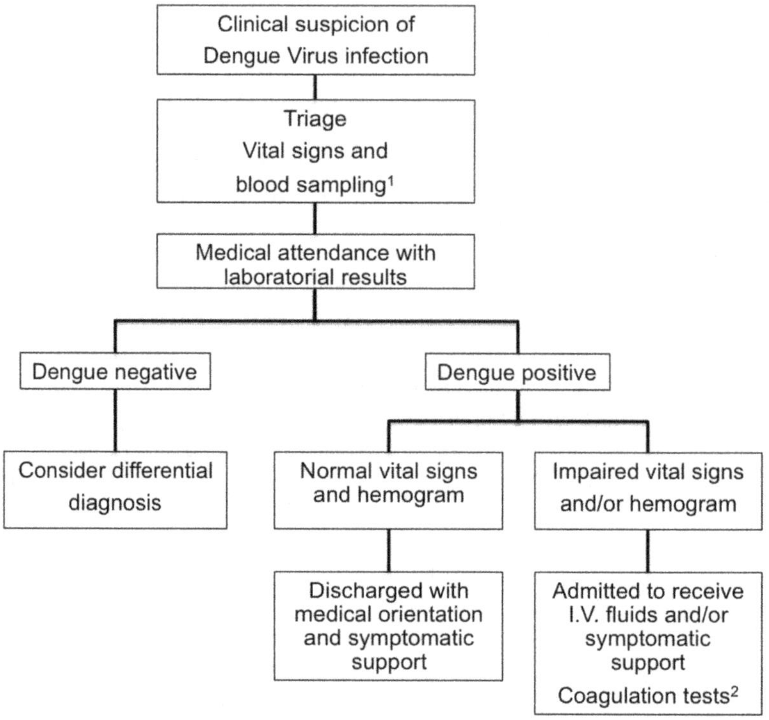

Fig. 2 Patient's flow chart attendance during dengue virus infection outbreak. Legend: [1]: blood samples for detection of dengue virus specific IgM/IgG and NS1 antigen, hemoglobin, hematocrit, white blood cell and platelet count. [2]: in the 53 patients with confirmed dengue virus infection and thrombocytopenia (platelet count <100 x 10^9/L), conventional coagulation tests (PT, TT, INR and aPTT), serum fibrinogen level, plasma d-dimer levels and rotational thromboelastometry (ROTEM®) were performed

thrombocytopenia (platelet count <100 x 10^9/L), conventional coagulation tests (PT, TT, INR and aPTT) (STA Compact; Stago®, Asnières-sur-Seine, France), serum fibrinogen level (Clauss method) (STA Compact; Stago®, Asnières-sur-Seine, France), plasma d-dimer level (STA Compact; Stago®, Asnières-sur-Seine, France) and rotational thromboelastometry (ROTEM®; Pentapharm Co., Munich, Germany) were performed.

Thromboelastometry

Thromboelastometry (ROTEM) assesses the viscoelastic properties of the clot and provides information on the speed of coagulation initiation, kinetics of clot formation, clot strength and breakdown [14, 15]. Blood samples of 3 ml were collected in citrate tubes (3.2%; Sarsted®, Wedel, Germany) and processed within a period of three hours for thromboelastometry analysis. The analyses were performed by pipetting 300 µl of citrated whole blood and 20 µl of 0.2 M calcium chloride with specific activators into a plastic cup [16]. Measurement of coagulation in ROTEM was performed after the vertical immersion of a plastic pin into the blood sample. The pin rotates slowly backwards and forwards through an angle of 4.75°. By generation of the first fibrin filaments between the pin and the wall of the test cup, the rotational range of the pin is reduced [13]. The increased restriction of the pin's movement is transferred to a graphical display, a plot that shows changes in the viscoelastic properties of the clot over time [15].

The following parameters were recorded during ROTEM analysis: clotting time [CT; seconds (sec)], which represents the beginning of the test until a clot firmness of 2 mm is detected, clot formation time (CFT; sec), until a clot firmness of 20 mm has been reached, alpha angle (degrees) represents the slope (tangent) between a CT of 2 mm and CFT of 20 mm, amplitude 10 (A10; mm), which represents the clot amplitude 10 min after the beginning of clotting and maximum clot firmness (MCF; mm), which represents the greatest amplitude of the thromboelastometric trace and reflects the "strength" of the clot [13–16]. We performed an extrinsically activated thromboelastometric test (EXTEM), a test that uses rabbit brain thromboplastin as an activator; an intrinsically activated thromboelastometric test (INTEM), a test that uses ellagic acid as an activator and a fibrin-based thromboelastometric test (FIBTEM), a test that assesses the fibrin-based clot using both extrinsic activation and addition of cytochalasin D to inhibit platelets' contribution to clot formation [13, 15].

Impaired ROTEM (hypocoagulability) was defined as a clot formation speed above the upper limit of the reference interval (CT INTEM >246 s or CT EXTEM >74 s) and/or (CFT INTEM >100 s or CFT EXTEM >148 s) and/or a MCF below the lower limit of the reference interval (INTEM MCF <52 mm or EXTEM MCF <49 mm) and/or alpha angle below the lower limit of the reference interval (INTEM alpha angle <70° or EXTEM alpha angle <63°) [13, 15]. Finally, impaired ROTEM on FIBTEM was defined as a MCF <9 mm [16]. Normal ROTEM was considered if CT, CFT, MCF and alpha angle were within the reference ranges (INTEM CT: 137–246 s, CFT: 40–100 s, alpha angle: 70–83° and MCF: 52–72 mm; EXTEM CT: 42–74 s, CFT: 46–148 s, alpha angle: 63–83° and MCF: 49–71 mm; FIBTEM MCF: 9–25 mm) [15, 16].

Statistical analysis

Categorical variables were presented as absolute and relative frequencies. Continuous variables were presented as mean values and standard deviation (SD) or median values with interquartile ranges (IQR) in case of non-normal distribution (tested by the Kolmogorov-Smirnov test). Continuous variables were compared using independent *t* test or Mann–Whitney *U* test in case of non-normal distribution.

Two-tailed tests were used and when $p < 0.05$, the test was considered statistically significant. The SPSS™ (IBM SPSS Statistics for Windows, Version 21.0. Armonk, NY: IBM Corp) and GraphPad Prism version 6.0 (GraphPad Software, La Jolla, California, USA) were used for statistical analyses.

Results

From April 6th to May 5th 2015, 4641 medical appointments were scheduled at the outpatient clinic. From those, 3003 were first consultations (Fig. 1). Dengue virus infections were confirmed in 68.9% (2069/3003) of patients while 10.8% (224/2069) of patients had DVI and thrombocytopenia. Out of those, fifty-three patients [53/224 (23.6%)] were consecutively enrolled in this study (Fig. 1).

The main characteristics of DVI patients included in this study are shown in Table 1. The median age of DVI patients was 32 (IQR, 21–43) years and approximately 60% were male. The majority of DVI patients [31/42 (73.8%)] had no significant previous medical history. Most DVI patients presented with fever and headache and were hemodynamically stable (Table 1). Onset of symptoms was acute (median, 4 days; IQR, 2–5), which is consistent with predominance of NS1 positive results [51/53 (96.2%)]. Bleeding manifestations such as epistaxis, gingivorrhagia, hematemesis, hematuria and melena were reported in only 14.3% (7/49) of patients (Table 1). A total of 5.8% (3/52) of patients required hospitalization.

Table 1 Main characteristics of participating patients. Values represent % (n/total) or median (interquartile range [IQR])

Characteristics	Values[a]
Age, years	32 (21–43)
Gender, male	60.4 (32/53)
Comorbidities	
None	73.8 (31/42)
Hypertension	16.7 (7/42)
HIV infection	2.4 (1/42)
Prostatic hyperplasia	4.8 (2/42)
Dyspepsia	2.4 (1/42)
Clinical presentation	
Fever	100.0 (53/53)
Headache	83.0 (44/53)
Rash	36.8 (14/38)
Vomiting	25.5 (13/51)
Bleeding manifestations[b]	14.3 (7/49)
Dehydration[c]	11.3 (6/53)
Axillary temperature	37.0 (36.1-37.7)
Systolic blood pressure	127 (115–133)
Diastolic blood pressure	80 (73–86)
Heart rate	93 (82–102)
Serologic diagnosis	
NS1	96.2 (51/53)
IgM	20.8 (11/53)
IgG	3.8 (2/53)
Prior DV infection[d]	9.8 (5/51)
Yellow Fever vaccination[e]	18.9 (7/37)
Days after onset of symptoms	4 (2–5)
Need of hospitalization[f]	5.8 (3/52)

HIV Human Immunodeficiency Virus, *NS1* non-structural protein-1, *IgM* Immunoglobulin M, *IgG* Immunoglobulin G; [a] Totals may not sum to 53, owing to missing values; [b] epistaxis, gingivorrhagia, hematemesis, hematuria and melena; [c] clinical signs in mucosa and skin assessed by medical attendant; [d] considered if patient acknowledge a prior diagnosis stated by medical service. [e]: considered if patient acknowledge as a positive previous vaccination status, [f]: Unknown in one patient (lost to follow-up)

Laboratorial characteristics

The main laboratorial characteristics of DVI patients are shown in Table 2. All DVI patients with thrombocytopenia [median (IQR) platelets count: 76 (62–88) x10^9/L] had normal coagulation tests such as PT, TT, INR and aPTT (Table 2).

Thromboelastometry

The INTEM and EXTEM analysis were abnormal in, respectively, 71.7% (38/53) and 54.7% (29/53) of DVI patients while FIBTEM was normal in 94.3% (50/53) of DVI patients (Table 3). DVI patients with impaired

Table 2 Laboratory and conventional coagulation tests result in dengue virus infection patients. Values are presented as median and interquartile range

Characteristics	
Hemoglobin (g/dL)	15.1(14.2-16.1)
Hematocrit (%)	42.9 (40.6-45.6)
White Blood Cells (x10^3/uL)	3.1 (2.7-4.5)
Neutrophil (%)	42.3 (31.0-48.0)
Neutrophil (x10^3/uL)	1.4 (1.0-1.8)
Platelets (x 10^9/L)	76 (62–88)
Prothrombin time (sec)	100 (90–100)
INR	1.0 (1.0-1.1)
Thrombin Time (sec)	18.2 (17.0-19.5)
aPTT (sec)	28.9 (26.0-32.5)
Fibrinogen (g/dl)	290 (267–323)
D-dimer (ng/ml)	1330 (800–1840)

INR international normalized ratio, *aPTT* activated partial thromboplastin time

(hypocoagulability) ROTEM in INTEM and EXTEM assays exhibited higher CFT, lower MCF and alpha angle than DVI patients with a normal ROTEM (Table 3).

Hypocoagulability was found in 28.6% (2/7) of DVI patients with minor bleeding manifestations in EXTEM and in 57.1% (4/7) patients in INTEM. Out of three patients who required hospitalization, two (66.6%) exhibited hypocoagulability in INTEM and one (33.3%) on EXTEM.

Conventional coagulation tests versus thromboelastometry

Comparisons between thromboelastometry and conventional coagulation tests are shown in Table 4. Compared to DVI patients with normal INTEM, DVI patients presenting with impaired INTEM exhibited lower platelet count, INR and plasma fibrinogen levels (Table 4). Dengue virus infection patients presenting with impaired EXTEM exhibited lower plasma fibrinogen levels and higher d-dimer, while platelets count, INR and aPTT did not differ between the groups (Table 4). Finally,

Table 4 Rotational thromboelastometry (ROTEM®) analysis and conventional coagulation tests. Values represent median (IQR)

Characteristics	Normal	Impaired	*P* value
INTEM, % (n/total)	28.3 (15/53)	71.7 (38/53)	
Platelets (x 10^9/L)	90 (77–94)	70 (57–84)	0.005[a]
INR	1.1 (1.0-1.3)	1.0 (1.0-1.1)	0.034[b]
aPTT (sec)	28.2 (26.0-31.8)	29.0 (26.0-33.3)	0.867[b]
Fibrinogen (g/dl)	321 (290–355)	278 (267–311)	0.021[b]
D-dimer (ng/ml)	950 (320–1510)	1410 (950–1900)	0.076[b]
EXTEM, % (n/total)	45.3 (24/53)	54.7 (29/53)	
Platelets (x 10^9/L)	82 (68–91)	69 (57–83)	0.052[a]
INR	1.0 (1.0-1.1)	1.0 (1.0-1.1)	0.390[b]
aPTT (sec)	30.3 (25.0-32.2)	28.1 (26.6-32.8)	0.816[b]
Fibrinogen (g/dl)	308 (278–354)	278 (264–300)	0.006[a]
D-dimer (ng/ml)	950 (705–1500)	1600 (1220–1990)	0.008[b]
FIBTEM, % (n/total)	94.3 (50/53)	5.7 (3/53)	
Platelets (x 10^9/L)	77 (62–88)	71 (64–95)	0.758[b]
INR	1.0 (1.0-1.1)	1.1 (1.0-1.1)	0.427[b]
aPTT (sec)	28.5 (26.0-31.8)	33.3 (26.7-33.4)	0.254[b]
Fibrinogen (g/dl)	291 (267–323)	278 (214–315)	0.520[b]
D-dimer (ng/ml)	1295 (790–1820)	1840 (1500–1980)	0.223[b]

INR international normalized ratio and *aPTT* activated partial thromboplastin time. *p* values with ([a]) independent *t* test and ([b]) Mann–Whitney *U* test

Table 3 Rotational thromboelastometry (ROTEM®) parameters in dengue virus infection patients. Values represent median (IQR)

Characteristics	All	Normal	Impaired	*P* value*
INTEM, % (n/total)	100.0 (53/53)	28.3 (15/53)	71.7 (38/53)	
Clotting time (sec)	177 (160–207)	166 (158–179)	180 (161–214)	0.114[b]
Clot formation time (sec)	144 (108–178)	98 (90–106)	166 (131–220)	<0.001[b]
Maximum clot firmness (mm)	48 (42–52)	53 (52–55)	45 (41–49)	<0.001[a]
Alpha angle (degrees)	69 (63–73)	74 (72–74)	66 (62–69)	<0.001[a]
Amplitude 10 (mm)	41 (37–45)	48 (47–50)	37 (33–42)	<0.001[a]
EXTEM, % (n/total)	100.0 (53/53)	45.3 (24/53)	54.7 (29/53)	
Clotting time (sec)	69 (65–78)	68 (61–74)	74 (66–84)	0.044[a]
Clot formation time (sec)	148 (126–198)	126 (114–140)	197 (163–269)	<0.001[b]
Maximum clot firmness (mm)	49 (44–55)	54 (52–56)	44 (40–48)	<0.001[a]
Alpha angle (degrees)	68 (63–72)	72 (68–74)	65 (56–69)	<0.001[b]
Amplitude 10 (mm)	41 (35–46)	46 (44–48)	36 (31–39)	<0.001[a]
FIBTEM, % (n/total)	100.0 (53/53)	94.3 (50/53)	5.7 (3/53)	
Maximum clot firmness (mm)	15 (13–18)	16 (14–18)	7 (7–8)	0.004[b]

*: Comparisons between normal and impaired groups. p values with ([a]) independent *t* test and ([b]) Mann–Whitney *U* test

conventional coagulation tests did not differ between DVI patients with normal or abnormal FIBTEM (Table 4).

Discussion

This study demonstrated that DVI patients with thrombocytopenia frequently exhibited hypocoagulability assessed by thromboelastometry while conventional coagulation tests (PT, TT, INR and aPTT) and plasma fibrinogen levels remained within reference range.

Our findings contrasted previous retrospective studies, which demonstrated that prolonged coagulation times are frequent and strongly associated with bleeding manifestations in DVI thrombocytopenic patients [8, 9, 17, 18]. For instance, Wills and colleagues demonstrated in DHF Vietnamese children that a prolonged aPTT >30 s and platelet count <50 x 10^9/L had an increased risk of bleeding [9]. They also suggested that thrombocytopenia is a mortality predictor in this population of patients [9]. The discrepancy between our findings and those reported by others could be explained, at least in part, by the differences in severity among DVI studied patients [2, 4].

Bleeding complications in DVI patients have been associated with a combination of thrombocytopenia, reduced thrombin formation and increased fibrinolysis [19, 20]. According to Nimmannitya, even extremely low platelet count, such as <20 x 10^9/L, does not increase bleeding risk except in prolonged shock states [21]. This is a very interesting observation since DVI patients frequently exhibited low platelets in association with impaired platelets function [4, 7, 19]. Platelets are crucial for primary hemostasis as they contribute to thrombus formation [10, 22]. Fibrinogen, the final substrate of coagulation and the ligand of platelet glycoprotein IIb-IIIa complex receptors, enhance platelets function [10, 16]. Therefore, we can assume that the low frequency of bleeding manifestations in thrombocytopenic DVI patients in our study can be explained, at least in part, by maintained plasma fibrinogen levels, as shown in FIBTEM analysis [13, 15].

It is likely that fibrinogen plays a key role in keeping clot strength in DVI patients during the first days of disease [10, 20, 22]. Fibrinogen, the factor I of coagulation system, is the most important numerically and functionally coagulation factor [12, 22]. Fibrinogen represents approximately ninety percent of the total amount of plasmatic coagulation factors and it is the first coagulation factor to fall below a critical value during bleeding and hemodilution [10, 20, 22, 23]. Nevertheless, the critical plasma fibrinogen level associated to increased severity of DVI patients due to major bleeding events, hospitalization and death, needs to be determined [3, 4, 9, 20].

Disseminated intravascular coagulation (DIC) is defined by the presence of four criteria: thrombocytopenia (platelets below 100 x10^9/L), high level of products of fibrin degradation (PDF), such as d-dimer, PT prolongation and low plasma fibrinogen level [24]. Our study demonstrated that patients in the first days of DVI already met at least two out of four criteria for DIC (low platelets and high PDF). Studies addressing hemostasis in DHF patients showed that all DHF patients manifested acute type of DIC [19, 20, 25]. Prolongation of aPTT and PT, decreased platelets count, plasma fibrinogen level, prothrombin, factor VIII, plasminogen and antithrombin III activities were observed transiently during acute phase of DHF [9, 20, 25] and they characterize hemorrhagic diathesis of DVI severe patients [3, 4, 20, 21, 25].

Viscoelastic tests allow early and individualized coagulation management in different scenarios, such as in trauma [26, 27], liver transplantation [13, 28], cardiac [15, 28] and neurologic surgeries [16, 29], post-partum hemorrhage [12, 27] and in critically ill patients [22, 26, 28]. Nevertheless, dengue treatment is based mainly on supportive care with fluids and electrolytes [2, 4, 30, 31]. Transfusion triggers and therapeutic goals are not consensus in DVI patients [2, 5, 30, 31]. A report of four DVI bleeding patients with severe DVI and thrombocytopenia in which desmopressin were administrated, showed clinical improvement and hemorrhage control [32]. Desmopressin is a hormone that stimulates release of Von Willebrand factor (vWF) by endothelial cells [10, 22]. The complex factor VIII (FVIII) and vWF improve platelets aggregation and clot stability [33]. Increased levels of vWF were demonstrated in DVI patients during the first days of disease [19, 33]. FVIII/vWF complex is likely to play a key hemostatic role during the early course of DVI [10, 22]. Endothelial activation may be responsible for extravascular plasma leakage and shock in severe DVI patients [2–5]. However, in the majority of DVI patients, inflammation and endothelial cell activation may represent a compensatory mechanism for thrombocytopenia, clot impairment and hypocoagulability during the early course of disease due to fibrinogen activation and increased vWF levels, which improve platelet aggregation [33–35].

Another key point in the treatment of DVI patients is the need of high I.V. volume expansion due to intense plasma leakage [2, 30, 31]. Thus, dilution coagulopathy may be present in DVI patients and further aggravate coagulation [2, 22, 34]. A thromboelastometry study showed clot impairment after fluid challenge infusions [36]. A fibrin polymerization deficit is assumed to be one of the major side effects of colloids and crystalloids on coagulation. However, impaired coagulation due to dilution coagulopathy is usually transient and can be partially reversed by fibrinogen concentrate transfusion [10, 36]. Moreover, colloids can also impair thrombus generation [22], decrease factor XIII-fibrin polymer interaction [36] and decrease platelet aggregability and adhesion [10, 11]. This could perpetuate a vicious circle of clot impairment in DVI patients with hypocoagulability secondary to a viral infection [37]. Therefore, we need to keep in mind the importance of individualizing volume expansion in DVI patients presenting with coagulopathy [31–34]. Therefore, a thromboelastometry-driven approach could represent an alternative strategy to manage complex cases of DVI associated with coagulopathy [37–39].

Our study has limitations. First, a small sample of DVI patients was included in this analysis. Nevertheless, to our knowledge, this was the first time DVI patients were analyzed with viscoelastic test such as thromboelastometry. Furthermore, most patients included in this report had primary DVI and were not severely ill, which might have affected and/or ameliorated their conventional coagulation tests results. Second, conventional coagulation tests abnormalities and bleeding disorders could be more pronounced in later stages during the course of disease and therefore not detected by our study. Third, dengue virus infection was confirmed by using immunochromatographic assays, which may lack sensitivity and specificity compared to real time polymerase chain reaction (PCR) or enzyme-linked immunosorbent assays (ELISA) for detection of IgM/IgG antibodies and NS1 antigen [40]. Finally, although Zika and Chikungunya viruses co-infections are well known today, they were unknown when this study was conducted [41]. Since diagnostic tools for Zika virus infection were not available in Brazil when the study was carried out, we cannot rule out Zika virus co-infection in our studied patients.

Conclusion

Outpatients with dengue virus infection and thrombocytopenia commonly exhibited impaired thromboelastometry despite normal conventional coagulation tests. That suggests viscoelastic tests might have a higher sensitivity to detect early coagulation abnormalities in this population of patients. Long-term outcomes and the question of whether or not transfusion resuscitation algorithms based on viscoelastic tests will improve outcomes in DVI patients with coagulopathy and bleeding needs to be further evaluated.

Abbreviations

A 10: Amplitude 10; aPTT: Activated partial thromboplastin time; CFT: Clot formation time; CT: Clotting time; DHF: Dengue hemorrhagic fever; DIC: Disseminated intravascular coagulation; DV: Dengue virus; DVI: Dengue virus infection; EXTEM: Extrinsically activated thromboelastometry test; FIBTEM: Fibrin-based thromboelastometry test; HR: Heart rate; INR: International normalized ratio; INTEM: Intrinsically activated thromboelastometry test; IQR: Interquartile range; IV: Intravenous; MCF: Maximum clot firmness; NS1: Non-structural protein-1; PDFs: Products of fibrin degradation; PT: Prothrombin time; ROTEM®: Rotational thromboelastometry test; SBP: Systolic blood pressure; SD: Standard deviation; TT: Thrombin time; vWF: Von Willebrand factor

Acknowledgements

The authors thank the nurses and laboratory technicians for their supportive care of patients during DVI outbreak. We thank Helena Spalic for proof-reading this manuscript.

Funding

Activator reagents for thromboelastometry analysis (INTEM, EXTEM and FIBTEM) were provided by MedLine®, TEM®, representation in São Paulo, Brazil.

Authors' contributions

FP designed the study, enrolled patients, recorded clinical data, performed laboratory and statistical analysis and drafted the manuscript; TDC and ARM contributed to the study design, enrolled patients, recorded clinical data, performed statistical analysis and revised the manuscript; AV and VA performed the laboratory analysis; JG, SS and MRL contributed to patients enrollment and reviewed the manuscript, EK contributed to study designed and manuscript production; RRR and ABC designed the study, analyzed the data and contributed to manuscript production. All authors revised and approved the final manuscript version.

Competing interests

The authors declare that they have no competing interests.

Consent for publication

Not applicable.

Author details

[1]Department of Intensive Care Medicine, Hospital Israelita Albert Einstein, Av. Albert Einstein, 627/701, 5° andar, São Paulo CEP: 05651-901, Brazil. [2]Hospital das Clinicas da Faculdade de Medicina da Universidade de São Paulo, São Paulo, Brazil.

References

1. Chen R, Vasilakis N. Dengue–quo tu et quo vadis? Viruses. 2011;3(9):1562–608.
2. Guzmán MG, Kouri G. Dengue: an update. Lancet Infect Dis. 2002;2(1):33–42.
3. Kurane I. Dengue hemorrhagic fever with special emphasis on immunopathogenesis. Comp Immunol Microb. 2007;30(5–6):329–40.
4. Srikiatkhachorn A. Plasma leakage in dengue haemorrhagic fever. Thromb Haemost. 2009;102(6):1042–9.
5. Guzman M. Dengue and dengue hemorrhagic fever in the Americas: lessons and challenges. J Clin Virol. 2003;27(1):1–13.
6. Chuang YC, Lin YS, Liu CC, Liu HS, Liao SH, Shi MD, et al. Factors contributing to the disturbance of coagulation and fibrinolysis in dengue virus infection. J Formos Med Assoc. 2013;112(1):12–7.
7. Hottz ED, Oliveira MF, Nunes PC, Nogueira RM, Valls-de-Souza R, Da Poian AT, et al. Dengue induces platelet activation, mitochondrial dysfunction and cell death through mechanisms that involve DC-SIGN and caspases. J Thromb Haemost. 2013;11(5):951–62.
8. Chua MN, Molanida R, de Guzman M, Laberiza F. Prothrombin time and partial thromboplastin time as a predictor of bleeding in patients with dengue hemorrhagic fever. Se Asian J Trop Med. 1993;24 Suppl 1:141–3.

9. Wills BA, Oragui EE, Stephens AC, Daramola OA, Dung NM, Loan HT, et al. Coagulation abnormalities in dengue hemorrhagic Fever: serial investigations in 167 Vietnamese children with dengue shock syndrome. Clin Infect Dis. 2002;35:277–85.
10. Brummel-Ziedins KE, Wolberg AS. Global assays of hemostasis. Curr Opin Hematol. 2014;21(5):395–403.
11. Favaloro EJ, Lippi G. Coagulation update: What's new in hemostasis testing? Thromb Res. 2011;127:S13–6.
12. Mallett SV, Armstrong M. Point-of-care monitoring of haemostasis. Anaesthesia. 2015;70 Suppl 1:73–7. e25-6.
13. McMichael MA, Smith SA. Viscoelastic coagulation testing: technology, applications, and limitations. Vet Clin Path. 2011;40(2):140–53.
14. Reikvam H, Steien E, Hauge B, Liseth K, Hagen KG, Storkson R, et al. Thrombelastography. Transfus Apher Sci. 2009;40(2):119–23.
15. Whiting D, DiNardo JA. TEG and ROTEM: technology and clinical applications. Am J Hematol. 2014;89(2):228–32.
16. Stensballe J, Ostrowski SR, Johansson PI. Viscoelastic guidance of resuscitation. Curr Opin Anesthesio. 2014;27(2):212–8.
17. Díaz-Quijano FA. Predictors of spontaneous bleeding in dengue patients: a systematic review of the literature. Invest Clin. 2008;49:111–22.
18. Diaz-Quijano FA, Villar-Centeno LA, Martinez-Vega RA. Predictors of spontaneous bleeding in patients with acute febrile syndrome from a dengue endemic area. J Clin Virol. 2010;49:11–5.
19. de Azeredo EL, Monteiro RQ, de-Oliveira Pinto LM. Thrombocytopenia in dengue: interrelationship between virus and the imbalance between coagulation and fibrinolysis and inflammatory mediators. Mediat Inflamm. 2015, Article ID 313842, 16 pages.
20. Orsi FA, Angerami RN, Mazetto BM, Quaino SK, Santiago-Bassora F, Castro V, et al. Reduced thrombin formation and excessive fibrinolysis are associated with bleeding complications in patients with dengue fever: a case–control study comparing dengue fever patients with and without bleeding manifestations. BMC Infect Dis. 2013, 3(1), article 350.
21. Nimmannitya S. Dengue hemorrahagic fever: disorders of hemostasia. Bangkok, Thailand: Proceeding International Congress of Hemotology, Asia-Pacific Division; 1999.
22. Hunt BJ. Bleeding and coagulopathies in critical care. N Engl J Med. 2014; 370(9):847–59.
23. Fries D, Martini WZ. Role of fibrinogen in trauma-induced coagulopathy. Brit J Anaesth. 2010;105(2):116–21.
24. Taylor FB, Toh CH, Hoots WK, Wada H. Towards definition, clinical and laboratory criteria, and a scoring system for disseminated intravascular coagulation. Thromb Haemost. 2001;86:1327–30.
25. Funahara Y, Sumarmo, Wirawan R. Features of DIC in dengue hemorrhagic fever. Bibl Haematol. 1983;49:201–11.
26. Ganter MT, Hofer CK. Coagulation monitoring: current techniques and clinical use of viscoelastic point-of-care coagulation devices. Anesth Analg. 2008;106(5):1366–75.
27. Schochl H, Nienaber U, Hofer G, Voelckel W, Jambor C, Scharbert G, et al. Goal-directed coagulation management of major trauma patients using thromboelastometry (ROTEM)-guided administration of fibrinogen concentrate and prothrombin complex concentrate. Crit Care. 2010; 14(2):R55.
28. Sniecinski RM, Levy JH. Bleeding and management of coagulopathy. J Thorac Cardiovasc Surg. 2011;142(3):662–7.
29. Perry DJ, Fitzmaurice DA, Kitchen S, Mackie IJ, Mallett S. Point-of-care testing in haemostasis. Brit J Haematol. 2010;150(5):501–14.
30. Rigau-Pérez JG, Clark GG, Gubler DJ, Reiter P, Sanders EJ, Vorndam AV. Dengue and dengue haemorrhagic fever. Lancet. 1998;352(9132):971–7.
31. Singhi S, Kissoon N, Bansal A. Dengue and dengue hemorrhagic fever: management issues in an intensive care unit. J Pediatr. 2007;83(2 Suppl):S22–35.
32. Pea L, Roda L, Moll F. Desmopressin treatment for a case of dengue hemorrhagic fever/dengue shock syndrome. Clin Infect Dis. 2001;33(9): 1611–2.
33. Neff AT, Sidonio Jr RF. Management of VWD. Hematology Am Soc Hematol Educ Program. 2014;2014(1):536–41.
34. Martina BE, Koraka P, Osterhaus AD. Dengue virus pathogenesis: an integrated view. Clin Microbiol Rev. 2009;22(4):564–81.
35. Ho TS, Wang SM, Lin YS, Liu CC. Clinical and laboratory predictive markers for acute dengue infection. J Biomed Sci. 2013, 20(1), article 75.
36. Kozek-Langenecker SA. Fluids and coagulation. Curr Opin Criti Care. 2015; 21(4):285–91.
37. Saner FH. Rotational thrombelastometry: a step forward to safer patient care? Crit Care. 2014;18(6):706.
38. Karon BS. Why is everyone so excited about thromboelastrography (TEG)? Clin Chim Acta. 2014;436:143–8.
39. Levy JH, Dutton RP, Hemphill 3rd JC, Shander A, Cooper D, Paidas MJ, et al. Multidisciplinary approach to the challenge of hemostasis. Anesth Analg. 2010;110(2):354–64.
40. Vickers IE, Harvey KM, Brown MG, Nelson K, DuCasse MB, Lindo JF. The performance of the SD BIOLINE Dengue DUO® rapid immunochromatographic test kit for the detection of NS1 antigen, IgM and IgG antibodies during a dengue type 1 epidemic in Jamaica. J Biomed Sci. 2015;22:55.
41. Zammarchi L, Tappe D, Fortuna C, Remoli ME, Günter S, Venturi G, et al. Zika virus infection in a traveler returning to Europe from Brazil, March 2015. Euro Surveill. 2015;20:(23).

3

Early diagnosis of dengue disease severity in a resource-limited Asian country

Philippe Cavailler[1,8*], Arnaud Tarantola[2], Yee Sin Leo[1,3], Andrew A. Lover[1,9], Anne Rachline[2], Moniboth Duch[4], Rekol Huy[5], Ai Li Quake[1], Yuvatha Kdan[4], Veasna Duong[6], Jeremy L. Brett[7,10] and Philippe Buchy[6,11]

Abstract

Background: Dengue is endemic throughout Cambodia, a country faced with significant health and economic challenges. We undertook a clinical study at the National Paediatric Hospital in Phnom Penh to evaluate clinical diagnostic parameters for dengue and predictors of disease outcome.

Methods: Between September 2011 and January 2013, all consecutive inpatients aged between 1 and 15 years and presenting with suspected dengue were enrolled. They were clinically assessed using both the 1997 and 2009 WHO dengue classifications. Specimens were collected upon admission and discharge and tested for dengue at Institut Pasteur in Cambodia.

Results: A total of 701 patients were screened. Of these, 79 % were dengue-confirmed by laboratory testing, and 21 % tested dengue-negative. A positive tourniquet test, absence of upper respiratory symptoms, leukopenia, thrombocytopenia, and elevated liver transaminases were independent predictors for laboratory-confirmed dengue among the children. The presence of several warning signs on hospital admission was associated with a concurrent laboratory-confirmed diagnosis of severe disease outcome.

Conclusions: The presence of two or more warning signs was associated with a concurrent laboratory-confirmed diagnosis of severe dengue at hospital admission. Thus, a cumulative score combining simple clinical parameters and first-line laboratory findings could be used to accurately predict dengue virus infection in pediatric populations, optimizing triage in settings with limited laboratory resources.

Background

Dengue is an acute febrile illness caused by one of four main dengue virus (DENV) serotypes (DENV-1, DENV-2, DENV-3 and DENV-4) and transmitted by *Aedes* spp. mosquitoes. Infection with DENV may remain asymptomatic or cause a spectrum of illnesses ranging from self-limiting influenza-like illness to life-threatening manifestations associated with plasma leakage and hemorrhage potentially leading to hypovolemic shock. DENV was first isolated in Cambodia in 1963. The disease is endemic, with peak epidemics observed each year during the rainy season.

Since 2000, the National Dengue Control Program of the Cambodian Ministry of Health (MOH) has reported an average of 103 cases per 100,000 population, with an annual case fatality rate ranging from 0.7 to 1.7 %. All four dengue serotypes have been found circulating in Cambodia with alternative predominance of serotypes DENV-2 and DENV-3. The DENV-1 represents from 5 to 20 % of all circulating viruses, depending on the year [1].

In resource-limited settings, the optimization of triage during dengue epidemics is crucial to avoid overwhelming health systems and to maximize the impact of available supportive treatments and resources. Therefore, in 2009, the World Health Organization (WHO) revised earlier guidelines to more accurately identify patients at risk of developing severe dengue and who may require hospitalization for closer clinical monitoring. Despite these guidelines, early diagnosis of dengue remains challenging for clinicians, as initial symptoms are generally indistinguishable from other endemic febrile illnesses in

* Correspondence: pcavailler@gmail.com
[1]Infectious Diseases Programme, Saw Swee Hock School of Public Health, National University of Singapore, Singapore, Singapore
[8]Current address: Agence de Médecine Préventive, 13 Chemin du Levant, Ferney-Voltaire 01210, France
Full list of author information is available at the end of the article

the tropics, and laboratory confirmation is not routinely available. Thus, there is currently no consensus on guidelines relying solely on clinical features to distinguish dengue from other febrile illnesses [2, 3]. While several prospective studies have described predictors for dengue diagnosis [4–6], none of these studies focused on the prediction of a concurrent laboratory-confirmed diagnosis of severe pediatric dengue at the time of hospital admission.

This study aims to describe the clinical spectrum of a large number of pediatric cases at a referral hospital in Phnom Penh, Cambodia, and to determine the clinical features predictive of laboratory-confirmed dengue infection. We also sought to determine, at hospital admission, the predictors of a concurrent laboratory-confirmed diagnosis of severe disease (Dengue Hemorrhagic Fever [DHF] as defined by the WHO 1997 guidelines [7] and Severe Dengue [SD] as defined by the WHO 2009 guidelines [8]).

Methods

The study was conducted at the internal medicine and emergency wards of the National Paediatric Hospital in Phnom Penh. All children aged 1 to 15 years who were hospitalized between September 2011 and January 2013 and presented with acute onset of fever (temperature of > 37.5 °C on admission or history of fever less than 7 days) were screened for eligibility using both the 1997 and the 2009 WHO guidelines criteria (Additional file 1: Eligibility Form). All patients with suspected dengue were enrolled after informed written consent was obtained from the patients' parents or guardians. Basic demographic, clinical and laboratory data were collected by trained clinicians at admission, using standardized Case Report Forms for all eligible patients (Additional file 2: CRF). Clinical information included the signs and symptoms listed in the 1997 and 2009 WHO case definitions. Basic laboratory data included the results of white blood cell and platelet counts, hematocrit and liver transaminases titers. The study was approved by the Cambodian National Ethics Committee for Health Research (approval number 123-NECHR, 22 August 2011).

Serum samples were collected at the time of admission during the acute febrile phase of dengue infection ("acute sample") and at the time of hospital discharge ("convalescent sample"), ideally at least 7 days after the collection of the acute sample to allow interpretation of hemagglutination inhibition test results. Other details of this study have been reported previously [9].

Paired serum specimens were tested using an immunoglobulin M (IgM)-antibody capture enzyme-linked immunosorbent assay (MAC-ELISA) and a hemagglutination inhibition (HI) assay. Because of possible cross-reactivity, all specimens were systematically tested for anti-dengue virus and anti-Japanese encephalitis virus IgM using an in-house MAC-ELISA and a HI assay. The acute sample was tested for viral ribonucleic acid (RNA) by a serotype-specific quantitative real-time RT-PCR (qRT-PCR) method [10]. In addition, virus isolation was performed by inoculating sera into C6/36 *Aedes albopictus* and Vero E-6 cell cultures, and the virus serotype was identified using a direct fluorescent antibody assay of monoclonal antibodies [11]. Patients with negative qRT-PCR and inconclusive serological testing were tested for NS1 antigen using an ELISA capture commercial kit (Panbio Dengue Early ELISA, Panbio©, Sinnamon Park, Australia).

A case was considered positive for dengue when laboratory tests met one or more of the following criteria [8, 12]: 1) Dengue viral RNA detected by qRT-PCR or virus isolated after inoculation into cell cultures; 2) Seroconversion of DENV-specific IgM detected by MAC-ELISA in paired acute and convalescent samples; 3) Four-fold increase of HI antibody titer between acute and convalescent sera; 4) Dengue NS1 antigen detection.

All statistical analyses were conducted using SPSS version 20 (PNSW, Chicago, IL, USA) and Stata 12.1 (StataCorp, College Station, Texas, USA). We performed univariate analysis to identify the features associated with dengue positivity and severe disease. For the analyses on the predictors for dengue virus infection, we included all variables from the clinical assessment and the results of baseline laboratory parameters conducted upon hospital admission. We then assessed the association between the presence of warning signs on admission and the concomitant laboratory-confirmed diagnosis of severe disease (dengue hemorrhagic fever [DHF], dengue shock syndrome [DSS], or severe dengue [SD]). Mantel-Haenszel test were used for the comparisons of proportions (Fisher's exact test if a cell had an expected frequency below five).

Multivariate logistic regression analysis was performed to identify variables independently associated with laboratory-positive dengue. The reference group included patients with a negative dengue laboratory confirmatory test. The initial logistic regression model included all covariates with a p-value of < 0.2 following univariate analysis. We then developed a score based on the results of the multivariate analysis; for each individual, each characteristic independently associated with dengue positivity was combined to provide an overall risk score. For each factor, categories with an odds ratio of ten or less relative to the baseline category were given a score of one, and categories with an odds ratio greater than ten were given a score of two. These scores were used to assess the ability to predict dengue infection via comparison of the sensitivity and specificity. Based on the procedures described in previous studies aiming to compare the performance of various clinical algorithms developed by WHO [13–15], the cut-off of each model was taken as the score that maximized the sum of the sensitivity and the specificity.

Receiver-Operator Characteristics (ROC) curves showing the Area Under the Curve (AUC) were generated to compare the overall ability of the different scores to predict dengue infection and concurrent laboratory-confirmed diagnosis of disease severity at hospital admission. Predicting accuracy was considered to be high if the AUC was > 0.9, moderate if in the range of 0.7 to 0.9, and low if between 0.5 and 0.7 [16].

Results

From September 2011 to January 2013, a total of 1115 admitted cases presenting with acute febrile illness were evaluated, of which 701 (59 %) were clinically suspected of being dengue-positive as per the 1997 or 2009 WHO guidelines. Of these 701 suspected cases, 79 % (558/701) were laboratory-confirmed dengue cases, and 21 % (143/701) were laboratory-negative and classified as Other Febrile Illnesses (OFI). Of the dengue laboratory-positive cases, 531 (95.2 %) were confirmed by PCR (520 DENV-1; eight DENV-2; one DENV-3; two DENV-4); 27 had a negative PCR result and were confirmed by another test: eight by IgM seroconversion, eight by a four-fold increase of HI titer, and 11 by NS1. Among the 558 laboratory-confirmed dengue cases, gender was found to be evenly distributed (49.5 % female and 50.5 % male). The median duration of hospital stay was 3 days (Inter-Quartile Range [IQR] 2–4). Age varied between 1 and 15 years, with a median of 7 years (IQR 5–10), and 18.3 % were under 5 years of age. The median onset of fever prior to admission was 4 days (IQR 4–5) and did not differ between dengue and non-dengue febrile illnesses (Table 1).

Using the 1997 WHO classification, 85 (15.2 %) of the dengue laboratory-confirmed cases would be classified as negative, 378 (67.7 %) as dengue fever (DF), 61 (10.9 %) as DHF, and 34 (6.1 %) as dengue shock syndrome (DSS). Using the 2009 WHO classification, 71 (12.7 %) of the dengue laboratory-confirmed cases would be classified as negative, 207 (37.1 %) as dengue without warning signs (WS), 240 (43.1 %) as dengue with WS, and 40 (7.2 %) as SD (Fig. 1).

Table 1 Demographics on admission of laboratory-positive and laboratory-negative patients, Dengue Surveillance Study ($N = 701$), National Paediatric Hospital, Phnom Penh, Sep. 2011–Jan. 2013

	DENV-Neg. $n = 143$	DENV-Pos. $n = 558$	*P*-value
Males (%)	50.0	50.5	>0.20
<5 years old (%)	24.5	16.7	0.09
Age: median [IQR]	7 [5–10]	7 [5–10]	>0.20
Onset of fever: median days [IQR]	4 [3–5]	4 [4–5]	0.29
Hospital stay: median days [IQR]	3 [3–4]	3 [2–4]	>0.20

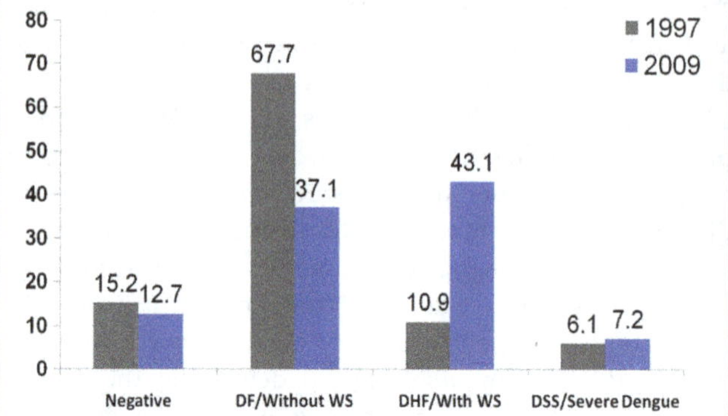

Fig. 1 Classification of cases according to the criteria of the WHO 1997/2009 case definitions for dengue, National Paediatric Hospital, Phnom Penh, Sep. 2011–Jan. 2013

Clinical features of dengue infection

The clinical features of both laboratory-confirmed and negative patients were compared using multivariate analysis (Additional file 3: Supplementary Data Analyses). When the results of liver transaminases were included, we found the following five variables to be independently associated with laboratory-confirmed dengue: positive tourniquet test (odds ratio [OR] 2.17, 95 % confidence interval [CI] 1.32–3.59); absence of upper respiratory infection (URI) symptoms (OR 2.53, 95 % CI 1.47–4.37); platelet count < 100,000 cells per mm^3 (OR 2.28, 95 % CI 1.32–6.37); leukocyte count < 4000 cells per mm^3 (OR 3.60, 95 % CI 2.04–6.37); and liver transaminases > 60 IU/mL (either AST or ALT; OR 2.31, 95 % CI 1.42–3.75). When we excluded the results of ALT/AST testing, as these tests may not always be available in resource-limited settings, the following six variables were associated with laboratory-confirmed dengue infection: nausea or vomiting (OR 1.81, 95 % CI 1.10–2.98); absence of URI symptoms (OR 2.59, 95 % CI 1.63–4.14); positive tourniquet test (OR 2.22, 95 % CI 1.43–3.44); liver enlargement (OR 2.97, 95 % CI 1.31–6.74); platelet count < 100,000 cells per mm^3 (OR 2.37, 95 % CI 1.48–3.82); and leukocyte count < 4000 cells per mm^3 (OR 2.96, 95 % CI 1.82–4.83).

Risk scores were developed based on the cumulative total of the variables independently associated with laboratory confirmation of dengue from logistic regression models. For both scoring systems (with and without ALT/AST results), the prediction with the best sensitivity and specificity for laboratory-confirmed dengue integrated three criteria (Additional file 3). Two clinical scoring algorithms were developed based on the results of these analyses.

Table 2 shows the comparative performance of the two clinical algorithms in predicting laboratory-confirmed dengue. The two clinical algorithms (either with or without AST/ALT results) had a low specificity (57.4 and

Table 2 Performance of clinical algorithms in the prediction of dengue, National Paediatric Hospital, Phnom Penh, Sep. 2011–Jan. 2013

	Model A (with ALT/AST)	Model B (no ALT/AST)
Sensitivity (95 % C.I.)	75.7 (71.4–79.6)	84.2 (80.9–87.2)
Specificity (95 % C.I.)	65.7 (56.4–65.3)	57.4 (48.9–75.4)
Sensitivity + Specificity	141.4	141.6
Positive Predictive Value	89.7	88.3
Negative Predictive Value	40.8	48.8
AUC (95 % C.I.)	0.71 (0.65–0.77)	0.69 (0.63–0.75)

65.7 %, respectively) but an acceptable level of sensitivity (84.2 and 75.7 %, respectively), with high positive predictive values. The ROC curves illustrate how these different models predict laboratory-confirmed dengue. The AUC was equal to 0.69 for the clinical algorithm without ALT/AST results, and to 0.71 for the algorithm with ALT/AST results.

Clinical features of DHF/DSS and severe dengue

We also explored the association between the presence of WS and the concurrent laboratory-confirmed diagnosis of DHF/DSS or SD at hospital admission. For both DHF/DSS and SD, the most frequent WS were clinical fluid accumulation (66 and 90 %, respectively), liver enlargement (55 and 65 %) and lethargy or restlessness (44 and 68 %). Table 3 describes the ability of the WS to predict laboratory-confirmed DHF/DSS or SD at hospital admission. Specificity was high for persistent vomiting (97 and 96 %, respectively), clinical fluid accumulation (96 and 91 %), and mucosal bleeding (92 and 90 %). Presentation of any WS was associated with a high sensitivity (92 %) but poor specificity in predicting severe outcomes. The presence of two or more WS at hospital admission yielded a sensitivity of 74 % and a specificity of 83 % in predicting a concurrent laboratory-confirmed diagnosis of DHF/DSS at hospital admission. The occurrence of three or more WS was associated with a sensitivity of 70 % and an increased specificity of 92 % for the prediction of a concurrent laboratory-confirmed diagnosis of SD at hospital admission.

The ROC curves (Figs. 2 and 3) illustrate the accuracy of these various models in predicting concurrent diagnosis of laboratory-confirmed DHF/DSS or SD at hospital admission, based on the total number of WS included in each model. For DHF/DSS, the highest predictive value was obtained when patients presented two or more WS upon admission (AUC = 0.78). For SD, predictive value was maximized when patients presented with at least three WS at admission (AUC = 0.81).

Discussion

We conducted a 16-month clinical study of pediatric inpatients in a single referral hospital in Phnom Penh, Cambodia. While all 701 children enrolled in the study had clinical suspicion of dengue on admission, dengue was biologically confirmed in only 558 (79.6 %). This enabled us to compare children with dengue and those with non-dengue febrile illnesses. This information is

Table 3 Performance of warning signs in the predictive diagnosis of dengue severe manifestations, National Paediatric Hospital, Phnom Penh, Sep. 2011–Jan. 2013

	DHF/DSS				Severe Dengue			
	Se	Sp	PPV[a]	NPV[b]	Se	Sp	PPV	NPV
Warning Signs								
Abdominal tenderness	43.2	77.0	43.2	86.8	40.0	74.6	10.9	94.1
Persistent vomiting	21.1	97.0	58.8	85.6	37.5	96.3	44.1	95.2
Clinical fluid accumulation	66.3	96.1	77.8	93.3	90.0	91.3	44.4	99.2
Mucosal bleeding	22.1	92.0	36.2	85.1	20.0	90.3	13.8	93.6
Lethargy/restlessness	44.2	83.3	35.3	87.9	60.0	81.6	20.2	96.3
Liver enlargement > 2 cm	55.8	82.0	39.0	90.0	65.0	78.7	19.1	96.7
Warning Signs Count								
• at least one	92.6	51.8	28.3	97.2	92.5	47.1	11.9	98.8
• at least two	73.7	82.9	47.0	93.9	80.0	77.4	21.5	98.0
• at least three	52.6	95.2	69.4	90.7	70.0	91.5	38.9	97.5
• at least four	22.1	98.3	72.4	86.0	42.5	97.7	58.6	95.7
• at least five	9.5	99.4	75.0	84.2	22.5	99.4	75.0	94.3
• All six are present	2.1	100.0	100.0	83.2	7.2	100.0	100.0	93.2

[a]*PPV* positive predictive value
[b]*NPV* negative predictive value

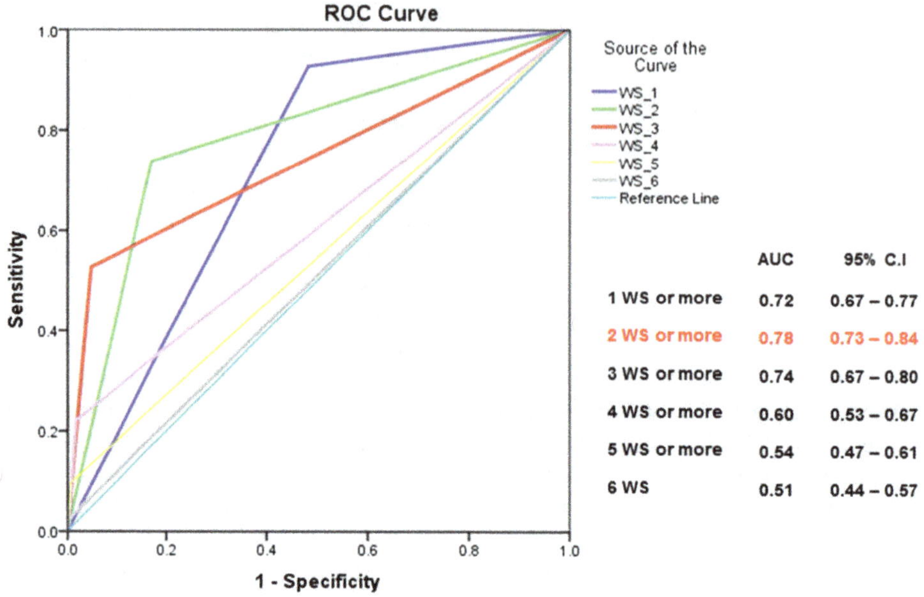

Fig. 2 Receiver operator characteristics (ROC) curves comparing the predictive accuracy for DHF, of various models integrating one or several warning signs and presenting the values of the Area Under Curve (AUC) coefficients. National Paediatric Hospital, Phnom Penh, Sep 2011–Jan. 2013

particularly useful in resource-limited settings where dengue diagnostic tests are not readily available.

The study period, from September 2011 to January 2013, covered two seasons of dengue epidemics. Although all four serotypes were circulating during this period, the predominant serotype was DENV-1 (98 %) in 2012–2013, which is consistent with data from the National Surveillance System (Institut Pasteur du Cambodge, personal communication).

Overall, at hospital admission, 17 % of patients would be clinically classified as DHF or DSS according to the 1997 WHO case definition criteria, while 7.2 % would be classified as SD based on the 2009 WHO case definition. This low proportion of patients presenting with severe outcomes is congruent with the low case fatality rate (0.7 %) observed in our hospital cohort and might reflect the quality of case management. In Cambodia, patients die traditionally at home, and family members usually

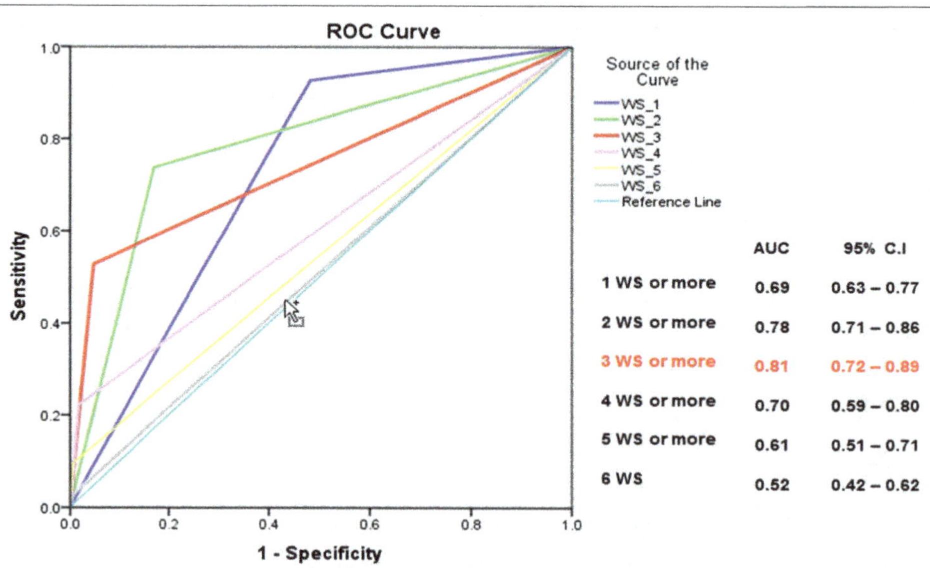

Fig. 3 Received-operator characteristics (ROC) curves comparing the predictive accuracy for Severe Dengue of various models integrating one or several warning signs, and presenting the values of the Area Under Curve (AUC) coefficients. National Paediatric Hospital, Phnom Penh, Sep. 2011–Jan. 2013

request that moribund relatives be discharged. For this reason, we conducted a post-discharge assessment in order to validate the vital status of a random sample of 20 study participants (from a total of 40 patients diagnosed with a severe form of dengue at admission) who resided outside Phnom Penh and presented with either DDS or SD at hospital admission. The heads of the villages confirmed that all 20 children were still alive at the time of the interview. The low case fatality rate observed in the study is encouraging. It is in line with the MOH's 2012–2013 National Strategic Plan, in which the National Dengue Control Program trained hospital teams to rationalize hospital care and improve case management of severe manifestations of dengue.

Similar to previous studies [17], we found that clinical algorithms had an acceptable sensitivity for the detection of dengue (76 to 81 %) but quite low specificity (57 to 66 %) in the epidemiological context of this study in Cambodia, where other pathogens mimicking the clinical presentation of DENV are present. Therefore, one important study objective was using clinical parameters to develop new clinical algorithms that better predict dengue. We found that a positive tourniquet test, leukopenia, thrombocytopenia and elevated transaminases were independent predictors of dengue infection; these findings are congruent with the results of other studies [5, 18, 19]. The presence of elevated liver enzymes was frequently observed in the early stages of both DF and DHF [20, 21]. We also found that the presence of URI symptoms was useful in ruling out dengue, as the absence of this criterion is highly sensitive (82.4 %) for the presence of dengue in this cohort. The inclusion of URI symptoms in our clinical algorithm is essential, since it helps discriminate between dengue and viral respiratory infections; this finding is important in the daily clinical setting and has already been highlighted by other authors [3, 4, 22].

Using the 2009 WHO classification, the presence of any WS at hospital admission leads to a concurrent laboratory-confirmed diagnosis of a severe form of dengue. WS are intended to help triage patients at risk of developing severe outcomes and needing hospital admission in order to initiate early management and intensive monitoring immediately upon admission [23], and the utility of this approach has been confirmed by recent studies conducted in Sri Lanka [24] and Singapore [25]. In Cambodia, we found that any one of the WS was associated with a high sensitivity (93 %) but a low specificity (47 %) in predicting concomitant laboratory-confirmed diagnosis of a severe form of dengue. In resource-limited settings, this might put additional pressure on an already overburdened healthcare system, especially during annual dengue epidemics. Thus, the presence of several WS would improve the specificity (up to 91 % with at least three WS present) in predicting severe disease at the expense of sensitivity and might be an appropriate strategy in countries like Cambodia.

This study adds further evidence for the usefulness of WS. The absence of any WS at hospital admission is strongly associated with non-severe dengue, even in the absence of laboratory confirmation of dengue. Such cases are routinely managed at the outpatient department. The presence of a single WS at admission was found to be insufficiently specific to predict a concurrent laboratory-confirmed diagnosis of a severe outcome of dengue. Therefore, our results strongly suggest that dengue-suspected cases with two or more WS should be admitted, since this predicts severe dengue with a sensitivity of 74 % and a specificity of 83 %.

This study has some limitations. First, the data were collected among inpatients at a referral pediatric hospital in Phnom Penh, whose patient population may be biased towards patients with more severe diseases than those of hospitals at peripheral health center level. Thus, these findings might not describe the full spectrum of dengue in Cambodia and, hence, might not be fully representative of areas with different dengue transmission patterns or serotypes, or where patients seek medical care later in the course of illness. Because of limited resources, it was not possible to run additional biological tests to investigate the etiologies of the other febrile illnesses. Further efforts should be made to validate the findings in other epidemiological contexts. Second, there were incomplete data for certain variables (i.e. results of the tourniquet tests and AST/ALT), although we have no reason to suspect that this introduced a bias. Third, because of limited resources, we were unable to test the 482 patients who did not fulfill the WHO criteria for dengue on admission and who represented a significant number of the patients with fever (40 %). It is likely we missed some dengue cases by relying solely on the WHO criteria. The median duration of hospitalization was short (3 days), and a significant number of patients did not have a convalescent sera collected. This could have caused misclassification of non-lab confirmed cases. DENV-1 was the predominant serotype identified during the study period, and it was not possible to explore the effects of other dengue serotypes; this might affect the generalizability of our results, which remain context-specific. Finally we analyzed clinical data at hospital admission, and because of sample size limitation, we were unable to analyze the predictors for the progression to severe disease following hospital admission. Finally, the limited number of recruited cases limits the possibility to conduct further stratified analysis by dengue serotypes or time periods. The complex interaction between climatic factors and the risk of dengue infection in this setting has already been highlighted [9].

Considering these limitations, and although dengue presentation can vary, the strength of this study is that it directly relates to the most severe aspects of dengue, which can cause not only morbidity but also mortality. Furthermore, our study took place over two seasons in a hospital receiving cases referred from many areas in the country. The inclusion criteria and study monitoring were rigorously applied; all patients were systematically and thoroughly assessed, and testing was performed in an internationally recognized laboratory. Finally, there were few missing data, and we have no reason to believe that missing data were not randomly distributed across the study records. The study also reinforces the need to educate clinicians on key parameters for triage and case management in a context where laboratory diagnosis may not be easily available.

Conclusions

We have described the clinical features of dengue among children in a referral hospital in Phnom Penh, Cambodia. Our study indicates that the addition of simple clinical parameters and first-line laboratory findings could be better used to predict concurrent laboratory-confirmed diagnosis of a severe form of dengue at hospital admission. While our findings remain context-specific, we demonstrate that the inclusion of multiple warning signs more accurately predicts a concomitant laboratory-confirmed diagnosis of severe disease at hospital admission, thereby optimizing triage in settings with limited laboratory resources. While some improvements can be achieved with these clinical parameters, access to dengue rapid diagnostic tests and basic laboratory testing should also be prioritized in resource-limited settings.

Acknowledgements
We are grateful to the personnel of the National Paediatric Hospital for their continuous support and hard work. We thank our study team based in Phnom Penh for their dedication and excellent work to ensure study performance, particularly Ms. Malen Chan and Ms. Heak Morina. We dedicate this study to the memory of Professor Chantha Ngan.

Funding
Funding for this study was provided by Sanofi-Pasteur. The funders had no role in the study design, data collection and data analysis. Decision to publish and preparation of the manuscript were made jointly by all the authors.

Authors' contributions
Concept, design, data acquisition, data analysis and data interpretation. AL, PB, PC: Concept, design, data analysis and data interpretation. YSL, RH, JB: Concept, design, data interpretation. AR: Concept, design, data acquisition. AT, MB, ALQ, YK, VD: Data acquisition; data analysis and data interpretation. Drafting or revising manuscript. PC, AT, AL, PB, JB, YSL: Drafting and revising. AR, MB, RH, ALQ, YK, VD: Revising. All authors read and approved the final manuscript.

Competing interests
Yee-Sin Leo was a medical advisor to Sanofi-Pasteur for a dengue vaccine trial. Jeremy Brett was a Sanofi-Pasteur employee. Philippe Buchy is currently an employee of GSK Vaccines. This does not alter the authors' adherence to all the BMC policies on sharing data and material.

Consent for publication
Not applicable.

Author details
[1]Infectious Diseases Programme, Saw Swee Hock School of Public Health, National University of Singapore, Singapore, Singapore. [2]Epidemiology Unit, Institut Pasteur du Cambodge, Phnom Penh, Cambodia. [3]Institute of Infectious Disease and Epidemiology, Tan Tock Seng Hospital, Singapore, Singapore. [4]National Paediatric Hospital, Phnom Penh, Cambodia. [5]National Dengue Control Program (NDCP), National Center for Parasitological, Entomology and Malaria Control, Ministry of Health, Phnom Penh, Cambodia. [6]Virology Unit, Institut Pasteur in Cambodia, Phnom Penh, Cambodia. [7]Medical Affairs Department, Sanofi Pasteur, Singapore, Singapore. [8]Current address: Agence de Médecine Préventive, 13 Chemin du Levant, Ferney-Voltaire 01210, France. [9]Current address: Global Health Group, University of California, San Francisco, USA. [10]Current address: Takeda Vaccines Pte Ltd., Singapore, Singapore. [11]Current address: GlaxoSmithKline vaccines, 150 Beach road, Singapore, Singapore.

References

1. Huy R, Buchy P, Conan A, Ngan C, Ong S, Ali R, Duong V, Yit S, Ung S, Te V, Chroeung N, Phaektra NC, Uok V, Vong S. National dengue surveillance in Cambodia 1980–2008: epidemiological and virological trends and the impact of vector control. Bull World Health Organ. 2010;88:650–7.
2. Farrar J, Focks D, Gubler D, Barrera R, Guzman MG, Simmons C, Kalayanarooj S, Lum L, McCall PJ, Lloyd L, Horstick O, Dayal-Drager R, Nathan MB, Kroeger A. Towards a global dengue research agenda. WHO/TDR Dengue Scientific Working Group. Trop Med Int Health. 2007;12(6):695–9.
3. Ramos MM, Tomashek KM, Arguello DF, Luxemburger C, Quinones L, Lang J, Munoz-Jordan JL. Early features of dengue infection in Puerto Rico. Trans R Soc Trop Med. 2009;103:878–84.
4. Gregory CJ, Santiago LM, Arguello DF, Hunsperger E, Tomashek KM. Clinical and laboratory features that differentiate dengue from other febrile illnesses in an endemic area–Puerto Rico, 2007–2008. Am J Trop Med Hyg. 2010; 82(5):922–9.
5. Kalayanarooj S, Vaughn DW, Nimmannitya S, Green S, Suntayakorn S, Kunentrasai N, Viramitrachai W, Ratanachu-eke S, Kiatpolpoj S, Innis BL, Rothman AL, Nisalak A, Ennis FA. Early clinical and laboratory indicators of acute dengue illness. J Inf Dis. 1997;176:313–21.
6. Tuan NM, Nhan HT, Chau NW, Hung NT, Tuan HM, Tram TV, Ha NL, Loi P, Quang HK, Kien DTH, Hubbards S, Chau TNBC, Wills B, Wolbers M, Simmons CP. Sensitivity and specificity of a novel classifier for the early diagnostic of dengue. PLoS Negl Trop Dis. 2015;9(4):e0003638.
7. WHO. Dengue haemorrhagic fever; guidelines for diagnosis, prevention, treatment and control. Geneva: World Health Organization; 2007.
8. WHO. Dengue guidelines for diagnosis, treatment, prevention and control. New edition. Geneva: World Health Organization; 2009.
9. Lover AA, Buchy P, Rachline A, Moniboth D, Huy R, Meng CY, Leo YS, Yuvatha K, Sophal U, Chantha N, Y B, Duong V, Goyet S, Brett JL, Tarantola A, Cavailler P. Spatial epidemiology and climatic predictors of paediatric dengue infections captured via sentinel site surveillance, Phnom Penh, Cambodia 2011–2012. BMC Public Health. 2014;14:658.
10. Hue KD, Tuan TV, Thi HT, Bich CT, Anh HH, et al. Validation of an internally controlled one-step real-time multiplex RT-PCR assay for the detection and quantification of dengue virus RNA in plasma. J Virol Methods. 2011;177(2): 168–73.
11. Gubler DJ. Application of serotype-specific monoclonal antibodies or identification of dengue viruses. In: Yunker C, editor. Arboviruses and arthropod cells in vitro. Boca Raton: CRC Press; 1986. p. 3–14.
12. Peeling RW, Artsob H, Pelegrino JL, Buchy P, Cardosa MJ, Devi S, Enria DA, Farrar J, Gubler DJ, Guzman MG, Halstead SB, Hunsperger E, Kliks S, Margolis HS, Nathanson CM, Nguyen VC, Rizzo N, Vázquez S, Yoksan S. Nat Rev Microbiol. 2010;8(12 Suppl):S30–8.

13. Vuylsteke B, Laga M, Alary M, Gerniers MM, Lebughe JP, Nzila N, Behets F, Van Dyck E, Piot P. Clinical algorithms for the screening of women for gonococcal and chlamydial infection: evaluation of pregnant women and prostitute in Zaire. Clin Infect Dis. 1993;17(1):82–8.
14. Mayaud P, Uledi E, Cornelissen J, ka-Gina G, Todd J, Rwakatare M, West B, Kopwe L, Manoko D, Grosskurth H, Hayes R, Mabey D. Risk scores to detect cervical infections in urban antenatal clinic attenders in Mwanza, Tanzania. Sex Transm Inf. 1998;74 Suppl 1:139–46.
15. Cornier N, Petrova E, Cavailler P, Dentcheva R, Terris-Preshold F, Janin A, Ninet B, Anguenot JL, Vassilakos P, Gerbase A, Mayaud P. Optimising the management of vaginal discharge in Bulgaria: cost effectiveness of four clinical algorithms with risk assessment. Sex Transm Inf. 2010;86(4):303–9.
16. Pepe MS. The statistical evaluation of medical tests for classification and prediction. New York: Oxford University Press; 2003.
17. Low JGH, Ong A, Tan LK, Chaterji S, Chow A, Lim WY, Lee KW, Chua R, Chua CR, Tan SWS, Cheung YB, Hibberd ML, Vasudevan SG, Ng LC, Leo YS, Ooi EE. The early clinical features of dengue in adults: challenges for early clinical diagnosis. PLoS Negl Trop Dis. 2011;5(5):e1191.
18. Phuong CXT, Nhan NT, Wills B, Kneen R, Ha NTT, Mai TTT, Huynh TTT, Lien DTK, Solomon T, Simpson JA, White NJ, Farrar J, the Dong Nai Paediatric Hospital Study Group. Evaluation of the World Health Organization standard tourniquet test and a modified tourniquet test in the diagnostic of dengue infection in Vietnam. Trop Med Int Health. 2002;7(2):125–32.
19. Hammond SN, Balmaseda A, Perez L, Tellez Y, Saborio SI, Mercado JC, Videa E, Rodriguez Y, Perez MA, Cuadra R, Solano S, Rocha J, Idiaquez W, Gonzalez A, Harris E. Differemces in dengue severity in infants, children and adults in a 3-year hospital-based study in Nicaragua. Am J Trop Med Hyg. 2005;73(6): 1063–70.
20. Wilder-Smith A, Earnest A, Paton N. Use of simple laboratory features to distinguish the early stage of severe acute respiratory syndrome from dengue fever. Clin Infect Dis. 2004;39:1818–23.
21. Lee LK, Gan VC, Lee VL, Tan AS, Leo YS, Lye DC. Clinical relevance and discriminatory value of elevated liver amino transferase levels for dengue severity. PLoS Negl Trop Dis. 2012;6:e1676.
22. Phuong CXT, Nhan NT, Kneen R, Thuy PTT, Thien CV, Nga NTT, Thuy TT, Solomon T, Stepniewska K, Wills B, the Dong Nai Study Group. Clinical diagnosis and assessment of severity of confirmed dengue infections in Vietnamese children: is the World Health Organization classification system helpful? Am J Trop Med Hyg. 2004;70(2):172–9.
23. Leo YS, Gan VC, Ng EL, Hao Y, Ng LC, Pok KY, Dimatatac F, Go CJ, Lye DC. Utility of warning signs in guiding admission and predicting severe disease in adult dengue. BMC Inf Dis. 2013;13:498.
24. Jayaratne SD, Atukorale V, Gomes L, Chang T, Wijesinghe T, Fernado S, Ogg GS, Malavige GN. Evaluation of the WHO revised criteria for classification of clinical disease severity in acute dengue infection. BMC Res Note. 2012;5:645.
25. Thein TL, Gan VC, Lye DC, Yung CF, Leo YS. Utilities and limitations of the World Health Organization 2009 warning signs for adult dengue severity. PLoS Negl Trop Dis. 2013;7(1):e2203.

4

Low sensitivity of the tourniquet test for differential diagnosis of dengue

Nathália Barbosa Furlan[1], Caroline Tukasan[1], Cássia Fernanda Estofolete[1,2], Maurício Lacerda Nogueira[2] and Natal Santos da Silva[1,2,3,4*]

Abstract

Background: The aim of this study was to evaluate the utility of the tourniquet test (TT) for dengue diagnosing. To our knowledge, no previous study with such a large sample, of this duration, with as many laboratory methods referenced, or relating the results of the TT to the 2009 WHO classification of severity has been conducted thus far.

Methods: In this study, we analyzed the records of 119,589 suspected dengue cases in a Brazilian city, with 30,670 confirmed cases. The Cohen's Kappa test was applied to evaluate the degree of agreement between the tests, and the sensitivity and specificity was calculated for the TT.

Results: Twenty-eight thousand six hundred thirty-five TT were performed. No association between the outcome of the TT and greater severity of infection, according to the 2009 guideline, was observed ($P = 0.28$); furthermore, relevant agreement with the final diagnosis ($\kappa = 0.01$; 95 % CI = 0.00 to 0.02) or individually with the IgM enzyme-linked immunoassay was not observed ($\kappa = 0.05$; 95 % CI = 0.04 to 0.06), and was even lower with PCR ($\kappa = 0.27$; 95 % CI = 0.06 to 0.49). Most importance of the TT was shown in relation to specificity (88.9 %; 95 % CI = 0.88 to 0.89) and negative predictive value (70.3 %; CI 95 % = 0.70 to 0.71).

Conclusions: TT was more effective in detecting cases that were truly negative than positive. These results suggest that the TT should not be used as diagnosis of dengue.

Keywords: Dengue, Tourniquet test, Diagnostic test for dengue

Background

The dengue virus (DENV) is the most important arbovirus in the world in terms of morbidity, mortality, and clinical implications [1]. Between 2.5 and 3.6 billion people, more than 50 % of the world's population, are currently living with the risk of infection. The incidence is even higher in tropical and subtropical countries where environmental conditions favor the proliferation of the *Aedes* mosquitoes [2–5]. However, this disease is also advancing into developed countries, where the occurrence of dengue has not been previously registered, such as the United States of America [6–8], Japan [9–11], and France [12].

* Correspondence: natalss@gmail.com
[1]Faculdade de Medicina, União das Faculdades dos Grandes Lagos, São José do Rio Preto, São Paulo, Brazil
[2]Laboratório de Pesquisas em Virologia, Faculdade de Medicina de São José do Rio Preto, São Paulo, Brazil
Full list of author information is available at the end of the article

Dengue is caused by four types of DENV: DENV-1, DENV-2, DENV-3, and DENV-4 [13]. More recently, a new serotype, DEN-5, was identified in serum samples collected during an epidemic of dengue in Malaysia in 2007, still under study [14]. All virus strains can lead to all forms of dengue infection, from asymptomatic to severe, or even fatal. However, it is unclear why some dengue cases progress to severe forms. Although there are controversies in the literature, sequential infections of different serotypes of DENV have an important role [15–17]. Still, even during epidemics in populations with high levels of antibodies against DENV, the proportion of severe dengue cases is low [18], suggesting that other risk factors are involved in the severity of the disease.

The main feature of the severe forms of the disease is increased vascular permeability resulting in plasma leakage from the intravascular compartment to the extravascular space [17, 19, 20]. Fluid loss, leading to hypovolemic shock, thrombocytopenia, coagulation abnormalities, and bleeding are also features of severe dengue disease [21]. The diagnosis of the infection is particularly difficult in mild forms of the disease, especially when differentiating dengue from other febrile illnesses. The risk of swift progression from mild to severe forms of dengue infection, which may require rapid resuscitation measures, demonstrates that accurate and early diagnosis through other methods is relevant in the absence of serologic and virologic confirmation [22–24].

In 1997, the World Health Organization (WHO) listed the tourniquet test (TT) as a criterion for dengue hemorrhagic fever, and that the positive test reflects both capillary fragility and thrombocytopenia [22]. Studies suggested that the test has a greater positivity rate in individuals with more severe forms of the disease but cannot exclude dengue infection [25, 26].

Evaluation of the utility of TT to diagnose or exclude dengue has been proposed in previous studies [20, 22, 27, 28], with mixed results. Thus, the aim of this study was to evaluate the use of TT in the screening of patients with suspected dengue and its severity, and to compare this test with routine diagnostic methods. Accordingly, we decided to use a relatively large sample over a considerably long time period. We also utilized many laboratory methods for reference, including the polymerase chain reaction (PCR), and simultaneously related results to the severity index set forth in the 2009 WHO classification.

Methods

We have used records from the Notifiable Diseases Information System (SINAN), a program of Brazil's Ministry of Health to collect notifications of all suspected dengue cases in the city of São José do Rio Preto, São Paulo, Brazil, whose population in 2010 was approximately 408,258 inhabitants. For this study, 119,589 cases notified between May 1998 and July 2012 were eligible, previous to the introduction of Zika and chikungunya virus in Brazil.

In addition to clinical evaluation by a physician, serum samples from all patients with suspected dengue were submitted to a diagnostic laboratory for the determination of dengue based on an IgM immunoglobulin enzyme-linked immunoassay (ELISA), non-structural protein 1 (NS1), or DENV PCR, depending on which test was being commonly used at the time of the case.

Case definition

For notification purposes, in accordance with the criteria of Brazil's Ministry of Health, suspected cases of dengue included all patients with acute febrile illness lasting up to seven days, accompanied by at least two of the following signs or symptoms: headache, retro-orbital pain, myalgia, arthralgia, prostration or rash associated with the presence of bleeding, positive epidemiological history, residence within a dengue transmission or *Aedes aegypti* endemic area in the last 15 days.

The clinical classification used retrospectively in this study for statistical purposes was based on the WHO guideline (2009) to distinguish between dengue and severe dengue. The first one is suspected in patients who live or have traveled to a dengue-endemic area, with fever and two or more of the following: nausea and/or vomiting, rash, pain (headache, retro-orbital pain, myalgia, and/or arthralgia), and a positive TT or leukopenia. Abdominal pain, persistent vomiting, fluid retention, mucosal bleeding, lethargy, hepatomegaly greater than 2 cm, increasing hematocrit, and rapid decrease in platelet count are suggestive of dengue and serve as warning signs of severe dengue. Severe dengue is characterized by severe plasma leakage leading to shock or respiratory distress, severe bleeding, impairment of organs with a pronounced increase of aminotransferases, altered consciousness level, or heart failure.

Statistical analysis

All reported cases (negative or positive for DENV) in which the TT was performed were evaluated, and this variable was studied in relation to the actual outcome, i.e., confirmed dengue on the basis of the conventional laboratory methods as described above. For cases in which the diagnosis of dengue was established, the percentage of positive TT results was evaluated over time and according to age.

A descriptive analysis of personal and serological variables was performed and related to a hemorrhagic manifestation as externalized bleeding and thrombocytopenia, defined as a platelet count of less than 100,000/mm^3.

The hypothesis that TT positivity would be associated with more severe scores of DENV infection was evaluated using nonparametric Mann-Whitney U tests. However, the Pearson's chi-square test (χ^2) was performed to check if there was a positive association between TT and thrombocytopenia in patients with suspected dengue. The Cohen's Kappa coefficient (κ) was applied to measure the degree of agreement between the TT and the final diagnosis, PCR results, and presence of IgM and NS1. To quantify the strength of this agreement, a scale used by Landis and Koch was proposed, where values lower than zero show poor agreement. Specifically, values less than zero indicate poor agreement, from 0 to 0.2 indicate slight agreement, 0.21 to 0.4 indicate fair agreement, 0.41 to 0.6 indicate moderate agreement, 0.61 to 0.8 indicate substantial agreement, and 0.81 to 1.0 indicate almost perfect agreement [29].

Later, the sensitivity and specificity, positive predictive value (PPV), negative predictive value (NPV), positive likelihood ratio, and negative likelihood ratio of the TT were also determined. All analyses were performed using SPSS software, version 19, and adopted a significance level of 5 % and a confidence interval of 95 %.

Results

We analyzed 119,589 participants, with an average age of 33.3 years, with considerable dispersion (±18.1 years); further, 65,595 (54.9 %) of the patients were female and 53,898 patients (45.1 %) were male (96 patients had no information about sex). The TT was performed in 28,635 patients (23.9 % of all notifications); 3252 (11.4 %) were positive and 25,383 cases (88.6 %) were negative.

At least one information about hemorrhagic manifestation was available for all patients undergoing to TT. The data shows that 17,123 (59.8 %) patients had not shown any hemorrhagic manifestations, while 11,512 (40.2 %) had one or more type of blood leakage (Table 1). However, information about thrombocytopenia was obtained in only 1930 (6.7 %) individuals. In these patients 906 (47.0 % of patients) had negative TT results without thrombocytopenia, 269 (13.9 %) had negative TT results with thrombocytopenia, 538 (27.9 %) had positive TT results without thrombocytopenia, and 217 (11.2 %) had positive TT results with thrombocytopenia. Therefore, there was a statistically significant difference between the TT results and the thrombocytopenia count of these patients ($\chi^2 = 8344$; $P = 0.004$).

The proportion of positive TT results in patients with dengue over the years shows an increasing trend until 2008, but a decrease in subsequent years (Fig. 1). This ratio was similar within age groups 0 to 14 years (11.2 %), 15 to 60 (12.1 %), and older than 60 years (11.4 %).

Of all cases with TT results, 921 (10.7 %) were dengue without warning signs, 7410 (86.4 %) were dengue with warning signs, 246 (2.9 %) were severe dengue, and 16 patients died. The hypothesis that there would be an association between the TT results and a greater severity score has not been confirmed with the Mann-Whitney test (U = 3,826,121; $P = 0.28$). For this analysis, only 8577 of the 30,670 confirmed cases of dengue had the TT performed, with 1026 (12.0 % of 8577) testing positive and 7551 (88.0 %) testing negative.

The TT had almost no concordance with the final diagnosis on the basis of the Cohen's Kappa coefficient (κ = 0.01, CI 95 % = 0.00 to 0.02), with IgM detection by ELISA (κ = 0.05; CI 95 % = 0.04 to 0.06), or with PCR (κ = 0.27, CI 95 % = 0.06 to 0.49) (Table 2). The comparison between the TT and the NS1 detection could not be carried out because only four individuals had these two tests performed simultaneously.

Based on the final diagnosis obtained, the TT had a sensitivity of 11.9 % (CI 95 % = 0.11 to 0.12), as opposed to a specificity of 88.9 % (CI 95 % = 0.88 to 0.89), indicating an ability to detect truly negative cases. In addition, it was observed that the ability of this test to predict if the patient was actually sick when the test was positive was significantly lower. That is to say, the PPV was only 31.6 % (CI 95 % = 0.31 to 0.32) while the NPV was 70.3 % (CI 95 % = 0.70 to 0.71), showing a greater ability to identify those individuals who really did not have dengue when the TT was negative. However, the positive likelihood ratio (1.08) shows that this does not practically change the chance of the TT results being truly positive in a population with dengue compared to a population without the disease. A similar result was also seen in the negative likelihood ratio (0.99), which showed that the likelihood of a negative test result in

Table 1 Hemorrhagic manifestations in patients undergoing tourniquet test

Hemorrhagic manifestation	Tourniquet test			
	Positive *N* (%)	Negative *N* (%)	Total *N* (%)	*p*-value
Epistaxis[a]				<0.001
Present	121 (17.5)	571 (82.5)	692 (100)	
Ausente	3032 (11.2)	23,954 (88.8)	26,986 (100)	
Petechiae[b]				<0.001
Present	701 (29.7)	1663 (70.3)	2364 (100)	
Absent	2445 (9,7)	22,694 (90.3)	25,139 (100)	
Exanthema[c]				<0.001
Present	1382 (18.8)	5984 (81.2)	7366 (100)	
Absent	1693 (8.3)	18,762 (91.7)	20,455 (100)	
Gingival bleeding[d]				<0.001
Present	76 (19.7)	309 (80.3)	385 (100)	
Absent	3073 (11.3)	24,181 (88.7)	27,254 (100)	
Metrorrhage[e]				<0.001
Present	34 (27.4)	90 (72.6)	124 (100)	
Absent	1673 (15.2)	9366 (84.8)	11,039 (100)	
Hematuria[f]				0.15
Present	16(18.2)	72(81.8)	88(100)	
Absent	2639(12.9)	17,880(87.1)	20,519(100)	
Gastrointestinal[g] bleeding				<0.001
Present	33 (25.6)	96 (74.4)	129 (100)	
Absent	2613 (12.8)	17,732 (87.2)	20,345 (100)	

Missing: there was no information for the respective hemorrhagic manifestations
p-value: Chi-square
[a]Missing: 957 (3.3 %)
[b]Missing: 1132 (4.0 %)
[c]Missing: 814 (2.8 %)
[d]Missing: 996 (3.5 %)
[e][Information about female] Missing: 4807(30.1 %)
[f]Missing: 8028 (28.0 %)
[g]Missing: 8161 (28.5 %)

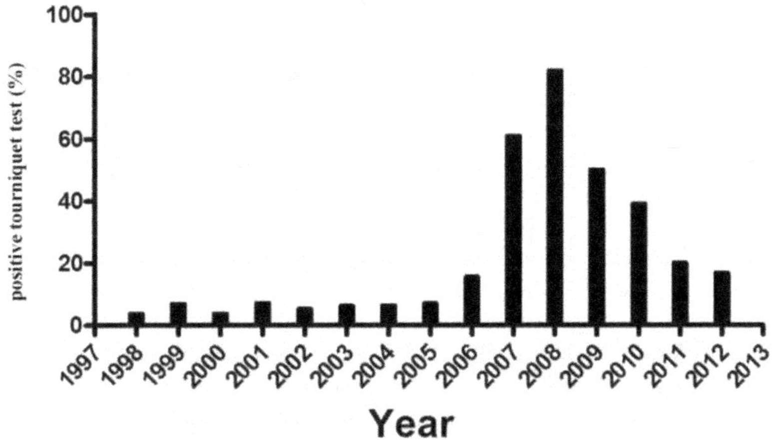

Fig. 1 Proportion of positive tourniquet test results between 1998 and 2012 in 25,383 dengue cases

patients with dengue was not different from those without the disease.

Discussion

The approach of the TT value as auxiliary method for diagnosing dengue as presented here is something unusual in the medical literature. The use of so many samples over such a long period of study, and the comparison of the results, including the dengue severity was never reported. About a quarter (28 635) of patients initially notified as suspected dengue fever (119,589) were evaluated by the TT, so a considerable amount of patients were not submitted to this test, perhaps as a consequence of difficulties in filling the notification form or due to non-realization of this test during the great outbreaks of the disease. In our investigation, there was a gradual increase in the percentage of positive TT results over the years, with a further decrease in the last five years of the study, with similar proportions of positive test results between age groups. No association between the TT results and greater severity (according to the 2009 guideline) was observed ($P = 0.28$). The TT results also failed to show relevant agreement with the final diagnosis ($\kappa = 0.01$; 95 % CI = 0.00 to 0.02), the ELISA-IgM results ($\kappa = 0.05$; 95 % CI = 0.04 to 0.06), and much less with the PCR results ($\kappa = 0.27$; 95 % CI = 0.06 to 0.49). This low concordance was also justified by the low sensitivity of the TT to diagnose dengue (11.9 %; 95 % CI = 0.11 to 0.12) and low PPV (31.6 %; 95 % CI = 0.31 to 0.32); nevertheless, it has shown most importance for specificity (88.9 %; 95 % CI = 0.88 to 0.89) and NPV (70.3 %; CI 95 % = 0.70 to 0.71).

Table 2 The degree of agreement between the results of the tourniquet test and those of various laboratory methods

	Tourniquet test			
	Positive *N* (%)	Negative *N* (%)	κ [a](CI 95 %)	Agreement
Final diagnosis			0.01 (0.00 to 0.02)	Slight
Positive	1026 (31.5)	7551 (29.7)		
Negative	2226 (68.5)	17,832 (70.3)		
Total	3252 (100.0)	25,383 (100.0)		
ELISA(IgM)			0.05 (0.04 to 0.06)	Slight
Positive	1016 (69.2 %)	7539 (53.4 %)		
Negative	453 (30.8 %)	6590 (46.6 %)		
Total	1469 (100.0)	14,129(100.0)		
PCR			0.27 (0.06 to 0.49)	Fair
Positive	20 (62.5 %)	15 (34.9 %)		
Negative	12(37.5 %)	28 (65.1 %)		
Total	32 (100.0)	43 (100.0)		

Comparison between tourniquet test and NS1 research could not perform because there were only four patients with both tests realized
[a]Cohen's Kappa coefficient (confidence interval of 95 %)

The wide clinical spectrum of infection by DENV and the possibility of progression from mild to more severe forms of dengue [30], which require early therapeutic measures and are related to higher mortality, demonstrate the need for alternative methods that can be correlated to this evolution and anticipate potential severity. WHO, in its 1997 guidelines, lists the TT as a criterion in the diagnosis of dengue hemorrhagic fever. In the 2009 guidelines, it is presented as a criterion for both mild and severe forms of the disease. However, studies differ in their use of the test for the diagnosis of infection by DENV and their correlation with severity. Although our findings are in agreement with those found by other authors regarding the TT's low sensitivity and high specificity [20, 22, 28, 31], there are findings whose values contradict ours, reporting a sensitivity of 83 % and specificity of 23.5 % when used in children in Malaysia [32], suggesting that children may exhibit a different pattern of TT positivity compared to other age groups. However, the finding of equal percentages of positive TT results in both children and adults leads us to disagree with this possibility, despite reports in the literature of different clinical manifestations in children (mainly bleeding) [33]. For other authors, the difference between sensitivity and specificity was practically equal, but with the PPV lower (45 and 55 %, respectively) than the NPV (64 and 69 %, respectively) [27].

Isolated, low PPV was found in our study with a low sensitivity and high specificity; however, Ho et al. [31] reported that PPV may reach 93.1 % when combined with leukopenia ($<4000/mm^3$), thrombocytopenia ($<150 \times 10^3/mm^3$), partial thromboplastin time (>38 s), elevated aminotransferases (AST/ALT >1.5), and low C-reactive protein (<20 mg/l) [30]. According to Gregory et al. (2011), the combination of a positive TT results and leukopenia ($<5000/mm^3$) identified 94 % of patients with dengue in the emergency room [34].

However, leukopenia may not present in the initial stages of dengue, which can delay the diagnosis of the disease when utilizing this method [35]. Therefore, the assessment isolated of the PPV, as well as the NPV, perhaps are not good parameters for evaluation, thus requiring additional laboratory data to make their validation stronger.

It must also be considered that the TT can be influenced by disease progression, age, gender [27], circulating strains, and virus circulation patterns over a determined period. This test can also yield a positive result for other pathological conditions with varying indexes, such as with typhoid fever and Japanese encephalitis [22], although the TT has lower sensitivity for these diseases than for dengue. In this study, 68.5 % of patients who had dengue confirmed by serological diagnosis showed a positive TT result. Understanding this condition could prevent infections with clinical presentations similar to dengue from being misdiagnosed and thus provide a better chance for accurate treatment in adequate time. Such evidence shows the complexity involved in the clinical diagnosis and management of dengue.

Due to the long period of study, the epidemiological conditions of dengue varied, both in relation to the circulating serotype and the number of co-circulating serotypes, which are factors that may be related to a positive TT result. According to the data in Fig. 1, a significant increase in the proportion of positive TTs can be noted until 2008, followed by a decrease. Between the introduction of DENV in the study area and 2008, we observed circulation of DENV-1, −2 and −3, with a maximum of two serotypes simultaneously. Since 2009, there was a reintroduction of DENV-1, followed by explosive outbreaks of DENV-1 and DENV-4 with about 20,000 suspected cases per year and the co-circulation of three serotypes. On the other hand, DENV-3 caused the major epidemics in 2006 and 2007, followed by a DENV-2 epidemic in 2008 [36–39]. Due to insufficient in the database, it was not possible to correlate the data from TTs with serotypes specifically, but the association between serotypes and genotypes may be related to this phenomenon. Moreover, we cannot rule out the possibility that the TT generates a false positive in the presence of other flaviviruses circulating in Brazil, particularly the Saint Louis encephalitis virus, which has been associated with a positive TT in our region [40, 41].

Indeed, in retrospective studies based on government epidemiological data or otherwise, the major limitation is that a lot of information cannot be reassessed, leading to additional reliability being placed on those individuals who collected and recorded information, such as the performance of the TT, which could not be directly supervised. However, it is relatively common that nurses, laboratory technicians, or trained doctors in Brazilian dengue-endemic areas manage dengue cases, which implies that the results are as realistic as possible. Additionally, inconsistent data, both in relation to reporting, such as white blood cell count, as well as the interpretation, were excluded from analysis in this study in order to minimize the effect of these limitations on the findings and conclusions.

Conclusions

Therefore, the TT was more effective in detecting cases that were truly negative than positive. These results suggest that the TT should not be used as diagnosis of dengue, however, if it is absolutely necessary to use it, as is the case in very poor dengue endemic areas where more sensitive and specific laboratory tests are not available, then it to be done with great caution for screening giving rise to suspicion of dengue cases.

Abbreviations

ALT: Alanine transaminase; AST: Aspartate transaminase; CI: Confidence interval; DENV: Dengue virus; ELISA: Enzyme-linked immunoassay; FAPESP: Fundação de Amparo à Pesquisa do Estado de São Paulo; NPV: Negative predictive value; NS1: Nonstructural protein 1;

PCR: Polymerase chain reaction; PPV: Positive predictive value; SINAN: Notifiable Diseases Information System; TT: Tourniquet test; WHO: World Health Organization; κ: Cohen's Kappa coefficient

Acknowledgements
We thank the Municipal Secretariat for Health of São José do Rio Preto for granting access to the database about dengue.

Funding
This work was supported by Fundação de Amparo à Pesquisa do Estado de São Paulo (FAPESP) [2013/21719-3] to MLN.

Authors' contributions
NBF, CT, and NSS conceived the study; NSS designed the study protocol; NBF, NSS, and CFE drafted the manuscript; MLN and NSS critically revised the manuscript for intellectual content. All authors read and approved the final manuscript. MLN and NSS are guarantors of the paper.

Competing interests
The authors declare that they have no competing interests.

Consent for publication
Not applicable.

Author details
[1]Faculdade de Medicina, União das Faculdades dos Grandes Lagos, São José do Rio Preto, São Paulo, Brazil. [2]Laboratório de Pesquisas em Virologia, Faculdade de Medicina de São José do Rio Preto, São Paulo, Brazil. [3]Laboratório de Modelagens Matemática e Estatística em Medicina, União das Faculdades dos Grandes Lagos, São José do Rio Preto, São Paulo, Brazil. [4]Laboratório de Modelagens Matemática e Estatística em Medicina, Faculdade de Medicina, União das Faculdades dos Grandes Lagos, Rua Dr. Eduardo Nielsem, 960 Jardim Novo Aeroporto, São Jose do Rio Preto, São Paulo CEP 15030-070, Brazil.

References

1. Tristao-Sa R, Kubelka CF, Zandonade E, et al. Clinical and hepatic evaluation in adult dengue patients: a prospective two-month cohort study. Rev Soc Bras Med Trop. 2012;45(6):675–81.
2. Srikiatkhachorn A, Rothman AL, Gibbons RV, et al. Dengue-how best to classify it. Clin Infect Dis. 2011;53(6):563–7.
3. Ferreira GL. Global dengue epidemiology trends. Rev Inst Med Trop Sao Paulo. 2012;54 Suppl 18:S5–6.
4. Thein TL, Leo YS, Fisher DA, et al. Risk factors for fatality among confirmed adult dengue inpatients in Singapore: a matched case-control study. PLoS One. 2013;8(11):e81060.
5. Zhang H, Zhou YP, Peng HJ, et al. Predictive symptoms and signs of severe dengue disease for patients with dengue fever: a meta-analysis. Biomed Res Int. 2014;2014:359308.
6. Radke EG, Gregory CJ, Kintziger KW, et al. Dengue outbreak in Key West, Florida, USA, 2009. Emerg Infect Dis. 2012;18(1):135–7.
7. Anez G, Rios M. Dengue in the United States of America: a worsening scenario? Biomed Res Int. 2013;2013:678645.
8. Teets FD, Ramgopal MN, Sweeney KD, Graham AS, Michael SF, Isern S. Origin of the dengue virus outbreak in Martin County, Florida, USA 2013. Virol Rep. 2014;1–2:2–8.
9. Arima Y, Matsui T, Shimada T, et al. Ongoing local transmission of dengue in Japan, August to September 2014. Western Pac Surveill Response J. 2014;5(4):27–9.
10. Kojima G. Autochthonous dengue fever imported to England from Japan, 2014. Emerg Infect Dis. 2015;21(1):182–4.
11. Kutsuna S, Kato Y, Moi ML, et al. Autochthonous dengue fever, Tokyo, Japan, 2014. Emerg Infect Dis. 2015;21(3):517–20.
12. Succo T, Leparc-Goffart I, Ferre JB, Roiz D, Broche B, Maquart M, Noel H, Catelinois O, Entezam F, Caire D, et al. Autochthonous dengue outbreak in Nimes, South of France, July to September 2015. Euro Surveill. 2016;21(21): 1 7.
13. Tumioto GL, Gregianini TS, Dambros BP, Cestari BC, Alves Nunes ZM, Veiga AB. Laboratory surveillance of dengue in Rio Grande do Sul, Brazil, from 2007 to 2013. PLoS One. 2014;9(8):e104394.
14. Mustafa MS, Rasotgi V, Jain S, Gupta V. Discovery of fifth serotype of dengue virus (DENV-5): a new public health dilemma in dengue control. Med J Armed Forces India. 2015;71(1):67–70.
15. Halstead SB. The Alexander D. Langmuir Lecture. The pathogenesis of dengue. Molecular epidemiology in infectious disease. Am J Epidemiol. 1981;114(5):632–48.
16. Burnett M. Dengue infections. J Spec Oper Med. 2013;13(2):64–8.
17. Lorono-Pino MA, Cropp CB, Farfan JA, et al. Common occurrence of concurrent infections by multiple dengue virus serotypes. Am J Trop Med Hyg. 1999;61(5):725–30.
18. Figueiredo MA, Rodrigues LC, Barreto ML, et al. Allergies and diabetes as risk factors for dengue hemorrhagic fever: results of a case control study. PLoS Negl Trop Dis. 2010;4(6):e699.
19. Halstead SB. Antibody, macrophages, dengue virus infection, shock, and hemorrhage: a pathogenetic cascade. Rev Infect Dis. 1989;11 Suppl 4:S830–9.
20. Mayxay M, Phetsouvanh R, Moore CE, et al. Predictive diagnostic value of the tourniquet test for the diagnosis of dengue infection in adults. Trop Med Int Health. 2011;16(1):127–33.
21. Srichaikul T, Nimmannitya S. Haematology in dengue and dengue haemorrhagic fever. Baillieres Best Pract Res Clin Haematol. 2000;13(2):261–76.
22. Cao XT, Ngo TN, Wills B, et al. Evaluation of the World Health Organization standard tourniquet test and a modified tourniquet test in the diagnosis of dengue infection in Viet Nam. Trop Med Int Health. 2002;7(2):125–32.
23. Bessoff K, Phoutrides E, Delorey M, Acosta LN, Hunsperger E. Utility of a commercial nonstructural protein 1 antigen capture kit as a dengue virus diagnostic tool. Clin Vaccine Immunol. 2010;17(6):949–53.
24. Ahmed NH, Broor S. Comparison of NS1 antigen detection ELISA, real time RT-PCR and virus isolation for rapid diagnosis of dengue infection in acute phase. J Vector Borne Dis. 2014;51(3):194–9.
25. Kalayanarooj S, Vaughn DW, Nimmannitya S, et al. Early clinical and laboratory indicators of acute dengue illness. J Infect Dis. 1997;176(2):313–21.
26. Kabra SK, Jain Y, Pandey RM, et al. Dengue haemorrhagic fever in children in the 1996 Delhi epidemic. Trans R Soc Trop Med Hyg. 1999;93(3):294–8.
27. Halsey ES, Vilcarromero S, Forshey BM, et al. Performance of the tourniquet test for diagnosing dengue in Peru. Am J Trop Med Hyg. 2013;89(1):99–104.
28. Antunes AC, Oliveira GL, Nunes LI, et al. Evaluation of the diagnostic value of the tourniquet test in predicting severe dengue cases in a population from Belo Horizonte, State of Minas Gerais, Brazil. Rev Soc Bras Med Trop. 2013;46(5):542–6.
29. Landis JR, Koch GG. The measurement of observer agreement for categorical data. Biometrics. 1977;33(1):159–74.
30. Srikiatkhachorn A, Gibbons RV, Green S, et al. Dengue hemorrhagic fever: the sensitivity and specificity of the world health organization definition for identification of severe cases of dengue in Thailand, 1994–2005. Clin Infect Dis. 2010;50(8):1135–43.
31. Ho TS, Wang SM, Lin YS, Liu CC. Clinical and laboratory predictive markers for acute dengue infection. J Biomed Sci. 2013;20:75.
32. Norlijah O, Khamisah AN, Kamarul A, Paeds M, Mangalam S. Repeated tourniquet testing as a diagnostic tool in dengue infection. Med J Malaysia. 2006;61(1):22–7.
33. Kittigul L, Pitakarnjanakul P, Sujirarat D, Siripanichgon K. The differences of clinical manifestations and laboratory findings in children and adults with dengue virus infection. J Clin Virol. 2007;39(2):76–81.
34. Gregory CJ, Lorenzi OD, Colon L, et al. Utility of the tourniquet test and the white blood cell count to differentiate dengue among acute febrile illnesses in the emergency room. PLoS Negl Trop Dis. 2011;5(12):e1400.
35. Barros LPS, Igawa SES, Jocundo SY, Junior LCB. Hematological and serological findings of individuals with suspicion of Dengue fever infection. Rev Bras Hematol Hemoter. 2008;30(5):363–6.
36. Colombo TE, Vedovello D, Araki CS, et al. Dengue-4 false negative results by Panbio(R) dengue early ELISA assay in Brazil. J Clin Virol. 2013;58(4):710–2.

37. Villabona-Arenas CJ, Mondini A, Bosch I, et al. Dengue virus type 3 adaptive changes during epidemics in Sao Jose de Rio Preto, Brazil, 2006–2007. PLoS One. 2013;8(5):e63496.
38. Drumond BP, Mondini A, Schmidt DJ, de Morais Bronzoni RV, Bosch I, Nogueira ML. Circulation of different lineages of Dengue virus 2, genotype American/Asian in Brazil: dynamics and molecular and phylogenetic characterization. PLoS One. 2013;8(3):e59422.
39. Mondini A, de Moraes Bronzoni RV, Nunes SH, et al. Spatio-temporal tracking and phylodynamics of an urban dengue 3 outbreak in Sao Paulo, Brazil. PLoS Negl Trop Dis. 2009;3(5):e448.
40. Terzian AC, Mondini A, Bronzoni RV, et al. Detection of Saint Louis encephalitis virus in dengue-suspected cases during a dengue 3 outbreak. Vector Borne Zoonotic Dis. 2011;11(3):291–300.
41. Mondini A, Cardeal IL, Lazaro E, et al. Saint Louis encephalitis virus, Brazil. Emerg Infect Dis. 2007;13(1):176–8.

5

A predictive model to differentiate dengue from other febrile illness

Eduardo Fernández[1], Marek Smieja[1,2,3], Stephen D. Walter[1] and Mark Loeb[1,2,3*]

Abstract

Background: Dengue is a major public health problem in tropical and subtropical countries and has a presentation similar to other febrile illnesses. Since laboratory confirmation is frequently delayed, the majority of dengue cases are diagnosed based on symptoms. The objective of this study was to identify clinical, hematological and demographical parameters that could be used as predictors of dengue fever among patients with febrile illness.

Methods: We conducted a retrospective cohort study of 548 patients presenting with febrile syndrome to the largest public hospitals in Honduras. Patients' clinical, laboratory, and demographic data as well as dengue laboratory detection by either serology or viral isolation were used to build a predictive statistical model to identify dengue cases.

Results: Of 548 patients, 390 were confirmed with dengue infection while 158 had negative results. Univariable analysis revealed seven variables associated with dengue: male sex, petechiae, skin rash, myalgia, retro-ocular pain, positive tourniquet test, and gingival bleeding. In multivariable logistic regression analysis, retro-ocular pain petechiae and gingival bleeding were associated with increased risk, while epistaxis and paleness of skin were associated with reduced risk of dengue. Using a value of 0.6 (i.e., 60% probability for a case to be positive based on the equation values), our model had a sensitivity of 86.2%, a specificity of 27.2%, and an overall accuracy of 69.2%; allowing for the diagnosis of dengue to be ruled out and for other febrile conditions to be investigated.

Conclusions: Among Honduran patients presenting with febrile illness, our analysis identified key symptoms associated with dengue fever, however the overall accuracy of our model was still low and specificity remains a concern. Our model requires validation in other populations with a similar pattern of dengue transmission.

Keywords: Dengue, Fever, Predictive model, Symptoms, Honduras

Background

Dengue is a vector-borne flavivirus infection transmitted by *Aedes* mosquitoes that poses a major public health threat in many tropical and subtropical regions [1–3]. Worldwide, dengue affects 50 million people annually and causes 20,000 to 25,000 deaths [1]. In Honduras, 66,814 cases were reported in 2010, with a case fatality rate of 3% [4]. Dengue cases in Honduras are concentrated in urban centers where the affected populations include both school age children and adults. In recent years the incidence has peaked between June and November, with epidemics observed every 24 to 36 months [4].

Clinical manifestations of dengue range from febrile illness to severe complications resulting in hospitalization and death. In its early stages, dengue resembles other febrile illness such as malaria, influenza, and leptospirosis, constituting a diagnostic challenge for clinicians in endemic countries [5]. Further complications to dengue diagnosis arise from the presence of overlapping manifestations such as the presence of hematuria, which can occur in cases of either falciparum malaria or dengue [6, 7]. The ability to differentiate between dengue and other conditions is of prime importance to clinicians in dengue endemic areas. An early diagnosis allows for the early monitoring of indicators that are associated with eventual severe disease.

A confirmatory diagnosis of dengue is made through laboratory diagnosis using serology (e.g., IgM titres, IgG seroconversion), antigen detection of non-structural

* Correspondence: loebm@mcmaster.ca
[1]Department of Clinical Epidemiology and Biostatistics, McMaster University, Hamilton, Ontario, Canada
[2]Department of Pathology and Molecular Medicine, McMaster University, Hamilton, Ontario, Canada
Full list of author information is available at the end of the article

protein (NS) in sera, or polymerase chain reaction (PCR) for dengue virus nucleic acids in blood. Of these laboratory methods, PCR is not available in many middle and low income countries. Similarly, antigen detection of NS is frequently unavailable or is not part of routine dengue confirmation. Although serology is available in many settings, there may be delays in obtaining results, and, in many areas, no laboratory testing is available at all.

Although there is no specific therapy, identifying dengue can help clinicians make better decisions; for example they can triage patients by knowing which patients need to be monitored for possible dengue complications. On the other hand, dengue diagnosis based solely on clinical presentation is challenging and can lead to misdiagnosis with the ensuing consequences for patients. In Honduras, for example, studies show that less than 50% of specimens tested in cases of suspected dengue are confirmed to be positive, with the remainder being negative or inconclusive [8, 9].

Previous reports exist of models for dengue, using symptoms, signs, and laboratory data to differentiate dengue from other febrile syndromes [10–16]. Demographic factors such as age and sex [12, 13]; clinical symptoms such as joint pain, vomiting, and myalgia [15]; and laboratory findings such leucopenia and thrombocytopenia [16], have all been reported as predictors for dengue. Limitations of these studies include a small sample size [11–14], lack of validation of the models [17], limited geographic representation [14, 15], and limited predictive ability of the results [17–19].

We conducted analyses using data that was systematically collected on a cohort of febrile patients seen at different health care facilities in Honduras. Using these data, we built and validated logistic regression models to identify clinical factors to predict laboratory confirmed dengue.

Methods

Data on signs and symptoms of patients who present with dengue is routinely collected in Honduras and submitted to the Honduran National Classification Committee for classification of cases. We used such data collected between June 2009 and June 2010 from patients who presented with fever and ≥ 2 symptoms to one of five hospitals and outpatient clinics located in Tegucigalpa and San Pedro Sula, the two largest cities in Honduras. These symptoms included headache, retro-ocular pain, myalgia, rash, anorexia and vomiting, any bleeding manifestation, including petechiae, ecchymosis, epistaxis, gingival bleeding, hematuria, heavy menstrual bleeding, and symptoms suggestive of capillary leakage, including abdominal pain, cold extremities, and sweating. Patients of all ages were included in our analyses, all were tested for dengue and all, if not hospitalized at presentation, were subsequently hospitalized. Patients were seen either at healthcare facilities that are part of the social security system (Instituto Hondureño de Seguridad Social) or not facilities that form part of the public health system. The former serves the insured employed population whereas the latter serves the general population with no restrictions.

General practitioners, nurses, and microbiologists at either the primary health care centres or at the tertiary hospitals completed a data collection form (for case classification) which included epidemiological and clinical information. Symptoms and signs were collected at first presentation while hematology and biochemical tests recorded were those at presentation and those repeated approximately one week later. Fever was defined as a temperature of > 37.5 degrees Celsius. Both objective measurements of fever and self-report of fever were included. Conditions with a febrile presentation, such as malaria, kidney infections, chronic hepatitis, leptospirosis, and respiratory infections were evaluated however complete information on the ultimate diagnosis for patients that tested negative for dengue was either not available or not recorded in the data collection form.

Blood samples were collected from patients for dengue laboratory confirmation. If a patient presented within 5 days of the first symptom onset, samples were processed for viral culture following guidelines from the U.S Centers for Disease Control and Prevention (CDC) [20]. If the blood sample was taken on the sixth day or later of onset of symptoms, a test for antibody detection was done using IgM antibody-capture enzyme-linked immunosorbent (IgM Mac ELISA) from Standard Diagnostic of Bio Venture Company (Gyeonggi-do, South Korea) [20, 21]. This commercial kit reports a sensitivity of 96.4% and specificity of 98.9% [21]. Serology and viral isolation were performed at the Honduras National Laboratory of Virology according to CDC guidelines and standardized techniques.

For hospitalized patients, our analysis was based on serial blood tests taken over the 3 days following admission, and using additional radiological or laboratory testing if available. The initial clinical diagnosis of the treating physician prior to laboratory confirmation was recorded and submitted to the Honduran National Classification Committee for classification as uncomplicated dengue or severe dengue i.e. dengue haemorrhagic fever or shock syndrome [8, 22].

All patients received a laboratory result for dengue (either positive or negative based on viral isolation or IgM). Complete information was obtained for 548 patients. Of 548 patients studied, 390 had laboratory evidence for dengue infection while 158 had negative results.

Predictor variables

We used the data collected at presentation to assess predictor variables for dengue by grouping these into three categories: 1) general symptoms, including fever, headache, retro-ocular pain, myalgia, rash, anorexia and vomiting; 2) bleeding manifestations, including petechiae, ecchymosis, hematemesis, melena, positive tourniquet, epistaxis (nose bleeding), gingival bleeding, hematuria, and heavy menstrual bleeding (metrorrhagia); and 3) symptoms and signs suggestive of capillary leakage, including abdominal pain, cold extremities, sweating, paleness of skin, serous membranes' effusion (pericardial, pleural effusion and ascites), and reduction of mean arterial pressure. Hematological results (leucocytes count, and hemoglobin and hematocrit values) were recorded if they were available for at least two consecutive days.

Power calculation

A sample size was not determined *a priori* since the study enrolled all patients admitted during the study period who had febrile illness and laboratory testing for dengue. Since petechiae are both readily identifiable and are commonly seen in dengue infection we based the study's power calculation on the predictive value of petechiae to differentiate dengue from other febrile illness [23]. Based on the 548 records (390 dengue-positive and 158 dengue-negative), assuming a prevalence of petechiae of 25% in non-dengue febrile illness and an alpha level of 0.05, the study had 80% power to detect a 1.5-fold increase risk of dengue given the presence of petechiae.

Data analysis

The chi-square test was used to detect significant differences between presenting signs and symptoms (recorded during admission and on the first day of the patient's stay, prior to being tested for dengue) and the laboratory tests results.

A logistic regression model was built using a forward step-wise selection. Variables with $p < 0.2$ were entered into the multivariable models. We decided *a priori* to include both age and sex in the analysis. Correlation among pairs of variables was assessed calculating values for tolerance and the variance inflation factor (VIF). Values for tolerance >0.2 and for VIF < 5 were considered as being compatible with a low collinearity. Variables that were statistically significant ($p < 0.05$) were kept in the final model.

Confidence intervals for the odds ratios, were calculated for each predictor. As part of the models' internal validation, the bootstrap method (i.e. resampling data) was used to estimate the accuracy of the estimators (standard error, confidence intervals and bias) [24–26]. The model was also validated using subsamples, each corresponding to one tenth of the sample and with nine tenths of the remaining sample used for a cross-validation. The subsamples were drawn using systematic sampling (including every tenth case for each subsample) without leaving any patient out of the procedure.

Additionally, as a sensitivity analysis, we created a dichotomous variable for the type of health care facility where patients had presented to either the social security system (accessible only to the insured employed population) or at public health clinics (open to the general population). This was done to account for potential centre effect, that is, differences between the two patient populations.

After building and validating logistic regression models, the sensitivity of the method was determined using the receiver operating characteristic (ROC) curve, which is a graphic plot illustrating the performance of a binary classifier system like the one used during this study.

Using the model equation, we then created a score from the equation by transforming the values assigned to each predictor to integers by multiplying by ten (avoiding decimal values). All statistical analysis were done using SPSS version 19 (IBM) [27].

Results

The final study sample consisted of 548 patients: 227 were female (41%); mean age 21 years of age (SD = 15.5 years). Of these patients, 295 (53.8%) were admitted to tertiary-level hospitals, 240 (43.8%) in hospitals providing care for insured workers, and 13 (2.4%) originally seen in regional and local health clinics and later admitted to hospital.

Complete clinical and demographic data was available for all 548 patients. However, information on the date of onset of symptoms was missing in 10% of the sample. The duration of signs or symptoms from date of onset is summarized in Table 1. For 495 patients for whom the date of onset of symptoms was available, the mean time for obtaining the dengue sample from onset of symptoms was 6 days (range 0–65 days).

Viral isolation by cell culture was done in 114 patients who presented within the first 5 days of symptoms, resulting in 9 (7.9%) positive isolates. Serology was done in the remaining 434 patients, 381 (87.8%) of whom were seropositive. Altogether, dengue laboratory testing revealed that 390 patients (71%) were positive (381 by serology and 9 by viral isolation).

The social security system submitted 239 blood samples and 203 (84.9%) tested positive. The public health system submitted 309 samples and 187 (60.5%) tested positive. In terms of type of test requested, viral isolation was requested in 14 patients by the social security

Table 1 Duration of signs and symptoms from date of onset of study patients

	0–3 days N (%)	4–6 days N (%)	≥7 days N(%)
Fever	54(100)	262(98.5)	172(98.3)
Headache	47(87.0)	229(86.1)	147(84.2)
Retroocular Pain	39(72.2)	200(75.2)	125(71.4)
Myalgias	46(85.2)	222(83.5)	151(86.3)
Arthralgias	40(74.1)	193(72.6)	136(77.7)
Skin rash	19(35.2)	92(34.6)	59(33.7)
Anorexia	38(70.4)	218(82.0)	142(81.1)
Petechiae	7(13.0)	73(27.4)	61(34.9)
Epistaxis	9(16.7)	53(19.9)	32(18.3)
Echymoses	1(1.9)	21(7.9)	21(12.0)
Gingival bleeding	2(3.7)	14(5.3)	9(5.1)
Pallor	25(46.3)	123(46.2)	86(49.1)

system and in 100 patients by the public health system, for a positivity of 28.6% (five cases) and 5% (five cases) respectively. Antibody determination was requested for 225 patients by the social security system and for 209 patients by the public health system, for a positivity of 88.4% (199 patients) and 87.1% (182 patients), respectively.

The mean hematocrit was 40.6 with a range from 17.4 to 40.6 while the mean platelet count at admission was 74,311 with a range from 113 to 61,600. The mean leukocyte count was 5066 (range 513 to 36,000).

Nine variables (petechiae, skin rash, myalgias, retro-ocular pain, tourniquet test, cold limbs, gingival bleeding, epistaxis, and skin paleness) had a p value < 0.2 and were thus considered for multivariable analysis (Table 2).

The following variables were independently associated with dengue in multivariable analysis: petechiae (OR 2.0, 95% CI: 1.3, 3.3), retro-ocular pain (OR 1.7, 95% CI: 1.1, 2.5), gingival bleeding (OR 3.7, 95% CI: 1.1, 13), epistaxis (OR 0.6, 95% CI: 0.4, 1.0), and skin paleness (OR 0.6, 95% CI: 0.4, 0.9) (Table 3). Statistics for collinearity were also applied and the values for tolerance were >0.7 and the VIF (variance inflation factor) was ≤1.3, which represent no significant collinearity among variables tested in the model.

Table 2 Variables associated with laboratory confirmed dengue among 548 febrile patients in univariable analysis

Variable	Positive Dengue No (%)	Odds ratio (95% CI)	*P* value
Male	168 (43.5)	1.28 (0.9 to 1.8)	0.20
Petechiae	120 (81.1%)	1.52 (1.0 to 2.3)	0.002
Skin rash	138 (76.7)	1.51 (1.0 to 2.3)	0.046
Myalgia	336 (72.6)	1.52 (0.93 to 2.47)	0.09
Retroocular pain	296 (74.6)	1.51 (1.0 to 2.3)	0.04
Positive Tourniquet test	26 (86.7)	2.75 (0.94 to 8.0)	0.05
Cold limbs	139 (66.8)	0.71 (0.5 to 1.0)	0.08
Gingival bleeding	24 (88.9)	3.4 (1.0 t 11.4)	0.04
Epistaxis	68 (63.6)	0.64 (0.41 to 1.01)	0.06
Paleness	174 (65.9)	0.61 (0.4 to 0.9)	0.009

The model had a sensitivity of 86.2% and a specificity of 27%, with a positive predictive value of 74.5% and a negative predictive value of 44.3%. The positive and negative likelihood ratios were 1.2 and 0.5, respectively, for an overall model accuracy of 69.2%. For the classification of cases (positive cases), the software's default threshold or cut-point was 0.5; however the specificity was extremely low (4.4%). Therefore, we increased the cut-point to 0.6 which reduced the overall model prediction (from 71.9 to 69.2%) but increased the specificity. In this cases the cut-point defined the level of acceptance of the cases as positive dengue, ROC was used to identify the best cut-point for the classification that provided a higher specificity while keeping a level of sensitivity higher than 85%.

Applying the bootstrap method, we found that p values from the subsamples were similar to those obtained in the entire sample, and the bias values were < 25% of the standard error values of the predictors of the subsamples.

Including the health care facility as a variable in the multivariable analysis, as a sensitivity analysis, yielded a model that included two clinical predictors with a positive association to confirmed dengue: petechiae (OR 1.80; 95% CI: 1.11 to 2.92) and gingival bleeding (OR 3.24,95% CI: 0.93,11.26). It also revealed paleness of skin as a negative association (OR 0.61; 95% CI: 0.41, 0.90). The health care facility was also a significant predictor for dengue (OR 3.42; 95%CI: 2.23, 5.26). Retroocular pain and epistaxis did not appear in this model and the odds ratios for the clinical predictors in this model had smaller odds ratios. At a cut point of 0.6, this alternative model correctly classified 69.9% of the patients, with a sensitivity of 84.1% and specificity of 34.8%, representing a slight improvement in overall classification and specificity but with a reduction in sensitivity over the previous model based only on clinical signs and symptoms. The model, which included health care facility, was also validated using the bootstrap test (data not shown). (Table 4).

Table 3 Final logistic regression model for predictors of dengue

Variable	Odds ratio (95% CI)	*P* value
Petechiae	2.0 (1.3 to 3.3)	0.003
Retroocular pain	1.7 (1.1 to 2.5)	0.01
Gingival bleeding	3.7 (1.1 to 13.0)	0.04
Epistaxis	0.6 (0.4 to 1.0)	0.045
Paleness	0.6 (0.4 to 0.9)	0.006

Table 4 Logistic regression model including health system

Variable	Odds ratio (95% CI)	*P* value
Petechiae	1.8 (1.1 to 2.9)	0.02
Gingival bleeding	3.2 (0.93 to 11.3)	0.06
Health system	3.4 (2.2 to 5.3)	<0.001
Paleness	0.6 (0.4 to 0.9)	0.01

In the analysis of ROC we found that the area under the curve was 0.663 (asymptotic 95% CI: 0.616, 0.710). The equation for the model was y = 0.694 + 0.718(petechiae) + 0.516 (retro-ocular pain) + .316(gingival bleeding) − 0.474 (epistaxis)- 0.535 (skin paleness). The results given by the ROC curve showed a logistic regression model with an area under the curve (AUC) of 0.65 (95% CI = 0.60, 0.70) and a standard error of 0.025, being statistically significant. The logistic regression model had a good overall prediction and this was confirmed through the ROC analysis.

Using the equation, a score was obtained by rounding up values of the equation to the close integer, with the next values. Therefore, petechiae = 7, retroocular pain = 5, gingival bleeding = 13 (all when the sign is present) and epistaxis = −5 and skin paleness = −5 (negative values for when they are present). When only positive predictors are present, the maximum score would be 25 whereas when only negative predictors are present the score would be −10. Intermediate values can be obtained with different combination of predictors.

The score was simplified using the values of the equation and reducing it to values 0 and 1 assigning 1 to those considered cases and 0 to non-cases. That is, signs and symptoms scores were added and a threshold value of 3 was selected to differentiate cases from non cases, (any value ≤ 3 was coded as 0 and values >3 were coded as 1). This resulted in 336 of the 390 positive correctly predicted, and 43 of the 158 negative patients predicted as no dengue cases. The sensitivity and specificity for this score were 86.2% and of 27%, respectively. The area under the curve was 0.567(asymptotic 95% CI were 0.512, 0.622) with a standard error of 0.028. The accuracy is still low if is intended to operationalize the equation for clinical personnel providing a rapid method to identify cases of dengue.

Discussion

Our logistic regression model found that five symptoms or signs helped differentiate dengue from other febrile illness: [1] petechiae, [2] retro-ocular pain, [3] gingival bleeding, [4] epistaxis and [5] skin paleness. Of these, the association was positive for the first three (likely to be present in dengue cases), and negative for the last two (epistaxis and pale skin), consistent with being less likely to be present in dengue cases.

Our analysis used similar variables to that of previous reported models, but in contrast to previous reports, we not only built and validated a model but created scoring system to assess the model. A cross-sectional study to differentiate dengue from non-dengue among patients attending the emergency department of a public hospital in Brazil was described in one report (10). Only conjunctival redness and leukocyte count were associated with dengue. The sensitivity and specificity of this model was 80.8 and 71.1% respectively but did not include validation techniques. Ramos et al. used surveillance data from Puerto Rico and reported that rash and either the absence of sore throat, nasal congestion, or cough had low (<50%) sensitivity for ruling out dengue in children (11). However, validation and construction of a predictive rule was not conducted. In another study from Puerto Rica using surveillance data, five variables (retro-orbital pain, rash, low platelet count, lack of sore throat, absence of cough) were used to build models that had AUC of 0.76. However, a cut-off point for diagnostic accuracy was not reported (13). In a study from Papa New Gunia, only facial flushing and male sex were associated with dengue in multivariable analysis (14). The AUC was 0.59 but no cut-off was used to predict cases. In a study from Nicaragua among children, fever, headache, retro-orbital pain, myalgia, arthralgia, rash, petechiae, positive tourniquet test, vomiting, leukopenia, platelets ≤150,000 cells/mL, poor capillary refill, cold extremities and hypotension.were associated wtth dengue. This study did not use the model to predict dengue in a validation set.

Including clinical signs in the model make intuitive sense and we consider it to be a strength. Petechiae and gingival bleeding, for example, represent subcutaneous or mucosal bleeding and are therefore readily noticeable by the patient and reported as such. Epistaxis can be frequently associated with respiratory conditions rather than with dengue, and in our sample most patients with epistaxis had a negative dengue test.

With respect to effect size, gingival bleeding had a higher odds ratio than other predictors but also had a wider confidence interval (OR 3.7, CI: 1.1, 13.0.) followed by petechiae, retro-ocular pain. Compared to other studies, our odds ratios were smaller for petechiae, retro-orbital pain and gingival bleeding but clearly represented a positive association with dengue positivity [10, 23, 28–34].

Unlike other studies that have found epistaxis and skin paleness positively associated with dengue [3, 10, 32, 34], our study identified an inverse association with both. Most of our patients with epistaxis had a negative dengue result. Mittal et al. reported that skin paleness or pallor was associated with advanced stages of dengue. In fact, 13.3% of their patients with dengue were described as having pallor [34].

Paleness of skin has been found associated to dengue presumably because of vascular events (bleeding, vasoconstriction) occurring when dengue evolves into severe forms. In Central America, as in other developing regions, paleness can be associated with chronic anemia and malnutrition but frequently the clinician is faced with limited laboratory resources and must resort to basic clinical evaluation to make a diagnosis.

Notably, proportionally more patients from the social security system hospitals were diagnosed correctly (84.9%) than those from the public health system (60.5%) as described in the results. The most likely explanation is that there were proportionately more patients in the public health system that had specimens sent for viral isolation at later time points (beyond 3 days) and that this resulted in a lower detection rate.

The model that included health care facility reduced the number of symptoms to three: petechiae, gingival bleeding and paleness of skin, keeping the same direction of association and similar effect size as the model without health system. The sensitivity of the model increased slightly to 84.1%, and the specificity to 34.8%, for an overall accuracy of 69.9%. Including the health care facility as a predictor increased the accuracy of the model but resulted in a reduction in the number of clinical predictors. Although this finding may suggest differences in the populations receiving care at different levels of the Honduran health system, it is most probably due to differences in the clinical judgment of treating physicians at those levels.

A strength of this study is that it was conducted during a period of active dengue transmission allowing for a sufficient number of patients to be assessed. One limitation is that our sample may have been characterized by an overrepresentation of symptoms deemed important to a subgroup of patients in the early stages of the syndrome, particularly with respect to pain (e.g. headache, retro-ocular pain). Also, the difference in the clinical diagnostic accuracy between health care facilities providing information is a factor to consider as this may represent different levels of experience with the disease. Another potential limitation is that our study was conducted when other viruses, such as Chikungunya and Zika, were not circulating. There is a possibility that this would have affected the predictive value of our model. Since we conducted an analysis using a database on suspected dengue, we did not have access to the final diagnosis of non-dengue cases.

Prior laboratory data in Honduras shows that around 40% of suspected cases with confirmed to be positive by laboratory testing [8, 9]. An important limitation of our study is that IgM testing was not conducted on all samples on days 4 and 5 [35]. We were also unable to differentiate between primary and secondary dengue and this could have affected results because of the predominance of different symptoms in primary versus secondary dengue. The fact that most patients were admitted after 5 days following symptom onset may limit generalizability. It is possible that our sample may have been biased by spectrum, with a representation of patients with more severe illness including symptoms of more severe disease which is observed in patients consulting the medical service but not in the community where milder disease is more frequent. The retrospective nature of our study is another limitation. To confirm the utility of this model it should be tested both during epidemic and inter-epidemic periods.

Conclusions

In conclusion, we demonstrate that a simple model may identify useful predictors to differentiate between dengue and other causes of febrile illness. The model should optimally be used with a method for rapid confirmatory testing. The use of such a model can define those cases more likely to be dengue and needing primarily a dengue test while other patients can be directed to a different management. The use of a score table as the one presented in the results can facilitate the effort of those working in the screening of febrile illness requiring hospitalization.

Acknowledgements
Not applicable

Funding
There was no specific grant supprt for this work.

Authors' contributions
EF, MS, SW, ML developed the concept and design of the study. EF collected the data. EF, MS, SW, ML contributed to the analysis. EF, MS, SW, ML drafted the manuscript, revised it critically, and gave final approval of the final versi6n of the manuscript to be published. EF, MS, SW, ML agree to be accountable for all aspects of the work in ensuring that questions related to the accuracy or integrity of any part of the work are appropriately investigated and resolved.

Competing interests
The authors declare that they have no competing interests.

Consent for publication
Not applicable.

Author details
[1]Department of Clinical Epidemiology and Biostatistics, McMaster University, Hamilton, Ontario, Canada. [2]Department of Pathology and Molecular

Medicine, McMaster University, Hamilton, Ontario, Canada. [3]Institute for Infectious Diseases Research, McMaster University, Hamilton, Ontario, Canada.

References

1. WHO. Dengue and dengue haemorrhagic fever. Geneva: World Health Organization; 2008. (updated March 2014; cited 2008 May 2008]; Factsheet No. 117]. Available from: http://www.who.int/mediacentre/factsheets/fs117/en/.
2. Gubler DJ. Dengue and dengue hemorrhagic fever: its history and resurgence as a global public health problem. In: Gubler DJK, G., editor. Dengue and dengue hemorrhagic fever. CAB International Press; 1997. p. 1–22.
3. Halstead SB. Pathogenesis of dengue: challenges to molecular biology. Science. 1988;239(4839):476–81.
4. PAHO. Health in the Americas 2012. Washington: Pan American Health Organization; 2012.
5. Rodriguez LE, Tomashek KM, Gregory CJ, Munoz J, Hunsperger E, Lorenzi OD, et al. Co-infection with dengue virus and pandemic (H1N1] virus (letter]. 2010, et al. Emerg Infect Dis (serial on the Internet]. 2010 May (date cited]. http://wwwnc.cdc.gov/eid/article/16/5/09-1920 Doi: 10.3201/eid1605.091920.
6. Wiwanitkit V. Concurrent malaria and dengue infection: a brief summary and comment. Asian Pac J Trop Biomed. 2011;1(4):326–7.
7. Kaushik RM, Varma A, Kaushik R, Gaur KJ. Concurrent dengue and malaria due to *Plasmodium falciparum* and *P. vivax*. Trans R Soc Trop Med Hyg. 2007;101(10):1048–50.
8. Secretaria de Salud. Boletin epidemiologico semanal. Tegucigalpa: Secretaria de Salud de Honduras, Direccion de Vigilancia de la Salud; 2005.
9. Mendez J, Fernandez EA. Taller sobre avances recientes en el control del *Aedes aegypti* basado en la comunidad: Honduras y Mexico. Merida, Yucatan. 1996.
10. Daumas RP, Passos SR, Oliveira RV, Nogueira RM, Georg I, Marzochi KB, et al. Clinical and laboratory features that discriminate dengue from other febrile illnesses: a diagnostic accuracy study in Rio de Janeiro, Brazil. BMC Infect Dis. 2013;13:77.
11. Ramos MM, Tomashek KM, Arguello DF, Luxemburger C, Quinones L, Lang J, et al. Early clinical features of dengue infection in Puerto Rico. Trans R Soc Trop Med Hyg. 2009;103(9):878–84.
12. Gregory CJ, Santiago LM, Arguello DF, Hunsperger E, Tomashek KM. Clinical and laboratory features that differentiate dengue from other febrile illnesses in an endemic area–Puerto Rico, 2007–2008. Am J Trop Med Hyg. 2010; 82(5):922–9.
13. Phuong HL, de Vries PJ, Nga TT, Giao PT, Hung le Q, Binh TQ, et al. Dengue as a cause of acute undifferentiated fever in Vietnam. BMC Infect Dis. 2006;6:123.
14. Senn N, Luang-Suarkia D, Manong D, Siba PM, McBride WJ. Contribution of dengue fever to the burden of acute febrile illnesses in Papua New Guinea: an age-specific prospective study. Am J Trop Med Hyg. 2011;85(1):132–7.
15. Biswas HH, Ortega O, Gordon A, Standish K, Balmaseda A, Kuan G, et al. Early clinical features of dengue virus infection in nicaraguan children: a longitudinal analysis. PLoS Negl Trop Dis. 2012;6(3):e1562.
16. Dietz VJ, Gubler DJ, Rigau-Perez JG, Pinheiro F, Schatzmayr HG, Bailey R, et al. Epidemic dengue 1 in Brazil, 1986: evaluation of a clinically based dengue surveillance system. Am J Epidemiol. 1990;131(4):693–701.
17. Potts JA, Rothman AL. Clinical and laboratory features that distinguish dengue from other febrile illnesses in endemic populations. Trop Med Int Health (Review]. 2008;13(11):1328–40.
18. Karande S, Gandhi D, Kulkarni M, Bharadwaj R, Pol S, Thakare J, et al. Concurrent outbreak of leptospirosis and dengue in Mumbai, India, 2002. J Trop Pediatr. 2005;51(3):174–81.
19. Deparis X, Murgue B, Roche C, Cassar O, Chungue E. Changing clinical and biological manifestations of dengue during the dengue-2 epidemic in French Polynesia in 1996/97–description and analysis in a prospective study. Trop Med Int Health. 1998;3(11):859–65.
20. Balmaceda A. Manual de procedimientos de tecnicas para el diagnostico del dengue: Organizacion Panamericana de la Salud, Salud DdDdSdSd. 2002.
21. Kuno G, Gomez I, Gubler DJ. An ELISA procedure for the diagnosis of dengue infections. J Virol Methods. 1991;33(1–2):101–13.
22. Dirección de Vigilancia de la Salud. Lineamientos de Vigilancia y Manejo Estandarizado de Pacientes con dengue. Tegucigalpa: Azer Impresos y Diseños; 2003. 40.
23. Kalayanarooj S, Vaughn DW, Nimmannitya S, Green S, Suntayakorn S, Kunentrasai N, et al. Early clinical and laboratory indicators of acute dengue illness. J Infect Dis. 1997;176(2):313–21.
24. Schlesselman JJ, editor. Case–control Studies: design, conduct, analysis. 1st ed. New York: Oxford University Press; 1982.
25. Hesterberg T, Moore DS, Monaghan S, Clipson A, Epstein R. Bootstrap Methods and Permutation tests. In: Moore DS, McCabe GP, editors. Introduction to the Practice of Statistics. New York: WH Freeman; 2005.
26. Efron B. Bootstrap Methods: Another look at the Jacknife. Ann Stat. 1979; 7(1):1–26.
27. SPSS I. SPSS for Windows (version 19]. Chicago: SPSS. Inc; 2010.
28. Phuong CX, Nhan NT, Kneen R, Thuy PT, van Thien C, Nga NT, et al. Clinical diagnosis and assessment of severity of confirmed dengue infections in Vietnamese children: is the world health organization classification system helpful? Am J Trop Med Hyg. 2004;70(2):172–9.
29. Chadwick D, Arch B, Wilder-Smith A, Paton N. Distinguishing dengue fever from other infections on the basis of simple clinical and laboratory features: application of logistic regression analysis. J Clin Virol. 2006;35(2):147–53.
30. Sawasdivorn S, Vibulvattanakit S, Sasavatpakdee M, Iamsirithavorn S. Efficacy of clinica diagnosis of dengue fever in paediatric age groups as determined by WHO case definition 1997 in Thailand. Dengue Bull. 2001;25:56–64.
31. Nunes-Araujo FR, Ferreira MS, Nishioka SD. Dengue fever in Brazilian adults and children: assessment of clinical findings and their validity for diagnosis. Ann Trop Med Parasitol. 2003;97(4):415–9.
32. Hammond SN, Balmaseda A, Perez L, Tellez Y, Saborio SI, Mercado JC, et al. Differences in dengue severity in infants, children, and adults in a 3-year hospital-based study in Nicaragua. Am J Trop Med Hyg. 2005;73(6):1063–70.
33. Diaz-Quijano FA, Martinez-Vega RA, Villar-Centeno LA. Early indicators of severity in dengue virus infection. Enferm Infecc Microbiol Clin. 2005;23(9): 529–32.
34. Mittal H, Faridi MM, Arora SK, Patil R. Clinicohematological profile and platelet trends in children with dengue during 2010 epidemic in north India. Indian J Pediatr. 2012;79(4):467–71.
35. Mishra B, Gupta PK, Dhiman V, Pujhari SK, Sharma M, Ratho RK. Clinical Applicability of Various Dengue Diagnostic Tests in Resource-Limited Endemic Settings. J Global Infect Dis. 2014;6(3):109–13. doi:10.4103/0974-777X.138504.

Patterns and causes of liver involvement in acute dengue infection

Samitha Fernando[1], Ananda Wijewickrama[5], Laksiri Gomes[1], Chameera T. Punchihewa[1], S. D. P. Madusanka[1], Harsha Dissanayake[2], Chandima Jeewandara[3], Hemantha Peiris[4], Graham S. Ogg[6] and Gathsaurie Neelika Malavige[1,6*]

Abstract

Background: Liver involvement in acute dengue infection is frequently observed and sometimes leads to acute liver failure, with fatal outcomes. Many factors are thought to contribute to liver dysfunction, including hypoxic injury due to decreased perfusion, direct damage by the virus and immune mediated injury. In this study, we sought to identify the pattern in the change in liver enzymes throughout the illness and its association with the degree of viraemia, onset and extent of plasma leakage and inflammatory mediators.

Methods: Serial daily blood samples were obtained from 55 adult patients with acute dengue from the time of admission to discharge and the liver function tests, viral loads and cytokines were assessed. The onset and extent of fluid leakage was measured by daily ultrasound examinations and all clinical and laboratory features were serially recorded.

Results: Aspartate transaminase (AST), alanine transaminase (ALT) and gamma glutamyl transferase (GGT) levels were elevated in patients with dengue infection throughout the illness. The highest AST levels were seen on day 6 of illness and both AST and GGT levels were significantly higher in patients with severe dengue (SD), when compared to those with non-severe dengue (NSD) on day 5 and 6 of illness. Three patients with SD had AST and ALT values of >1000/IU in the absence of any fluid leakage or a rise in the haematocrit (≥20 %). The peak of the AST levels and the lowest serum albumin levels were seen 24 h before the maximum fluid leakage and 24 h after the peak in viraemia. Both serum IL-10 and IL-17 levels were elevated during early illness and were significantly higher in those with SD when compared to NSD.

Conclusion: Dengue associated liver injury appears to peak around day 6 and 7. Therefore, liver function tests done at earlier dates might not reflect the extent of liver involvement in acute infection. Since severe liver involvement can occur in the absence of fluid leakage, after the peak viraemia, and since it is associated with high IL-17 and IL-10 levels, possible immune mechanisms leading to hepatic damage should be investigated.

Keywords: Dengue, Liver injury, Transaminases, Viral loads, Immune mediated, Fluid leakage

Background

Dengue viral infections are one of the most rapidly evolving vector borne infections, which now affects 125 countries, causing approximately 100 million apparent infections each year [1]. It is predicted that the transmission of dengue will be more intensified in dengue endemic countries, and due to climate change and other factors, the infection may spread to countries that are currently not significantly affected by dengue in Europe and America [1]. Currently there is no specific antiviral or any other drug that is effective in the treatment of acute dengue infection.

Infection with the DENV results in asymptomatic disease or an undifferentiated viral fever like illness in the majority of infected individuals. However, in others, it may result in dengue fever (DF), dengue haemorrhagic fever (DHF) leading to shock (DSS), or the expanded dengue syndrome [2]. Involvement of the liver leading to hepatic dysfunction is a well-recognized complication of dengue [3–5]. Dengue associated acute liver failure has a high mortality due to

* Correspondence: gathsaurie.malavige@ndm.ox.ac.uk
[1]Department of Microbiology, Centre for Dengue Research, Faculty of Medical Sciences, University of Sri Jayewardenepura, Nugegoda 10250, Sri Lanka
[6]MRC Human Immunology Unit, Weatherall Institute of Molecular Medicine, Oxford NIHR Biomedical Research Centre and University of Oxford, Oxford OX3 9DS, UK
Full list of author information is available at the end of the article

complications such as encephalopathy, severe bleeding, renal failure and metabolic acidosis [3, 4]. Although dengue associated acute liver failure is thought to occur due to liver injury as a result of prolonged shock, it is also known to occur in the absence of shock [4].

Varying degrees of liver involvement are seen during acute dengue infection and are thought to result from hepatocyte apoptosis directly by the virus, hypoxic damage due to impaired liver perfusion resulting from fluid leakage, oxidative stress or immune mediated injury [6–8]. Studies done in mouse models have proposed that dengue associated liver injury can be both viral induced or immune mediated. The dengue virus (DENV) has been shown to readily infect hepatocytes in mouse models, and HepG2 and Huh7 hepatoma cell lines [9–11]. In both mouse models and hepatoma cell lines, apoptosis of hepatocytes was shown to be due to both direct viral infection and also cytokine induced [12]. It has been shown that in dengue mouse models, that both IL-22 and IL-17 were associated with severe clinical disease, and particularly liver injury [13]. In addition, liver involvement was found to be significantly reduced following IL-17 receptor blockade [13]. Again in dengue mouse models, early infiltration of the liver by natural killer cells followed by T cells was observed, and was found to associate with apoptosis of hepatocytes [14]. Cytokine mediated liver damage has also been proposed as a mechanism, as high levels of IP-10 and IL-10 were found to associate with high liver transaminase levels in children with dengue [15]. Many believe that dengue associated liver dysfunction is probably due to reduced perfusion associated hypoxic injury as a consequence of a severe vascular leak [2].

However, since the frequency of liver involvement associated with dengue is increasing and since isolated liver involvement in the absence of shock and other dengue associated complications (expanded dengue syndrome) is also increasing [2], it has become important to identify the causes of liver involvement in dengue, including the kinetics in changes in liver function tests associated with acute dengue infection. Therefore, in this study, we serially studied a cohort of adult dengue patients with severe dengue (SD) and non-severe dengue (NSD), who did not develop shock during the course of their illness, and investigated the changes in liver enzymes during the natural course of the illness and determined the degree of liver damage in association with the degree of viraemia, the onset and extent of vascular leak and changes in inflammatory mediators.

Methods

Patients

Fifty five adult patients with acute dengue infection were recruited from the Infectious Diseases Hospital of Sri Lanka in year 2015 from January to August, following informed written consent. Those who were known to have chronic liver disease, chronic renal disease, pregnant individuals, those on a steroid dose of >40 mg/day for over 7 days and those who had been given NSAIDs for the treatment of dengue prior to admission, were excluded from the study. None of the patients were given any drugs except for the recommended dose of paracetamol. Only those whose duration from onset of illness was ≤5 days were recruited. The day in which the patient first developed fever was considered as day one of illness. As one of the main aims of this study was to determine the timing of liver injury with changes in viral load, vascular leak and increase in inflammatory mediators, the clinical features along with these parameters were recorded daily. Blood samples were obtained daily at 10 am from the day of recruitment until discharge from the hospital. As the maximum duration of illness in this cohort was 9 days, no samples were analysed beyond day 9 of illness. The number of patients assessed at each time point is given in Additional file 1: Table S1.

Clinical features such as fever, blood pressure, pulse pressure and the urine output were measured at least 4 times a day. Serial recordings of liver function tests, viral loads, the extent of fluid leakage and serum cytokine levels were done daily. In order to determine the relationship between plasma leakage and liver derangements, we carried out serial ultrasound scans of all patients to define the onset and extent of fluid leakage. Ultrasound scanning was done in the supine position to assess the peritoneal fluid in the hepatorenal angle, subdiaphragmatic position, in paracolic gutters and in the pelvis. In order to determine the fluid in the pleural cavity the patient was kept seated upright on the examination bed for 2 min for all the pleural fluid to gravitate in to costodiaphragmatic recesses and then the patient was scanned from the back of the chest with hands raised up and crossed at the back of the head. Fluid was measured at the mid and posterior axillary lines and in seated-up position. Fluid accumulation in the peritoneal cavity was assessed by a semi quantitative manner, with classification of ascites as minimal, mild, moderate, severe and massive by looking for the presence of fluid in five areas of the abdomen namely right upper quadrant (perihepatic and morrison's pouch), left upper quadrant (perisplenic), right paracolic gutter, left paracolic gutter and pelvis.

Severity of dengue infection was classified according to the 2009 WHO guidelines [16]. Accordingly, patients who had detectable fluid in the pleural or abdominal cavities by ultrasound scanning, or who had liver transaminases above >1000/IU were grouped as having SD. Those who had dengue with warning signs or without warning signs were classified as having non severe dengue (NSD). Signs of severe dengue were characterized by the presence of cold clammy skin, along with a narrowing of pulse pressure ≤ 20 mmHg were classified as having shock as per WHO 2009 guidelines.

Confirmation of dengue infection and dengue antibody assays

Acute dengue infection was confirmed in the serum samples using the NS1 early dengue ELISA (Panbio, Australia) and by determining viral loads (see below). In order to determine if the patients had a primary or secondary dengue infection, the commercial capture-IgM and IgG enzyme-linked immunosorbent assay (ELISA) (Panbio, Brisbane, Australia) was used. The ELISA was performed and the results were interpreted according to the manufacturers' instructions. This ELISA assay has been validated as both sensitive and specific for primary and secondary dengue virus infections [17, 18].

Determining viral loads in serial blood samples

As we wished to determine the changes in viral loads in patients with SD and non-SD during the course of the illness, RNA was extracted from all serial serum samples using QIAamp Viral RNA Mini Kit (Qiagen, USA) according to the manufacturer's protocol. The RNA was reverse transcribed into cDNA in GeneAmp PCR system 9700 using High Capacity cDNA reverse transcription kit (Applied Biosystems, USA) according to the manufacturer's instructions. Reaction conditions were 10 min at 25 °C, 120 min at 37 °C, 5 min at 85 °C and final hold at 4 °C.

Multiplex quantitative real-time PCR was performed as previously described using the CDC real time PCR assay for detection of the dengue virus [19]. This assay was modified to quantify the DENV apart from quantitative analysis. Oligonucleotide primers and a dual labeled probe for DEN 1,2,3,4 serotypes were used (Life technologies, India) based on published sequences [19]. The probe was dual-labeled with the probe and the QSY quencher. The DENV serotype specific primers were labeled as follows: DENV-1 with JUN, DENV-2 with ABY, DENV-3 with FAM, DENV-4 with VIC. The reactions consisted of 20 μl volumes and contained the following reagents, TaqMan multiplex master mix (containing mustag dye), 900 nM of each primer, 250 nM of each probe, 2 μl of cDNA and nuclease free water (Applied Biosystems, USA). The reaction was performed in an Applied Biosystems7500, 96-well plate detection system. Following initial denaturation for 20 s at 95 °C, the reaction was carried out for 40 cycles of 3 s at 95 °C and 30 s at 60 °C. The threshold cycle value (Ct) for each reaction was determined by manually setting the threshold limit. Viral quantification (PFU/ml) of unknown samples was performed using the standard curve.

Generating standard curves for quantification of the DENV

For generation of standard curves the four DENVs were grown in C6/36 cell lines supplemented with L15 media at 28 ° C. The virus supernatants were harvested at day 7 following infection and were immediately used to infect vero81 cell lines to determine the infective virus particles by plaque assays. The plaque assay was carried out on vero81 monolayer and the virus culture supernatants were serially diluted and inoculated in triplicate. Undiluted sample from the virus culture supernatant was used as the positive control and culture media as the negative control. After 5 days of incubation at 37 °C in 5 % CO2 incubator, the plaques were developed and counted. Virus concentration was calculated as PFU/ml. Following quantification of the viruses, the standard curves were generated as serial dilutions from 10^6 to 10^1 of pfu/ml of each virus serotype. In order to quantify the virus in clinical samples the unknowns were compared to known values in the standard curves of each virus and the viral loads expressed as pfu/ml (Additional file 2: Figure S1).

Assays for determining the liver profile

Assessment of the liver profile was done on all serial blood samples on a daily basis, obtained from the time of recruitment to discharge from hospital. Liver function tests to assess liver cell damage: aspartate transaminase (AST), alanine transaminase (ALT); tests to assess synthetic functions: serum albumin; tests to assess conjugative functions: conjugated and unconjugated bilirubin and tests to assess intrahepatic and hepatobiliary cholestasis: gamma glutamyl transferase (GGT) and alkaline phosphatase (ALP) were done using automated biochemical analyzer (Thermo scientific clinical chemistry analyzer-Indiko, United States).

Quantitative ELISA for detection of cytokines

IL-10 and IL-17 levels were determined in serial serum samples, which were collected daily from the time of admission to discharge, using the human IL-10 enzyme linked immunosorbent assay (ELISA) PRO kit (Mabtech, Sweden) and LEGEND MAX™ Human IL-17A ELISA Kit (BioLegend, USA). The ELISAs were performed and results were interpreted according to the manufacturer's instructions.

Statistical analysis

Statistical analysis was performed using Graph PRISM version 6. Differences in the serial values of liver enzymes, viral loads and cytokine values in patients with NSD and SD were done using multiple unpaired t tests. Corrections for multiple comparisons were done using Holm-Sidak method and the statistical significant value was set at 0.05 (alpha). The association between the extent of liver injury and clinical parameters, viral loads and inflammatory mediators was done using Spearman correlation.

Results

Based on the WHO 2009 guidelines, 33 patients had NSD and 22 had SD. None of the patients developed shock

[16]. Three patients who developed SD had diabetes and one had hypertension while 2 patients with NSD had diabetes and one had hypertension. The clinical features of the 33 patients (mean age 33.60, SD ± 13.26) with NSD and 22 patients with SD (mean age 30.36, SD ± 14.23) are shown in Table 1. Of the 22 patients with SD, 3 of them did not have any evidence of fluid leakage but were classified as having SD as their liver transaminases were elevated >1000/IU. 10 patients with SD were given dextran boluses and 4 of them were given blood transfusions, although none of them developed shock. The haematological and biochemical parameters of these patients are shown in Tables 2 and 3. Although 5 patients with NSD developed bleeding manifestations, these were mild bleeding manifestations and as the patients did not have any evidence of fluid leakage, by ultrasound scanning or by a rise in the haematocrit, they were categorized as having NSD.

Patterns of changes in liver transaminase levels during the course of the illness

As elevation of liver transaminases commonly occurs during dengue infections, we sought to investigate the kinetics of liver transaminases in acute dengue infection and the relationship in the rise in these enzymes with viraemia, onset of fluid leakage and changes in inflammatory mediators. Both AST and ALT levels rose during the course of illness and AST peaked at day 6 of illness, while ALT peaked at day 7. After peaking at day 6 and 7 the AST and ALT levels rapidly declined (Fig. 1a and b). The AST levels were much higher in patients with SD than in those with NSD with the differences most prominent on day 5 ($p = 0.04$) and day 6 ($p = 0.006$) (Fig. 1a). The mean AST levels on day 6 (mean 263.44, SD ± 34.1 IU) were more than two fold when compared to the mean AST values on day 4 (mean 123.4, SD ± 41.8 IU) in patients with SD. The differences in ALT levels in patients with SD and NSD were not prominent (Fig. 1b). AST: ALT ratio has been considered as a better indicator of the type of liver injury than changes in AST or ALT alone [20, 21]. We found that the AST: ALT ratio was >2 in patients with SD and NSD, although the ratios were higher in those with DHF (Fig. 1c). As expected the AST levels positively correlated with other indicators of liver disease such as ALT (Spearmans correlation = 0.61, $p < 0.0001$), GGT (Spearmans correlation = 0.57, $p < 0.0001$), total bilirubin (Spearmans correlation =0.27, $p < 0.0001$) and also with IL-10 (Spearmans correlation = 0.15, $p = 0.04$).

Table 1 Clinical characteristics of patients with SD and NSD

Clinical findings	NSD ($n = 33$)	SD ($n = 22$)
Duration of fever		
3–5 days	25 (75.75 %)	15 (68.18 %)
6–8 days	8 (24.24 %)	6 (27.27 %)
>8 days	0	1 (4.54 %)
Vomiting	9 (27.27 %)	11 (50 %)
Abdominal pain	12 (36.36 %)	16 (72.72 %)
Hepatomegaly	5 (15.15 %)	15 (68.18 %)
Bleeding manifestations	5 (15.15 %)	7 (31.81 %)
Pleural effusion	0	15 (68.18 %)
Ascites	0	19 (86.36 %)
Shock	0	0

Table 2 Haematological changes in patients with SD and NSD

Laboratory features	NSD ($n = 33$)	SD ($n = 22$)
Lowest platelet count		
<20,000 cells/mm^3	1 (3.03 %)	15 (68.18 %)
20,000 to 50,000	12 (36.36 %)	7 (31.81 %)
50,000–100,000	15 (45.45 %)	0
>100,000	15 (45.45 %)	0
Lowest Lymphocyte count		
<750	13 (39.39 %)	12 (54.54 %)
750–1500	19 (57.57 %)	9 (40.90 %)
>1500	1 (3.03 %)	0

Table 3 Biochemical findings in patients with SD and NSD

Biochemical findings	NSD ($n = 33$)	SD ($n = 22$)
AST (IU/L)		
<40	5 (15.15 %)	0
40–160	15 (45.45 %)	6 (27.27 %)
>160	13 (39.39 %)	16 (72.72 %)
ALT (IU/L)		
<40	7 (21.21 %)	3 (13.63 %)
40–160	23 (69.96 %)	11 (50 %)
>160	3 (9.09 %)	8 (36.36 %)
Albumin (g/L)		
<35	18 (54.54 %)	22 (100 %)
≥35	14 (42.42 %)	0
Total protein (g/L)		
<64	21 (63.63 %)	21 (95.45 %)
≥64	12 (36.36 %)	1 (4.54 %)
Alkaline phosphatase (IU/L)		
<128	31 (93.93 %)	18 (81.81 %)
≥128	2 (6.06 %)	4 (18.18 %)
Total bilirubin (μmol/L)		
<20	31 (96.87 %)	21 (95.45 %)
>20	1 (3.12 %)	1 (4.54 %)
Gamma glutamyl transferase (u/L)		
normal value for sex	9 (27.27)	2 (9.09 %)
>normal value for sex (female ≤ 38 and male ≤55)	24 (72.72 %)	20 (90.9 %)

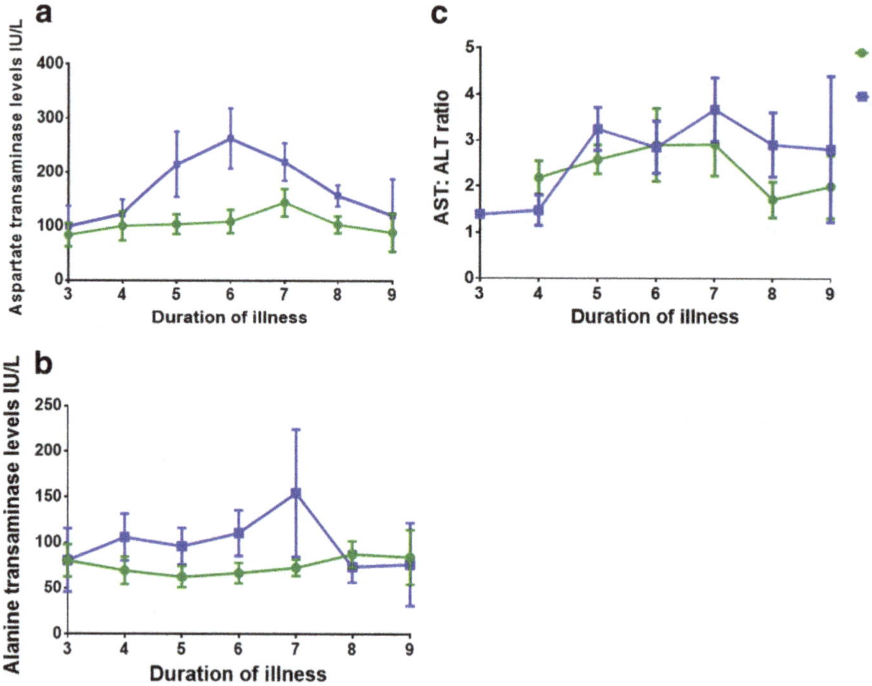

Fig. 1 Changes in serum transaminase levels throughout the course of illness in patients with acute dengue infection. **a**: Changes in serum aspartate transaminase levels (AST) in patients with SD ($n = 22$) and NSD ($n = 33$). The lines indicate the means and standard error of mean (SEM). **b**: Changes in serum alanine transaminase levels (ALT) in patients with SD ($n = 22$) and NSD ($n = 33$). The lines indicate the means and standard error of mean (SEM). **c**: Changes in AST and ALT ratios in patients with SD ($n = 22$) and NSD ($n = 33$). The lines indicate the means and standard error of mean (SEM)

Changes in serum gamma glutamyl transferase (GGT) levels and alkaline phosphatase (ALP) levels

Although GGT is not specific to the liver, it has widely been used as a test to assess the liver profile. High levels are found with cholestasis, excessive alcohol intake, pancreatitis, diabetes and many other conditions [22]. Since it is also known to be elevated in oxidative stress [22], and since oxidative stress is thought to play a role in the pathogenesis of dengue [8, 23], we sought to investigate the changes of GGT in patients with acute dengue. We found that GGT levels were elevated throughout the course of infection in patients with both SD and NSD (Fig. 2a). The levels were significantly higher on day 6 ($p = 0.02$) and day 7 ($p = 0.03$) in patients with SD when compared to those with NSD. Twenty (90.9 %) of the patients with SD (12 males and 8 females) and 24 (72.7 %) of patients with NSD (15 males and 9 females) had elevated GGT levels.

ALP is not a liver specific enzyme and is found in many tissues such as bone, intestine and placenta apart from the liver [24]. ALP is generally elevated in hepatobiliary diseases that result in cholestatis [24]. Although 2 patients with NSD and 4 patients with SD had a mild elevation of ALP levels, all other patients had normal ALP levels throughout the course of illness, which suggests that cholestasis is unlikely to occur in dengue induced liver disease (Fig. 2b).

Changes in bilirubin, serum albumin, plasma leakage and viraemia during the course of acute dengue

Elevation of serum bilirubin occurs due to defects in cholestasis and biliary effects. However, in acute liver disease, it is considered to be a more sensitive marker than ALT in determining the extent of liver injury [25, 26]. However, we found that the total serum bilirubin levels were only marginally high in one patient with SD and one with NSD. These patients also had normal conjugated and unconjugated bilirubin levels, further supporting that cholestatis or biliary stasis, did not significantly occur in dengue associated liver disease.

Low serum albumin levels have been associated with severe dengue and were more frequent among those who had fatal dengue [27, 28]. As expected the serum albumin levels were significantly lower in patients with SD, especially during day 5 ($p = 0.04$), day 6 ($p = 0.06$) and day 7 ($p = 0.04$), while the values were normal in those with NSD (Fig. 3a). Interestingly, the lowest serum albumin levels were seen 2 days before the maximum peak in the fluid leakage (Fig. 3b). It is generally believed that liver dysfunction sometimes leading to acute liver failure is due to reduced hepatic perfusion secondary to prolonged shock [2]. However, it has been known to occur in the absence of shock [4]. Three of the patients in our cohort had severe liver impairment (liver transaminases >1000/IU) in the

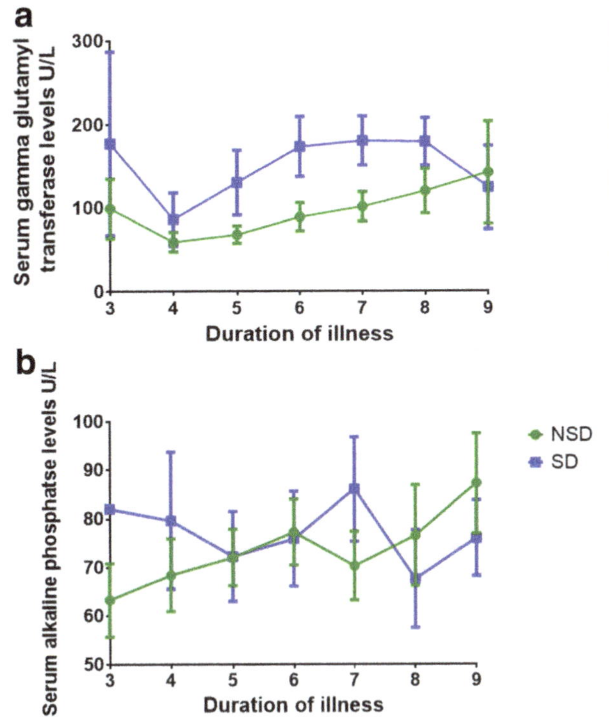

Fig. 2 Changes in serum GGT and ALP levels throughout the course of illness in patients with acute dengue infection. **a**: Changes in serum GGT levels in patients with SD ($n = 22$) and NSD ($n = 33$). The lines indicate the means and standard error of mean (SEM). **b**: Changes in serum ALP levels in patients with SD ($n = 22$) and NSD ($n = 33$). The lines indicate the means and standard error of mean (SEM)

complete absence of any evidence of fluid leakage or a significant rise in the haematocrit. However, in those with SD, the maximum rise in AST and ALT levels occurred the day before the pleural effusions were largest (Fig. 3c). However, the rise in GGT levels mirrored the increase in the pleural effusions.

As studies done on HepG2 cell lines have shown that the DENV directly induced apoptosis of HepG2 cells [29], we proceeded to determine the relationship between the kinetics of viraemia with the changes in the patterns of liver enzymes. We found that the rise in liver transaminases and GGT occurred 24–48 h after the decline in the viraemia (Fig. 3d). Also, there was no association between the extent of viraemia and the extent of the rise in liver transaminases, GGT or a reduction in serum albumin levels. However, the viral loads inversely correlated with the lowest lymphocyte count observed in these patients (Spearman's correlation = −0.6, $p < 0.0001$).

Changes in IL-10 and IL-17 levels and extent of liver involvement

Our previous studies and others have shown that elevated IL-10 is associated with severe dengue [30, 31], and therefore, we sought to investigate the changes in IL-10 levels throughout the clinical disease and its association with liver damage. We found that IL-10 levels were elevated in the early course of the illness with IL-10 values being significantly higher on day 5 of illness in patients with SD ($p = 0.03$), when compared to those with NSD (Fig. 4a). As seen in our previous studies, we found that IL-10 inversely correlated with the lowest lymphocyte counts (Spearman's correlation =0.58, $p < 0.0001$). However, except with being associated with AST levels (Spearman's correlation =0.14, $p = 0.04$), IL-10 did not associate with any other liver enzyme or clinical parameter.

It has been shown in dengue mouse models that both IL-22 and IL-17 are associated with severe clinical disease and in particularly liver injury [13]. Therefore, we determined the kinetics of changes in IL-17 in acute dengue and its association with liver injury. We found that similar to IL-10, IL-17 was significantly elevated during the early phase of dengue infection. IL-17 levels were significantly elevated in patients with SD on day 4 ($p = 0.02$) and day 5 ($p = 0.02$) when compared to those with NSD (Fig. 4b). IL-17 levels correlated with serum IL-10 levels (Spearmans correlation =0.26, $p = 0.0002$), viral loads (Spearmans correlation = 0.26, $p = 0.005$) and ALT (Spearmans correlation =0.16, $p = 0.02$).

Discussion

In this study, we have determined the changes in liver enzymes over the course of acute dengue infection and also the relationship of liver involvement with the degree of viraemia, onset and extent of fluid leakage and levels of cytokines. We found that all patients with SD (but who did not have shock) had some degree of liver involvement, while only 15.1 % of those with NSD did not have any liver involvement.

ALT and AST are considered as indicators of liver cell injury as they are released into the circulation following liver cell injury [25]. Although ALT is also found in low concentrations in skeletal muscle, brain and intestinal tissue, it is predominantly considered to be a liver specific enzyme [25]. In contrast, AST is released following damage to liver, cardiac and skeletal muscle [25]. We found that the rise in AST was more prominent than the rise in ALT levels in patients with SD, which probably suggests that other sources apart from the liver could also be contributing to the rise in serum AST levels. Importantly, the mean AST levels rose more than twofold from day 4 to day 6 of onset of illness, and the three patients whose liver transaminases were >1000/IU, had AST levels around 200–250 IU during day 4 of illness. Therefore, determining liver transaminase levels on day 4 or day 5 (day of admission) alone might very much underestimate the level of liver injury during acute dengue infection.

In this study, we also assessed the changes in GGT, ALP, serum bilirubin and serum albumin levels and none

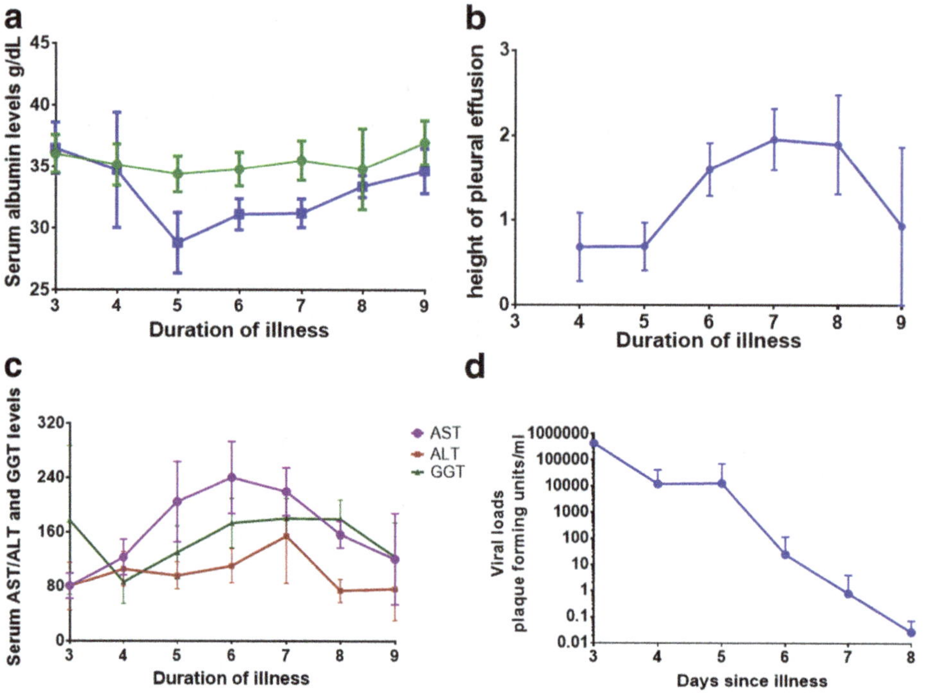

Fig. 3 Association of liver damage with extent of fluid leakage and viraemia. **a**: Changes in serum albumin levels in patients with SD ($n = 22$) and NSD ($n = 33$). The lines indicate the means and standard error of mean (SEM). **b**: Extent of pleural effusion in patients with SD ($n = 15$, as 3 patients with SD did not have any leakage). The values indicate the height of pleural effusion in cm, over the course of illness. **c**: Changes in serum AST, ALT and GGT levels in patients with SD ($n = 22$). **d**: Changes in viral loads in patients with SD ($n = 22$)

of the patients had significant elevations in ALP or serum bilirubin, which suggests that there was minimal cholestasis. Although GGT is also considered to be a marker of cholestasis, it can be elevated due to several other causes including oxidative stress. Oxidative stress has shown to occur in dengue infections, which has been shown to associate with severity of illness [8, 32]. It has been shown that glutathione, which is the main substrate of GGT was reduced in DENV infected cells [33]. Since the GGT levels tend to increase when cellular glutathione levels fall, the increase in GGT levels in dengue could be due to reduction of glutathione levels as a result of oxidative stress [22].

Post mortem studies done in patients who had a fatal outcome have shown that the liver is congested with liver cell necrosis and apoptosis predominantly, in midzonal and centrilobular areas, macrovascular steatosis and councilman bodies, with little inflammation [7, 34, 35]. Centrilobular liver cell necrosis is a typical feature of hypoxic hepatitis, which is the type of liver injury observed in situations of prolonged shock [36]. Although acute liver failure has been reported in many patients with prolonged shock due to dengue [3], acute liver failure has also occurred in the absence of shock [4]. In our cohort of patients with SD, the only 3 patients who had liver transaminases elevated of >1000 IU did not have ultrasound evidence of fluid leakage or any rise in the haematocrit. In addition, 39.4 % of patients with NSD, who did not have any evidence of fluid leakage had more than fourfold rise in their levels of liver transaminases. Therefore, it appears that although hypoxic injury due to reduced hepatic perfusion is probably a cause of liver injury in dengue, other causes such as viral induced liver cell apoptosis and immune mediated damage could also play a role.

Studies done on IL-22 knock out mice have shown that IL-17 plays an important role in the pathogenesis of dengue and also stimulated neutrophil recruitment to the liver, which was found to associate with the severity of liver damage [13]. IL-17 blockade was associated with reduced dengue severity and reduced liver transaminase levels [13]. Although this study shows that IL-17 produced by γδT cells was pathogenic and IL-22 produced by natural killer cells played a protective role, another study in a dengue mouse model showed that early infiltration by NK cells was associated with apoptosis of liver cells [14]. In our cohort of patients, we found that both IL-10 and IL-17 were significantly elevated during early illness, before the patients developed vascular leakage or significant liver injury. Both cytokines were significantly elevated in patients with SD, when compared to NSD, but this difference was not observed after day 5. ALT, which is a liver specific transaminase, was significantly associated with IL-17 levels. Although, our data do not show that IL-17

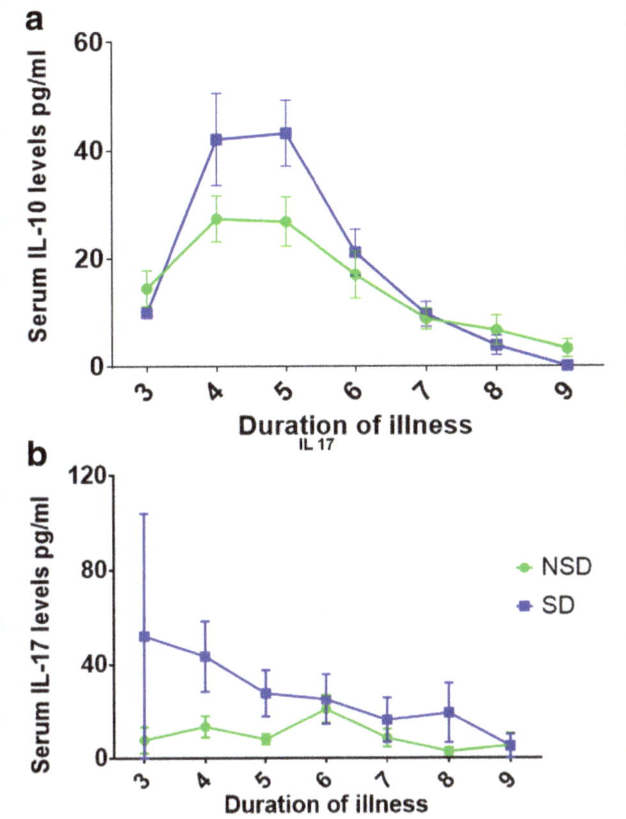

Fig. 4 Changes in cytokine levels throughout the course of illness. **a**: Changes in serum IL-10 levels in patients with SD ($n = 22$) and NSD ($n = 33$). The lines indicate the means and standard error of mean (SEM). **b**: Changes in serum IL-17 levels in patients with SD ($n = 22$) and NSD ($n = 33$). The lines indicate the means and standard error of mean (SEM)

or IL-10, are in fact responsible for the liver injury in dengue, the findings suggest that it would now be important to investigate their role in more detail in acute dengue infection.

Conclusion

In summary, our results show that varying degree of acute liver injury are common in dengue viral infections, but did not associate with the degree of viraemia or the onset or extent of fluid leakage. Since the rise in liver transaminase and GGT levels peaked around day 5–7, assays of liver function tests done around day 4–5 (on admission), may significantly underestimate the degree of liver damage. Since both IL-10 and IL-17 were significantly associated with SD, and high levels were seen very early in the illness, their role in the pathogenesis of dengue and dengue liver injury should be further investigated.

Abbreviations

ALP, alkaline phosphatase; ALT, alanine transaminase; AST, aspartate transaminase; DENV, the dengue virus; GGT, gamma glutamyl transferase; NSD, non severe dengue; PCR, polymerase chain reaction; SD, severe dengue

Funding

Funding was provided by the Centre for Dengue Research, University of Sri Jayewardenepura, Sri Lanka; National Science Foundation (RG/2014/HS/22) and the Medical Research Council, UK and NIHR Biomedical Research Centre Programme.

Authors' contributions

Conceived and designed the experiments: GNM, AW, HP and GSO. Involved in patient recruitment, serial ultra sound scans and sample collection: SF, AW, CTP, SDPM, HD. Performed the experiments: SF, LG, CJ. Contributed reagents/materials/analysis tools: GNM. Wrote the paper: GNM, SF, GSO. All authors read and approved the final manuscript and have given consent to publish.

Competing interests

None.

Consent for publication

Not applicable.

Author details

[1]Department of Microbiology, Centre for Dengue Research, Faculty of Medical Sciences, University of Sri Jayewardenepura, Nugegoda 10250, Sri Lanka. [2]Department of Anatomy, Faculty of Medical Sciences, University of Sri Jayewardenepura, Nugegoda 10250, Sri Lanka. [3]Department of Family Medicine, Faculty of Medical Sciences, University of Sri Jayewardenepura, Nugegoda 10250, Sri Lanka. [4]Department of Biochemistry, Faculty of Medical Sciences, University of Sri Jayewardenepura, Nugegoda 10250, Sri Lanka. [5]Infectious Diseases Hospital, Angoda, Sri Lanka. [6]MRC Human Immunology Unit, Weatherall Institute of Molecular Medicine, Oxford NIHR Biomedical Research Centre and University of Oxford, Oxford OX3 9DS, UK.

References

1. Messina JP, Brady OJ, Pigott DM, Golding N, Kraemer MU, Scott TW, Wint GR, Smith DL, Hay SI. The many projected futures of dengue. Nature Rev. 2015;13(4):230–9.
2. WHO. Comprehensive guidelines for prevention and control of dengue fever and dengue haemorrhagic fever. SEARO, New Delhi, India: World Health Organization; 2011.
3. Malavige GN, Ranatunga PK, Jayaratne SD, Wijesiriwardana B, Seneviratne SL, Karunatilaka DH. Dengue viral infections as a cause of encephalopathy. Indian J Med Microbiol. 2007;25(2):143–5.
4. Trung DT, le Thao TT, Hien TT, Hung NT, Vinh NN, Hien PT, Chinh NT, Simmons C, Wills B. Liver involvement associated with dengue infection in adults in Vietnam. AmJTrop Med Hyg. 2010;83(4):774–80.
5. Jayaratne S, Atukorale V, Gomes L, Chang T, Wijesinghe T, Fernando S, Ogg GS, Malavige GN. Evaluation of the WHO revised criteria for classification of clinical disease severity in acute adult dengue infection. BMC Res Notes. 2012;5:645.
6. Diamond MS, Edgil D, Roberts TG, Lu B, Harris E. Infection of human cells by dengue virus is modulated by different cell types and viral strains. J Virol. 2000;74(17):7814–23.
7. Martina BE, Koraka P, Osterhaus AD. Dengue virus pathogenesis: an integrated view. Clin Microbiol Rev. 2009;22(4):564–81.
8. Gil L, Martinez G, Tapanes R, Castro O, Gonzalez D, Bernardo L, Vazquez S, Kouri G, Guzman MG. Oxidative stress in adult dengue patients. AmJTrop Med Hyg. 2004;71(5):652–7.
9. Cabrera-Hernandez A, Thepparit C, Suksanpaisan L, Smith DR. Dengue virus entry into liver (HepG2) cells is independent of hsp90 and hsp70. J Med Virol. 2007;79(4):386–92.

10. El-Bacha T, Midlej V, da Silva Pereira AP, da Costa Silva L, Benchimol M, Galina A, Da Poian AT. Mitochondrial and bioenergetic dysfunction in human hepatic cells infected with dengue 2 virus. Biochim Biophys Acta. 2007;1772(10):1158–66.
11. Franca RF, Zucoloto S, da Fonseca BA. A BALB/c mouse model shows that liver involvement in dengue disease is immune-mediated. Exp Mol Pathol. 2010;89(3):321–6.
12. Sreekanth GP, Chuncharunee A, Sirimontaporn A, Panaampon J, Srisawat C, Morchang A, Malakar S, Thuwajit P, Kooptiwut S, Suttitheptumrong A. Role of ERK1/2 signaling in dengue virus-induced liver injury. Virus Res. 2014;188:15–26.
13. Guabiraba R, Besnard AG, Marques RE, Maillet I, Fagundes CT, Conceicao TM, Rust NM, Charreau S, Paris I, Lecron JC. IL-22 modulates IL-17A production and controls inflammation and tissue damage in experimental dengue infection. Eur J Immunol. 2013;43(6):1529–44.
14. Sung JM, Lee CK, Wu-Hsieh BA. Intrahepatic infiltrating NK and CD8 T cells cause liver cell death in different phases of dengue virus infection. PLoS One. 2012;7(9):e46292.
15. Ferreira RA, de Oliveira SA, Gandini M, Ferreira LD, Correa G, Abiraude FM, Reid MM, Cruz OG, Kubelka CF. Circulating cytokines and chemokines associated with plasma leakage and hepatic dysfunction in Brazilian children with dengue fever. Acta Trop. 2015;149:138–47. doi:10.1016/j.actatropica.2015.04.023. Epub 2015 May 2.
16. WHO. Dengue guidelines for diagnosis, prevention and control, New edition edn. South East Asian Region of the WHO: Southeast Asian Office of the WHO World Health Organisation; 2009.
17. Vaughn DW, Nisalak A, Solomon T, Kalayanarooj S, Nguyen MD, Kneen R, Cuzzubbo A, Devine PL. Rapid serologic diagnosis of dengue virus infection using a commercial capture ELISA that distinguishes primary and secondary infections. AmJTrop Med Hyg. 1999;60(4):693–8.
18. Sang CT, Cuzzubbo AJ, Devine PL. Evaluation of a commercial capture enzyme-linked immunosorbent assay for detection of immunoglobulin M and G antibodies produced during dengue infection. Clin Diagn Lab Immunol. 1998;5(1):7–10.
19. Santiago GA, Vergne E, Quiles Y, Cosme J, Vazquez J, Medina JF, Medina F, Colon C, Margolis H, Munoz-Jordan JL. Analytical and clinical performance of the CDC real time RT-PCR assay for detection and typing of dengue virus. PLoS Negl Trop Dis. 2013;7(7):e2311.
20. Clark JM. The epidemiology of nonalcoholic fatty liver disease in adults. J Clin Gastroenterol. 2006;40 Suppl 1:S5–10.
21. Fontana RJ, Lok AS. Noninvasive monitoring of patients with chronic hepatitis C. Hepatology. 2002;36(5 Suppl 1):S57–64.
22. Whitfield JB. Gamma glutamyl transferase. Crit Rev Clin Lab Sci. 2001; 38(4):263–355.
23. Olagnier D, Peri S, Steel C, van Montfoort N, Chiang C, Beljanski V, Slifker M, He Z, Nichols CN, Lin R. Cellular oxidative stress response controls the antiviral and apoptotic programs in dengue virus-infected dendritic cells. PLoS Pathog. 2014;10(12):e1004566.
24. Van Hoof VO, De Broe ME. Interpretation and clinical significance of alkaline phosphatase isoenzyme patterns. Crit Rev Clin Lab Sci. 1994;31(3):197–293.
25. Ozer J, Ratner M, Shaw M, Bailey W, Schomaker S. The current state of serum biomarkers of hepatotoxicity. Toxicology. 2008;245(3):194–205.
26. Bauer M, Press AT, Trauner M. The liver in sepsis: patterns of response and injury. Curr Opin Crit Care. 2013;19(2):123–7.
27. Villar-Centeno LA, Diaz-Quijano FA, Martinez-Vega RA. Biochemical alterations as markers of dengue hemorrhagic fever. AmJTrop Med Hyg. 2008;78(3):370–4.
28. Amancio FF, Heringer TP, de Oliveira CC, Fassy LB, de Carvalho FB, Oliveira DP, de Oliveira CD, Botoni FO, Magalhaes Fdo C, Lambertucci JR. Clinical Profiles and Factors Associated with Death in Adults with Dengue Admitted to Intensive Care Units, Minas Gerais, Brazil. PLoS One. 2015;10(6):e0129046.
29. Nagila A, Netsawang J, Suttitheptumrong A, Morchang A, Khunchai S, Srisawat C, Puttikhunt C, Noisakran S, Yenchitsomanus PT, Limjindaporn T. Inhibition of p38MAPK and CD137 signaling reduce dengue virus-induced TNF-alpha secretion and apoptosis. Virol J. 2013;10:105.
30. Malavige GN, Gomes L, Alles L, Chang T, Salimi M, Fernando S, Nanayakkara KD, Jayaratne S, Ogg GS. Serum IL-10 as a marker of severe dengue infection. BMC Infect Dis. 2013;13(1):341.
31. Perez AB, Garcia G, Sierra B, Alvarez M, Vazquez S, Cabrera MV, Rodriguez R, Rosario D, Martinez E, Denny T. IL-10 levels in Dengue patients: some findings from the exceptional epidemiological conditions in Cuba. J Med Virol. 2004;73(2):230–4.
32. Soundravally R, Sankar P, Hoti SL, Selvaraj N, Bobby Z, Sridhar MG. Oxidative stress induced changes in plasma protein can be a predictor of imminent severe dengue infection. Acta Trop. 2008;106(3):156–61.
33. Tian Y, Jiang W, Gao N, Zhang J, Chen W, Fan D, Zhou D, An J. Inhibitory effects of glutathione on dengue virus production. Biochem Biophys Res Commun. 2010;397(3):420–4.
34. Guzman MG, Alvarez M, Rodriguez R, Rosario D, Vazquez S, Vald SL, Cabrera MV, Kouri G. Fatal dengue hemorrhagic fever in Cuba, 1997. Int J Infect Dis. 1999;3(3):130–5.
35. Aye KS, Charngkaew K, Win N, Wai KZ, Moe K, Punyadee N, Thiemmeca S, Suttitheptumrong A, Sukpanichnant S, Prida M. Pathologic highlights of dengue hemorrhagic fever in 13 autopsy cases from Myanmar. Hum Pathol. 2014;45(6):1221–33.
36. Henrion J. Hypoxic hepatitis. Liver Int. 2012;32(7):1039–52.

Increased sensitivity of NS1 ELISA by heat dissociation in acute dengue 4 cases

Sibelle Nogueira Buonora[1*], Flavia Barreto dos Santos[2], Regina Paiva Daumas[3], Sonia Regina Lambert Passos[1], Manoela Heringer da Silva[2], Monique Rocha de Lima[2] and Rita Maria Ribeiro Nogueira[2]

Abstract

Background: Dengue is an acute febrile illness considered the major arboviral disease in terms of morbidity, mortality, economic impact and dissemination worldwide. Brazil accounts for the highest notification rate, with circulation of all four dengue serotypes. The NS1 antigen is a dengue highly conserved specific soluble glycoprotein essential for viral replication and viability that can be detected 0 to 18 days from the onset of fever (peak first 3 days). It induces a strong humoral response and is known as a complement-fixing antigen. Lower NS1 test sensitivity occurs in secondary dengue infections probably due to immune complex formation impairing antigen detection by ELISA.

Methods: We compared the sensitivity of NS1 ELISA in heat dissociated and non-dissociated samples from 156 RT-PCR confirmed acute dengue-4 cases from 362 prospectively enrolled patients.

Results: Secondary infections accounted for 83.3% of cases. NS1 ELISA was positive in 42.5% and indeterminate in 10. 2% of dengue-4 cases. After heat dissociation, 7 negative and 16 indeterminate samples turned positive, increasing the overall test sensitivity to 57.7%.

Conclusions: Although it is time consuming and requires the use of specific laboratory equipment, NS1 ELISA combined with heat dissociation could be a slightly better alternative for triage in suspected dengue cases.

Keywords: NS1 ELISA, Accuracy, Dengue diagnosis, Immune complex dissociation, DENV-4

Background

Dengue is an acute febrile illness considered the major worldwide arboviral disease, in terms of morbidity, mortality, economic impact and dissemination [1]. Dengue occurs in all non-polar continents [2] and is an important public health concern in tropical and subtropical regions mainly in Asia and Americas [3, 4]. Estimates account for 390 million dengue infections per year of which 96 million present clinical manifestations [5]. The disease is endemic in 100 countries and approximately 40% of the world population is at risk of dengue infection [1]. By the end of the 20th century, Brazil became the country with the highest notification rate, accounting for 98.5% of the American continent's reported cases and the highest fatality rate in the sub region [1]. Since 2008, all four dengue serotypes (DENV-1 to DENV-4) can be found in the country [6].

NS1 Ag is a dengue highly conserved specific soluble glycoprotein essential for viral replication and viability that can be detected in dengue patients from day 1 up to 18 days after fever onset [7] with peak sensitivity in the first 3 days of fever onset [8]. It induces a strong humoral response and is known as a complement-fixing antigen [9].

Previous studies have evaluated the usefulness and the accuracy NS1 tests [10–14]. According to da Costa et al. the main factors influencing the diagnostic accuracy are the type of infection (primary versus secondary), viral serotype, geographical origins of samples, and the timing of sample collection [12].

Low NS1 test sensitivity in secondary dengue infections may be attributed to high levels of IgG in anamnestic response with immune complex formation impairing antigen detection by ELISA [9, 15]. Some studies have also noticed lower NS1 sensitivity in DENV-4 compared to

* Correspondence: sibellebuonora@gmail.com
National Institute of Infectious Diseases Evandro Chagas, Laboratory of Clinical Epidemiology, Oswaldo Cruz Foundation, Av. Brasil, 4036 sala 201 A – Manguinhos, Rio de Janeiro CEP: 21040-361, Brazil
Full list of author information is available at the end of the article

other serotypes, in both primary and secondary dengue [12, 13]. Furthermore, immune complex dissociation techniques have proven to be important for the early diagnosis of HIV infections and most recently DENV [9, 16]. A study conducted in Rio de Janeiro with DENV-4 cases analyzed acid treatment/neutralization and heat dissociation, with a better performance for the latter [9]. In the present study, we compared the sensitivity of NS1 ELISA in heat dissociated and non-dissociated samples from acute DENV-4 patients.

Methods

This study is part of a prospective cross-sectional pragmatic diagnostic study of clinical and diagnostic algorithms for dengue diagnosis conducted at Rio de Janeiro, Brazil during the 2013 dengue epidemic season (March and April). We used the Standards for Reporting of Diagnostic Accuracy Study (STARD) Guideline [17]. Eligible adult patients who presented to a public outpatient unit (Unidade de Pronto Atendimento-UPA 24H) within 72 h of a febrile illness without an evident source of infection were interviewed and examined by the investigators. At the time the study was carried out there were no evidences that other Flaviviruses, such as Zika were circulating in Rio de Janeiro [18].

Blood samples were collected and sera stored at -70 °C until the tests. The index test (Platelia™ Dengue NS1 Ag-ELISA), specific IgG and confirmatory RT-PCR were all performed at the Flavivirus Regional Reference Laboratory, IOC, FIOCRUZ.

The Platelia™ Dengue NS1 Ag-ELISA (Bio-Rad Laboratories, Marnes-La-Coquette, France) was performed in all samples according to the manufacturer's instructions and described elsewhere, briefly the test is based on a one-step sandwich format microplate enzyme

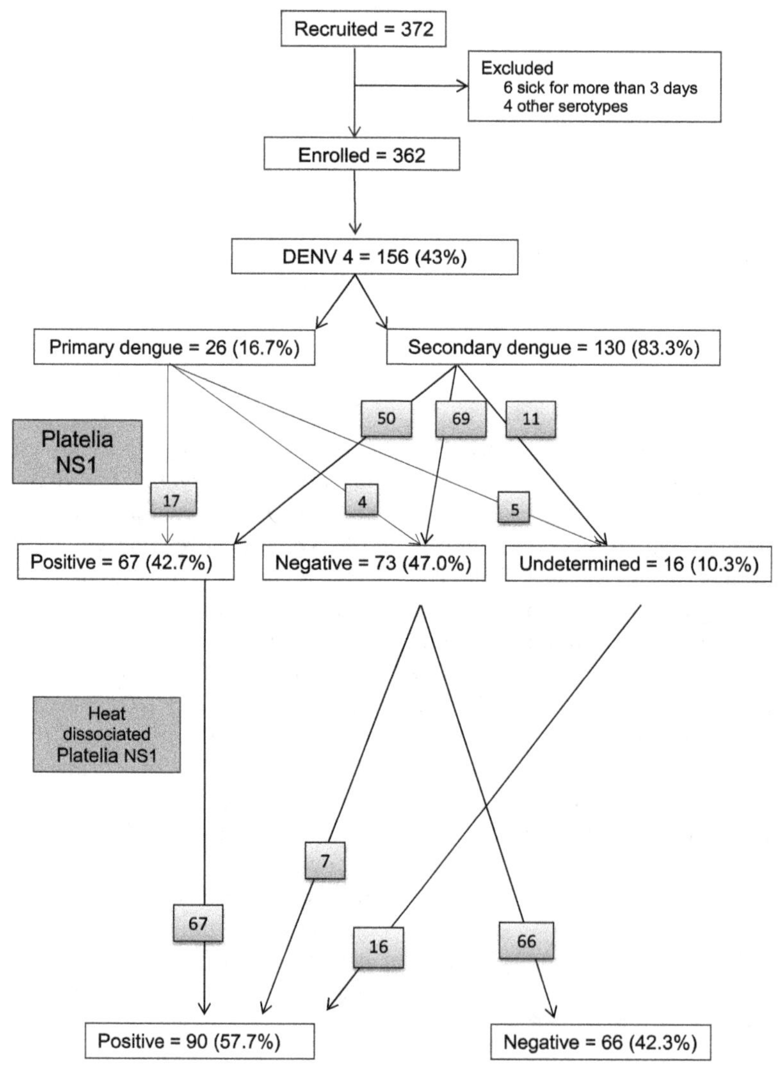

Fig. 1 STARD [17] diagram DENV-4 patients in Rio de Janeiro, 2013

Table 1 DENV-4 NS1 performance according to type of nfection and method, Rio de Janeiro, 2013

Platelia™ Dengue NS1 Ag-ELISA	Results	Type of infection		Total N = 156
		Primary N = 26	Secondary N = 130	
Non-dissociated	Positive	17 (65.4%)	50 (38.4%)	67 (43.0%)
	Negative	4 (15.3%)	69 (53.3%)	73 (46.8%)
	Indeterminate	5 (19.2%)	11 (8.3%)	16 (10.2%)
Heat dissociated	Positive	22 (84.6%)	68 (52.3%)	90 (57.7%)
	Negative	4 (15.4%)	62 (47.7%)	65 (42.3%)

immunoassay to detect DENV NS1 antigen in human serum [10].

The same samples were further submitted to the heat dissociation method when 50 μL of the serum was added to 100 μL of RNA/DNAse free water and heated in a boiling water bath for five minutes, as described previously [9].

We defined as secondary cases those patients who presented positive IgG results within 72 h onset of disease [19]. The Dengue Virus IgG DxSelect™ ELISA (Focus Diagnostics, California, USA) was performed according to the manufacturer's instructions in all samples to diagnose secondary dengue cases.

The viral RNA detection by RT-PCR was performed according to the technique described elsewhere [20]. Laboratory personnel were blinded to other laboratory data such as Platelia™ Dengue NS1 Ag-ELISA, IgG and RT-PCR when executing a specific test. DENV infections by other serotypes were excluded. Exploratory analysis was performed using SPSS© v 17.0 (SPSS Inc., Chicago, Illinois). The MedCalc© 14.8.1 program was used to calculate 95% confidence intervals (CI) for the Platelia™ Dengue NS1 Ag-ELISA sensitivity.

Results

A total of 372 ambulatory patients were enrolled, with 10 exclusions (six presenting symptoms for more than 3 days and four due to infections to other DENV serotypes. The remaining 362 patients had their clinical profile previously described [21]. Briefly, 55.6% were female, the median age was 33 years old (ranging from 18 to 83) and the median time from the onset of illness was two days.

The RT-PCR identified DENV-4 in 42.8% (156/362) of the cases. From those, 16.7% (26/156) were classified as primary infection cases and 83.3% (129/156), as secondary ones, Fig. 1.

The NS1 ELISA performance as described by the manufacturer's protocol in the 156 DENV-4 cases resulted in 43.0% (67/156) of positive cases, 46.8% (73/156) negative and 10.2% (16/156) indeterminate (Table 1). After the heat dissociation process, all 67 DENV-4 positive cases remained positive; 7 negative all 16 indeterminate cases became positive, as also described by Lima et al [9]. These results could jeopardize the theory of IgG immune complex formation; however the increase in sensitivity in those cases might occur due to an increased detection of monomeric NS1 forms [22].

Discussion

In our study, the overall sensitivity of the NS1 test in DENV-4 cases was 47.8%, quite similar to the 46.6% obtained by Lima [9], but lower than the 58% sensitivity obtained in da Costa's meta-analysis [12], Table 2. This low overall sensitivity may be caused by the South American virus polymorphism lower overall viremia and lower NS1 secretion [12, 13]. The differences in the sensitivities in primary and secondary infections in our case before heat dissociation 80.9% vs 42.0% were also found in da Costa's meta-analysis (94.6% vs 66%) [12]. Even attenuating the influence of secondary infections by heat dissociation, the sensitivities obtained were still low.

Table 2 Sensitivity of Platelia™ Dengue NS1 Ag-ELISA in acute DENV-4, Rio de Janeiro, 2013

	Platelia™ Dengue NS1 Ag-ELISA		Sensitivity (95% CI)	*p*-value
Overall sensitivity	Non-dissociated		47.8 (39.3 – 56.4)	$p < 0.001$
	Heat dissociated		57.7 (49.5 – 65.5)	
Type of infection	Primary	Non-dissociated	80.9 (58.1 – 94.6)	$p < 0.001$
		Heat dissociated	84.6 (65.1 – 95.6)	
	Secondary	Non-dissociated	42.0 (33.0 – 51.4)	$p < 0.001$
		Heat dissociated	52.3 (43.3 – 61.1)	

We demonstrated significant sensitivity increases after dissociation in both types of DENV-4 infections in agreement with other studies that used unspecific dengue serotype acid dissociated NS1 samples [15, 23].

This study has advantages since it was prospectively executed, the samples were clinically and laboratorially well characterized, and collected during a single outbreak in one outpatient unit increasing the chance of genotypic similarity, quite different from the previous study which was carried out during a 17 month period when genotypic heterogeneity is possible [9]. We were able to demonstrate the advantages of incorporating heat dissociation to the Platelia™ Dengue NS1 Ag-ELISA kit in order to increase its sensitivity, mostly in settings where circulating DENV-4 can be an issue. The study limitation was the lack of heterogeneity of viral strains that impairs the generalization of the results in other epidemic settings.

Conclusions

Although time expending and the requirement of specific laboratory equipment the NS1 ELISA combined to heat dissociation could be a slightly better alternative for accurate dengue diagnosis.

Abbreviations

CI: Confidence interval; CNPq: Brazilian National Council of Scientific and Technological Development; DENV-1: Dengue virus serotype 1; DENV-4: Dengue virus serotype 4; DNA: Deoxyribonucleic acid; ELISA: Enzyme-linked immunosorbent assay; FIOCRUZ: Oswaldo Cruz Foundation; IgG: Immunoglobulin G; IOC: Instituto Oswaldo Cruz; NS1: Nonstructural protein-1; RNA: Ribonucleic acid; RT-PCR: Reverse transcriptase-polymerase chain reaction.; STARD: Standards for Reporting of Diagnostic Accuracy Study; UPA 24H: Unidade de Pronto Atendimento

Acknowledgements

We wish to acknowledge the assistance of the following: Diana Rodrigues and Fernanda Quintella, graduate students for data collection and analysis. We would also like to thank Cleber do Carmo for statistical assistance.

Funding

This study was funded by the Conselho Nacional de Desenvolvimento Científico e Tecnológico- CNPq through CNPq/PROEP 402068/2012-2 grant and CNPq/REBRATS 401366/2013 grant. SRLP is funded through CNPq 311414/2013-3 grant. The sponsors were not involved in the design, sample collection and handling, analysis, data interpretation or conclusions.

Authors' contributions

SNB, SRLP and RPD conceived of the study, participated in its design and coordination and helped to draft the manuscript. RMRN, MRL, MHS and FBS carried out the immunoassays, rapid immunochromatographic test, viral characterization and writing the manuscript. All authors read and approved the final manuscript.

Competing interests

The authors declare that they have no competing interests.

Author details

[1]National Institute of Infectious Diseases Evandro Chagas, Laboratory of Clinical Epidemiology, Oswaldo Cruz Foundation, Av. Brasil, 4036 sala 201 A – Manguinhos, Rio de Janeiro CEP: 21040-361, Brazil. [2]Oswaldo Cruz Institute, Instituto Oswaldo Cruz – Pavilhão Hélio e Peggy Pereira, Flavivirus Laboratory, Oswaldo Cruz Foundation, Avenida Brasil, 4365, Manguinhos, Rio de Janeiro CEP: 21040-900, Brazil. [3]Germano Sinval Faria Teaching Primary Care Center, National School of Public Health, Oswaldo Cruz Foundation, Rua Leopoldo Bulhões, 1480 - Bonsucesso, Rio de Janeiro CEP: 21041-210, Brazil.

References

1. WHO. Dengue: diagnosis, treatment, prevention and control. Geneva; 2009. http://www.who.int/neglected_diseases/resources/9789241547871/en/. Accessed 15 Jan 2015.
2. Simmons CP, Farrar JJ, Nguyen v V, Wills B. Dengue. N Engl J Med. 2012; 366(15):1423–32.
3. Gubler DJ. The global pandemic of dengue/dengue haemorrhagic fever: current status and prospects for the future. Ann Acad Med Singapore. 1998; 27(2):227–34.
4. Schatzmayr HG. Dengue situation in Brazil by year 2000. Mem Inst Oswaldo Cruz. 2000;95 Suppl 1:179–81.
5. Bhatt S, Gething PW, Brady OJ, Messina JP, Farlow AW, Moyes CL, et al. The global distribution and burden of dengue. Nature. 2013;496(7446):504–7.
6. Messina JP, Brady OJ, Scott TW, Zou C, Pigott DM, Duda KA, et al. Global spread of dengue virus types: mapping the 70 year history. Trends Microbiol. 2014;22(3):138–46.
7. Xu H, Di B, Pan YX, Qiu LW, Wang YD, Hao W, et al. Serotype 1-specific monoclonal antibody-based antigen capture immunoassay for detection of circulating nonstructural protein NS1: Implications for early diagnosis and serotyping of dengue virus infections. J Clin Microbiol. 2006;44(8):2872–8.
8. Duong V, Ly S, Lorn Try P, Tuiskunen A, Ong S, Chroeung N, et al. Clinical and virological factors influencing the performance of a NS1 antigen-capture assay and potential use as a marker of dengue disease severity. PLoS Negl Trop Dis. 2011;5(7), e1244.
9. Lima MR, Nogueira RM, Filippis AM, Nunes PC, Sousa CS, Silva MH, et al. A simple heat dissociation method increases significantly the ELISA detection sensitivity of the nonstructural-1 glycoprotein in patients infected with DENV type-4. J Virol Methods. 2014;204:105–8.
10. Lima MR, Nogueira RM, Schatzmayr HG, dos Santos FB. Comparison of three commercially available dengue NS1 antigen capture assays for acute diagnosis of dengue in Brazil. PLoS Negl Trop Dis. 2010;4(7), e738.
11. Lima MR, Nogueira RM, de Filippis AM B, dos Santos FB. Comparison of two generations of the Panbio dengue NS1 capture enzyme-linked immunosorbent assay. Clin Vaccine Immunol. 2011;18(6):1031–3.
12. da Costa VG, Marques-Silva AC, Moreli ML. A meta-analysis of the diagnostic accuracy of two commercial NS1 antigen ELISA tests for early dengue virus detection. PLoS One. 2014;9(4), e94655.
13. Pal S, Dauner AL, Mitra I, Forshey BM, Garcia P, Morrison AC, et al. Evaluation of dengue NS1 antigen rapid tests and ELISA kits using clinical samples. PLoS One. 2014;9(11), e113411.
14. Sea VR, Cruz AC, Gurgel RQ, Nunes BT, Silva EV, Dolabella SS, et al. Underreporting of Dengue-4 in Brazil due to low sensitivity of the NS1 Ag test in routine control programs. PLoS One. 2013;8(5), e64056.
15. Koraka P, Burghoorn-Maas CP, Falconar A, Setiati TE, Djamiatun K, Groen J, et al. Detection of immune-complex-dissociated nonstructural-1 antigen in patients with acute dengue virus infections. J Clin Microbiol. 2003;41(9):4154–9.
16. Schüpbach J, Böni J. Quantitative and sensitive detection of immune-complexed and free HIV antigen after boiling of serum. J Virol Methods. 1993;43(2):247–56.
17. Bossuyt PM, Reitsma JB, Bruns DE, Gatsonis CA, Glasziou PP, Irwig LM, et al. Toward complete and accurate reporting of studies of diagnostic accuracy. The STARD initiative. Am J Clin Pathol. 2003;119(1):18–22.
18. Brasil P, Calvet GA, Siqueira AM, Wakimoto M, de Sequeira PC, Nobre A, et al. Zika Virus Outbreak in Rio de Janeiro, Brazil: Clinical Characterization, Epidemiological and Virological Aspects. PLoS Negl Trop Dis. 2016;10(4), e0004636.
19. Lima MRQ, Nogueira RM, Santos FB. Dengue diagnosis: commercially available kits and laboratory support. In: Clinical insights: dengue: transmission, diagnosis & surveillance. 1st ed. London: Future Medicine Ltd; 2014. p. 27–47.

20. Lanciotti RS, Calisher CH, Gubler DJ, Chang GJ, Vorndam AV. Rapid detection and typing of dengue viruses from clinical samples by using reverse transcriptase-polymerase chain reaction. J Clin Microbiol. 1992; 30(3):545–51.
21. Buonora SN, Passos SR, do Carmo CN, Quintela FM, de Oliveira DN, dos Santos FB, et al. Accuracy of clinical criteria and an immunochromatographic strip test for dengue diagnosis in a DENV-4 epidemic. BMC Infect Dis. 2016;16(1):37.
22. Falconar AK, Young PR. Immunoaffinity purification of native dimer forms of the flavivirus non-structural glycoprotein, NS1. J Virol Methods. 1990;30(3):323–32.
23. Lapphra K, Sangcharaswichai A, Chokephaibulkit K, Tiengrim S, Piriyakarnsakul W, Chakorn T, et al. Evaluation of an NS1 antigen detection for diagnosis of acute dengue infection in patients with acute febrile illness. Diagn Microbiol Infect Dis. 2008;60(4):387–91.

8

Role of *Aedes aegypti* (Linnaeus) and *Aedes albopictus* (Skuse) in local dengue epidemics in Taiwan

Pui-Jen Tsai[1*] and Hwa-Jen Teng[2]

Abstract

Background: *Aedes* mosquitoes in Taiwan mainly comprise *Aedes albopictus* and *Ae. aegypti*. However, the species contributing to autochthonous dengue spread and the extent at which it occurs remain unclear. Thus, in this study, we spatially analyzed real data to determine spatial features related to local dengue incidence and mosquito density, particularly that of *Ae. albopictus* and *Ae. aegypti*.

Methods: We used bivariate Moran's I statistic and geographically weighted regression (GWR) spatial methods to analyze the globally spatial dependence and locally regressed relationship between (1) imported dengue incidences and Breteau indices (BIs) of *Ae. albopictus*, (2) imported dengue incidences and BI of *Ae. aegypti*, (3) autochthonous dengue incidences and BI of *Ae. albopictus*, (4) autochthonous dengue incidences and BI of *Ae. aegypti*, (5) all dengue incidences and BI of *Ae. albopictus*, (6) all dengue incidences and BI of *Ae. aegypti*, (7) BI of *Ae. albopictus* and human population density, and (8) BI of *Ae. aegypti* and human population density in 348 townships in Taiwan.

Results: In the GWR models, regression coefficients of spatially regressed relationships between the incidence of autochthonous dengue and vector density of *Ae. aegypti* were significant and positive in most townships in Taiwan. However, *Ae. albopictus* had significant but negative regression coefficients in clusters of dengue epidemics. In the global bivariate Moran's index, spatial dependence between the incidence of autochthonous dengue and vector density of *Ae. aegypti* was significant and exhibited positive correlation in Taiwan (bivariate Moran's index = 0.51). However, *Ae. albopictus* exhibited positively significant but low correlation (bivariate Moran's index = 0.06). Similar results were observed in the two spatial methods between all dengue incidences and *Aedes* mosquitoes (*Ae. aegypti* and *Ae. albopictus*).
The regression coefficients of spatially regressed relationships between imported dengue cases and *Aedes* mosquitoes (*Ae. aegypti* and *Ae. albopictus*) were significant in 348 townships in Taiwan. The results indicated that local *Aedes* mosquitoes do not contribute to the dengue incidence of imported cases.
The density of *Ae. aegypti* positively correlated with the density of human population. By contrast, the density of *Ae. albopictus* negatively correlated with the density of human population in the areas of southern Taiwan. The results indicated that *Ae. aegypti* has more opportunities for human–mosquito contact in dengue endemic areas in southern Taiwan.

Conclusions: *Ae. aegypti*, but not *Ae. albopictus*, and human population density in southern Taiwan are closely associated with an increased risk of autochthonous dengue incidence.

Keywords: Dengue fever, *Aedes* mosquitoes, Breteau index, Global bivariate Moran's I, Geographically weighted regression

* Correspondence: puijentsai@gmail.com
[1]Center for General Education, Aletheia University, New Taipei City 25103, Taiwan, ROC
Full list of author information is available at the end of the article

Background

Dengue fever (DF) is a serious mosquito-borne viral infectious disease, mostly distributed in tropical regions [1]. DF epidemics were first recognized nearly simultaneously in Asia, Africa, and North America in the 1780s [2]. Later, DF epidemics were mostly reported in Southeast Asia, particularly after the end of World War II [3]. DF epidemics became more frequent and extended to Latin America in the early 1980s [4]. Dengue virus (DENV), with a nearly ubiquitous distribution in tropical regions, was more recently introduced in Europe [5]. In DENV circulation areas, 3.97 billion people are estimated to have a risk of dengue infections [6]. Moreover, approximately 50 million clinical cases annually occur in more than 100 countries worldwide [7]. Of these, 2.5 % of dengue cases become more severe and progress into dengue hemorrhagic fever (DHF) and/or dengue shock syndrome (DSS). These severe forms of the disease are responsible for high morbidity and fatal outcomes. Approximately 5 % of patients with DHF or DSS are estimated to die, predominantly children younger than 15 years old [8]. However, in recent years, severe dengue cases have tended to increase among adults in some areas [9]. DENV is the etiological agent of DF, DHF, and DSS. A sylvatic cycle that serves as an enzootic cycle involving monkeys and jungle mosquitoes may be present [10]. A study reported that the currently circulating DENV-1 may have resulted from a spillover of ancestral sylvatic strains [11]. DENV is one of the 70 members of the genus Flavivirus of the family Flaviviridae, which consists of four closely related but genetically distinct antigenic serotypes, namely DENV-1, -2, -3, and -4, originally classified based on their serological characteristics [12]. Each DENV serotype elicits neutralizing antibodies in infected humans, resulting in lifelong immunity against the corresponding virus serotype [3]. DENV can infect various tissues in mosquito vectors, particularly the midgut and salivary glands [13].

The mosquitoes *Aedes aegypti* and *Ae. albopictus* [14] are vectors of several globally critical arboviruses including DENV [15], yellow fever virus [16], chikungunya virus [17], and Zika viruses [18]. *Ae. aegypti* originated in Africa, where its ancestral form was a zoophilic tree-hole mosquito named *Ae. aegypti formosus* [19]. The domestic form of *Ae. aegypti* is genetically distinct with discrete geographic niches [20]. It has been hypothesized that harsh conditions coupled with the onset of the slave trade resulted in the introduction of *Ae. aegypti* into the new world from Africa, from where it subsequently spread into tropical and subtropical regions of the world [19]. *Ae. albopictus*, originally a zoophilic forest species from Asia [21], spread to islands in the Indian and Pacific Oceans [22]. During the 1980s, *Ae. albopictus* rapidly expanded into Europe, the United States, Brazil, and Central Africa [23–25].

Taiwan is geographically located in a region that spans both tropical and subtropical climates (22–25°N and 120–122°E). Although both *Ae. aegypti* and *Ae. albopictus* are prevalent in Taiwan, they have different distributions [26, 27]. *Ae. albopictus* is extensively distributed at elevations of less than 1500 m throughout the island, whereas *Ae. aegypti* appears only in the south below the Tropic of Cancer (i.e., 23.5°N). The Taiwan Centers for Disease Control (CDC) reported similar results based on surveys of the dengue vector *Ae. aegypti* conducted in Taiwan during 1988–1996 and 2003–2004 [27]. However, the reason behind the absence of *Ae. aegypti* in northern Taiwan remains unclear. This absence may be attributable to the sensitivity of *Ae. aegypti* to lower winter temperatures in the north, resulting in their limited distribution in Taiwan [28]. The same observations were reported in the temperate and subtropical regions of Argentina (e.g., the city of Resistencia, Chaco). The mortality rate of *Ae. aegypti* eggs due to lower winter temperatures was 48.6 % [29]. DF is a travel-related disease in Taiwan because travelers can carry DENV from endemic areas into the island [30–33]. After the transport of this virus into the island, it is passed on to *Aedes* mosquitoes, which can cause an outbreak of DF. Historical epidemics of dengue in Taiwan were documented in 1902, 1915, and 1922 in Penghu Islet (i.e., Penghu County); 1924 and 1927 in southern Taiwan; 1931 in Tainan; and 1942–1943, island-wide [34]. A reason for these epidemics was the high prevalence of water storage tanks among households during wartime and the entry of dengue patients from epidemic or endemic countries into Southeast Asia. The virus was silent for almost 37 years until 1981, when the DEN-2 DF epidemic occurred on the islet of Hsiao-LiuChiu (i.e., Liouciou Township), which is located off southern Taiwan [35]. However, it did not cause an epidemic in mainland Taiwan. A DENV-1 epidemic occurred in 1987–1988 in southern Taiwan. In 1987–2002, the epidemic patterns of dengue in Taiwan cycled with small-scale outbreaks occurring nearly every 3 years and large-scale epidemics occurring nearly every 10 years [36]. However, since 2002, the Taiwan CDC have recorded nine outbreaks with more than 1000 cases of DF and/or DHF/DSS in 2002, 2006, 2007, 2009, 2010, 2011, 2012, 2014, and 2015, respectively [37]. With a few exceptions, these outbreaks occurred in the south of Taiwan where *Ae. aegypti* is prevalent and coexists with *Ae. albopictus*. The relationship between vectors and autochthonous dengue incidence in terms of geographical correlation has not yet been quantitatively assessed. Therefore, the role of *Aedes* mosquitoes (i.e., *Ae. aegypti* and *Ae. albopictus*) in local dengue epidemics has largely been neglected in spatial research. Therefore, this study investigated the role of *Aedes* mosquitoes in the occurrence of autochthonous dengue and the effects of human population density on the distribution of *Aedes* mosquitoes in Taiwan.

Methods

Surveillance of *Aedes* mosquitoes in the main island of Taiwan

The mosquito data set used in this study was a part of national routine entomological surveillance of dengue and the original data collected in a 3-year project of Taiwan CDC through 2009-2011 [27]. In brief, a sample of 100 mosquito larvae was collected from each of the 7,019 subtownships (i.e., villages or communities; the smallest administrative units in this study) in the main island of Taiwan between 2009 and 2011. In the villages, the mosquito larvae sampling frequency ranged from 1 to 130 over the 3 years, and the mean sampling frequency was 23. All samples were sent to the CDC for laboratory analysis. All mosquito classification data from the 7,019 villages were categorized into 365 townships. In this study, we focused on the main island of Taiwan for detecting spatial contiguity and pattern consistency. Thus, we excluded townships belonging to outlying islands and investigated a total of 348 townships (Wutai Township, which is located in a remote mountainous area, was the only township on the main island of Taiwan that was not investigated; Fig. 1). The incidence rates of *Ae. albopictus* in each township were calculated using the number of confirmed *Ae. albopictus* larvae as a numerator and a total of confirmed *Aedes* larvae as a denominator. The incidence rates of *Ae. aegypti* were calculated using the same formula.

The Breteau index (BI) is defined as the number of positive containers per 100 houses inspected [38]. We used averaged BI values to represent the dengue vector density in a given area. BI data for the period between 2009 and 2011 were obtained from the CDC. A total of 115,690 BI records for the villages were archived into 348 townships and were used for calculating the average BI. For each township, the BI of *Ae. albopictus* was calculated by multiplying the incidence rate of *Ae. albopictus* with the average BI, and the BI of *Ae. aegypti* was calculated using the same formula.

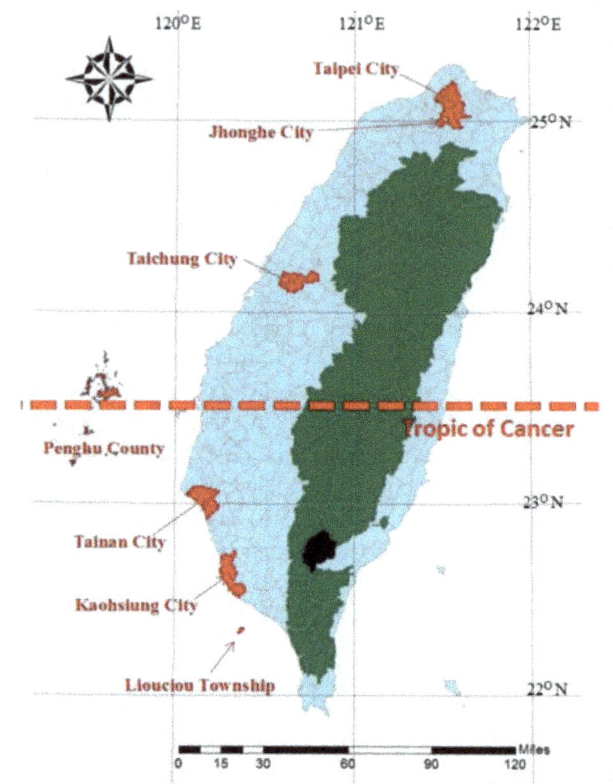

Fig. 1 Map of townships in the study area throughout the main island of Taiwan and excluded studied areas of Penghu County and Liouciou Township. A total of 348 studied areas consisted of 294 townships on plain regions (blue and red boxes) and 54 aboriginal townships in mountainous regions (green box), except Wutai Township (black box)

Data collection for confirmed dengue cases

The data of confirmed imported and autochthonous DF cases were obtained from the Taiwan National Infectious Disease Statistics System of the CDC [37]. Because DF is a notifiable disease, blood samples from patients with suspected DF symptoms are collected and sent to the CDC for laboratory confirmation. Patients who had any of the following condition will be considered to have DENV infection: (i) positive virus isolation; (ii) positive result of real-time polymerase chain reaction; (iii) positive result of higher titers of dengue-specific IgM and IgG antibody in which cross-reaction to Japanese encephalitis had been excluded; or (iv) positive seroconversion or 4-fold rise in dengue-specific IgM or IgG antibody in the convalescent phase and positive result in the NS1 antigen test [32, 39].

Data were obtained for the period between 2009 and 2011. According to the definition of the CDC, epidemiological questions regarding the travel history, incubation period, and first day of illness of patients confirmed as having DF were used to identify the possible origin of dengue infection. Laboratory-confirmed dengue cases with a travel history to endemic countries within 14 days before the date of dengue onset were defined as "dengue cases imported to Taiwan" [39]. The remaining confirmed dengue cases were defined as autochthonous cases. Ethical approval for this study was not required because we used public domain data. We evaluated 348 townships on the main island of Taiwan. The demographic data used in this study were obtained from the

Ministry of the Interior [40]. Between 2009 and 2011, the incidence rate of imported and autochthonous dengue cases and the average ratio of all confirmed dengue cases were calculated for each township [37]. The incidence rate was calculated as the number of confirmed dengue cases divided by the total human population in that township.

Global Moran's I Statistic

Global Moran's spatial autocorrelation was used to assess the correlation among neighboring observations and to identify patterns and levels of spatial clustering in neighboring districts [41]. Moran's statistic [42], similar to the Pearson correlation coefficient, was calculated using the following formula:

$$I = \frac{N}{S_O}\sum_i\sum_j w_{ij}\frac{(x_i-\overline{x})(x_j-\overline{x})}{\sum_i(x_i-\overline{x})^2} \quad (1)$$

where N is the number of districts, w_{ij} is the element in the spatial weight matrix corresponding to the observation pair i and j, and x_i and x_j observations for the areas i and j, *respectively,* with the mean $\overline{x}$, and

$$S_O = \sum_i\sum_j w_{ij}. \quad (2)$$

Because weights were row standardized ($\Sigma w_{ij} = 1$), the first step in the spatial autocorrelation analysis was to construct a spatial weight matrix that contained information on the neighborhood structure for each location. Adjacency was defined as immediately neighboring administrative districts, including the district itself. Non-neighboring administrative districts were assigned a weight of zero. Spatial contiguity for polygons was defined as the property of sharing a common boundary or vertex. Contiguity analysis is a crucial method for assessing unusual features in connectivity distribution [43]. Queen's contiguity can be used to compensate for spatial contiguity by incorporating both the Rook and Bishop relationships into a single measure [44]. The administrative districts considered in this study were highly irregular in both shape and size. The first-order queen polygon contiguity method was the most appropriate for quantifying the spatial weights matrix for the analysis of connectivity. On the basis of this approach, spatial weight or connectivity matrices were determined and used in conjunction with the global Moran's calculations described further.

Moran's I values may range from −1 (dispersed) to +1 (clustered). A Moran's I value of 0 suggests complete spatial randomness. A random permutation procedure recalculates a statistic many times by reshuffling data values among map units to generate a reference distribution. The obtained calculated statistic, based on the observed spatial pattern, is then compared to the reference distribution, and a pseudo significance level (pseudo p value) is computed. To verify that the Moran's I value significantly differed from the expected value, we used a Monte Carlo randomization test with 9,999 permutations to obtain significant values. The data values were reassigned among the N locations, providing a randomized distribution against which the observed value could be judged. If the observed I value was within the tails of this distribution, a significant spatial autocorrelation was present in the data and a pseudo p value was smaller than 0.05; thus, the assumption of independence among the observations could be rejected [45].

Global bivariate Moran's I statistic

The global bivariate Moran's I statistic quantifies the spatial dependency between the two variables X_l and X_k in a same location i [46]. This yields a counterpart of a univariate Moran-like spatial autocorrelation, defined as follows:

$$I_{kl} = \frac{Z_k W Z_l}{n} \quad (3)$$

Where n is the number of observations, $z_k = [x_k-\overline{x}_k]/\sigma_k$ and $z_l = [x_l-\overline{x}_l]/\sigma_l$, which have been standardized such that the mean is zero and standard deviation equals one. W is the row-standardized spatial weight matrix. The weight matrix defines the neighbor set for each observation with non-zero elements for neighbors and zero for the others. The significance of this bivariate spatial correlation can be typically assessed using a randomization (or permutation) approach.

In this case, observed values for one of the variables are randomly reallocated to locations (centroids of townships), and the statistic is recomputed for each such random pattern. The resulting empirical reference distribution can aid in evaluating how extreme the observed statistic is relative to its distribution under spatial randomness to produce a Moran's I scatter plot. The Moran's I scatter plot visualizes a spatial autocorrelation statistic as the slope of the regression line with the spatial lag (a weighted average of the value of a variable in the neighboring locations) on the vertical axis and the original variable on the horizontal axis [46].

The same analysis is true for the bivariate Moran's I scatter plot. The slope of the linear regression through this scatter plot equals the statistic in equ. (3), yielding an interpretation of the spatial lag because inverse distance neighboring values will be used for the spatial weight matrix.

Because the Z variables are standardized, the sum of squares used in the denominator of equ. (3) is constant and is equivalent to n, irrespective of whether Z_k or Z_l is used. Therefore, the focus is on the linear association of a variable Z_k at a location i (Z_{ki}) with the corresponding spatial lag of the other variable $[W_{zl}]_i$. This concept was derived from bivariate spatial correlation and therefore centers on the extent to which values of the variable Z_k observed at a given location k exhibit a systematic association with another variable Z_l observed at the neighboring location *i* [47].

Global bivariate Moran's I values may range from −1 to +1. A Moran's I value of −1, 0, and 1 indicates perfect negative spatial dependence between variables, no correlation between variables, and perfect positive spatial dependence between variables, respectively. A random permutation procedure recalculates a statistic numerous times by reshuffling data values among map units to generate a reference distribution. The obtained calculated statistic based on the observed spatial pattern was then compared to this reference distribution, and a pseudo significance level (pseudo *p* value) was computed. To verify that the Moran's I value significantly differed from the expected value, we applied a Monte Carlo randomization test with 9,999 permutations to obtain significant values. Data values were reassigned among the N locations, providing a randomized distribution against which the observed value may be judged. If the observed Moran's I value was within the tails of this distribution, significant spatial dependence was present in the data, and if there the pseudo *p* value was less than 0.05, then the assumption of independence among the observations could be rejected. Global Moran's I statistic and Global bivariate Moran's I statistic were calculated using GeoDa 1.4.6 [48].

Geographically weighted regression

Geographically weighted regression (GWR) is a type of a local statistic that can produce a set of local parameter estimates demonstrating the variation of a relationship over space and then enable examination of the spatial pattern of the local estimates to gain some understanding of possible hidden causes for the pattern. GWR provides a local model of the variable or process by fitting a regression equation to every feature in the dataset. GWR constructs these separate equations by incorporating the response and explanatory variables of features falling within the bandwidth of each target feature. The shape and size of the bandwidth is dependent on the user input for the kernel type, bandwidth method, distance, and number of neighbor parameters [49].

GWR [49, 50] extends the traditional regression framework (such as the ordinary least squares model; OLS) by enabling local, rather than global, parameters to be estimated so that the model is rewritten as follows:

$$y_i = \beta_o(u_i, v_i) + \sum_j \beta_j(u_i, v_i)x_{ij} + \varepsilon_i \tag{4}$$

where y_i is the response variable, u_i and v_i are the coordinates for each location *i*, β_0 (u_i, v_i) is the intercept for location *i*, β_j (u_i, v_i) is the continuous function β_j (*u*, *v*) at location *i*, x_{ij} is the ith observation of attribute x at location *j*, and ε_i is the error term for location *i*.

The weight assigned to each observation is based on a distance-decay function centered on observation *i*.

The estimator for the GWR model is similar to the weighted least squares global model, except that the weights are conditioned on location *u* relative to the observations in the dataset and thus change for each location. The estimator is expressed as follows:

$$\hat{\beta}(u) = \left(X^T W(u) X\right)^{-1} X^T W(u) y \tag{5}$$

W(*u*) is a square matrix of weights relative to the position *u*. A particular location can be indexed (u_j,v_j) in the study area. *XTW*(*u*)*X* is the geographically weighted variance-covariance matrix, and *y* is the vector of the response variable value.

The *W*(*u*) matrix contains the geographical weights in its leading diagonal and zero in its off-diagonal elements.

$$\begin{bmatrix} w_1(u) & 0 & 0 & 0 \\ 0 & w_2(u) & 0 & 0 \\ 0 & 0 & \cdots & 0 \\ 0 & 0 & 0 & w_n(u) \end{bmatrix} \tag{6}$$

The distance-decay function, which may take various forms, is modified by a bandwidth setting at a distance at which the weight rapidly approaches zero. In the area in which the present study was conducted, the sample points raised from the polygon centroids were not regularly placed, but were clustered. A convenient way of implementing the adaptive bandwidth specification is to select a kernel that allows the same number of sample points for estimations.

The weight can be calculated using the fixed spatial kernel and the value set for any observation with a distance exceeding the bandwidth to zero. The bi-square function can be expressed as follows:

$$w_{ij} = \left(1 - \left({}^{d_{ij}}/_{h}\right)^2\right)^2 \tag{7}$$

where w_{ij} is a continuous function of d_{ij}, d_{ij} is the distance from the location *i* to *j*, w_{ij} is zero when $d_{ij} > h$ (*h* represents a quantity known as the bandwidth). This is a near-Gaussian function with the useful property of the weight being zero at a finite distance.

When the values for a particular explanatory variable cluster spatially, problems with local multicollinearity

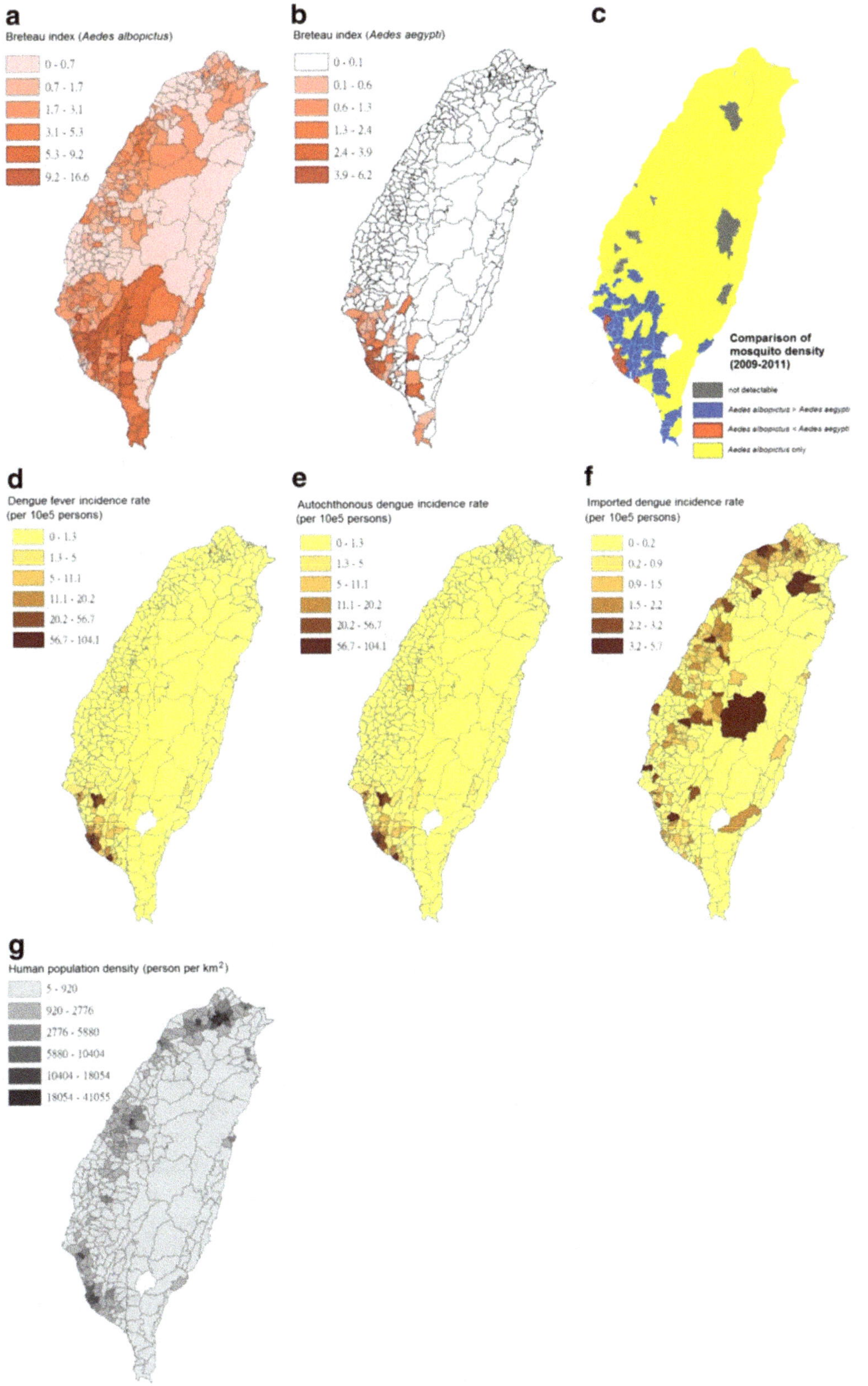

Fig. 2 (See legend on next page.)

(See figure on previous page.)
Fig. 2 Maps of dengue fever incidence, *Aedes* mosquito density, and human population density in 348 townships in Taiwan during 2009–2011. **a** Breteau index (BI) of *Ae. albopictus* during 2009–2011. **b** BI of *Ae. aegypti* during 2009–2011. **c** Comparison between *Ae. albopictus* and *Ae. aegypti* density. **d** Incidence rates of all dengue fever (DF) cases during 2009–2011. **e** Incidence rates of autochthonous DF cases during 2009–2011. **f** Incidence rates of imported DF cases during 2009–2011. **g** Human population density during 2009–2011

likely occur. The condition number in the output feature class indicates when results are unstable due to local multicollinearity. In general, results of features having a condition number of >30 should be interpreted with caution. Problems with local collinearity can prevent both the Akaike information criterion (AIC) and cross validation (CV) bandwidth methods from resolving an optimal distance or number of neighbors.

The bandwidth was chosen by minimizing the AIC score, calculated as follows:

$$AIC_c = 2nlog_e(\hat{\sigma}) + nlog_e(2\pi) + n\left\{\frac{\text{n} + \text{tr(S)}}{\text{n-2-yr(S)}}\right\} \quad (8)$$

where n is the sample size, $\hat{\sigma}$ is the estimated standard deviation of the error, and tr(S) is the trace of the hat matrix. The AIC method has the advantage of accounting for variation in the degrees of freedom among models centered on different observations. The optimal bandwidth was determined by minimizing the corrected AIC, as described by Fotheringham et al. [49].

GWR models produce a set of local regression results, including local intercepts, regression coefficients, residuals, R squared, and condition numbers, which can be mapped to show their spatial variability. GWR models were employed and mapped using ArcMap 10.

In a global model, whether regression coefficients significantly differ from zero is typically examined. This can be accomplished using a t test: the t statistics and their associated p values. A coefficient whose estimated value is found to be not significantly different from zero is associated with a variable whose variation does not contribute to the mode. Variables with nonsignificant regression coefficients can be eliminated from the model. The situation with GWR is slightly more complex. If one set of coefficients is associated with each regression point and with one set of standard errors, then potentially hundreds or thousands of tests would be required to determine whether coefficients are locally significant. The assumption behind the tests indicates that five in every hundred tests would be significant if a significance level of 0.05 is used [51].

The Benjamini-Hochberg (B-H) procedure for controlling the false discovery rate (FDR), which consistently modifies the significance level for each test, was suitably used to test the significance of local regression coefficients of GWR [51, 52]. Thissen et al. (2002) reported a rapid and easy method to calculate the FDR of the B-H procedure by using Microsoft Excel [52]. The B-H approach controls the FDR by sequentially comparing the observed p value for each family of multiple test statistics, in order from the largest to the smallest, to a list of computed B-H critical values [pB-H(i)]. The critical value on the list is determined for each test statistic, indexed by i, by linear interpolation between $\alpha/2$ (for the largest observed p value) to $(\alpha/2)/\text{m}$, where m is the family size (for the smallest of the p values). The last value is the Bonferroni critical value; thus, the reason for the gain in power of B-H relative to Bonferroni is clear. In the B-H approach, only the smallest of the m observed p values are compared with the Bonferroni critical value. All other p values are calculated using less stringent criteria [52]. The local regression coefficient is estimated to be significant if the p value is less than the B-H critical value; otherwise, it is deemed nonsignificant. The results of the significant determination of local regression coefficients were mapped using ArcMap 10.

General statistics

We used Yate's correction for chi-square tests [53] to analyze the variation in the incidence pattern (imported and autochthonous cases) among the 9 dengue outbreak years.

Results

Figure 2 presents a map showing the geographical distribution of the BIs of *Ae. albopictus* and *Ae. aegypti* per district; comparison of the density of *Ae. albopictus* and *Ae. aegypti*; incidence rates of DF, autochthonous dengue, and imported dengue cases; and density of human population between 2009 and 2011.

Table 1 lists the results of the global autocorrelation statistics for the variables of BI of *Ae. albopictus*; BI of *Ae. aegypti*; incidence rates of DF, autochthonous dengue, and imported dengue cases; and density of human population. The results of the global Moran's test for all the variables were statistically significant, having a pseudo p value of less than 0.05 and indicating spatial heterogeneity (clustered).

According to the results of the global autocorrelation statistics, all the studied variables indicated spatial heterogeneity, which refers to the uneven distribution of a trait, event, or relationship across a region. The research methods of spatial dependence (e.g., global bivariate Moran's I analysis) and spatial regression (e.g., GWR) were examined to investigate the relationship between

Table 1 Global autocorrelation analysis of the studied variables in Taiwan during 2009–2011

Variable	Moran's index	Z(I)	Pseudo *p* value	Description
Aedes albopictus (Breteau Index)	0.5718	17.46	0.0001	Clustered
Aedes aegypti (Breteau Index)	0.5818	18.03	0.0001	Clustered
dengue fever incidence rate	0.5587	17.75	0.0001	Clustered
autochthonous dengue incidence rate	0.5587	17.65	0.0001	Clustered
imported dengue incidence rate	0.1475	4.499	0.0002	Clustered
human population density	0.6623	20.54	0.0001	Clustered

Z(I) a value greater than 1.96 is considered statistically significant

the variables of *Aedes* mosquitoes and dengue incidences as well as between human population density and *Aedes* mosquitoes, which were implemented using eight types of combinations (Table 2). Global bivariate Moran's I analysis was used to indicate variations in spatial distribution of data patterns and in cases where the correlation of two variables was investigated. The results of global bivariate Moran's I analysis are listed in Table 2, with significance values based on a permutation approach and a corresponding p value of <0.05. Figure 3 depicts the corresponding global bivariate Moran's I scatter plot. The slopes of the regression line in eight scatter plots equaled to Moran's I indicator in Table 2 and differed from zero, indicating significant spatial correlation among the studied variables.

Condition numbers indicate when results are unstable because of local multicollinearity and the sensitivity of a linear equation solution to small changes in matrix coefficients. The condition number included in the GWR output indicates when local collinearity is a problem. A condition number of >30 is not reliable. In this study, condition numbers were calculated using the GWR analysis, as presented in Figs. 4f, 5f, 6f, 7f, 8f, 9f, 10f and 11f. The values ranged from 1 to 7.5. All the outcomes of fitting the GWR models were reliable.

The maps in Fig. 4 are presented as local intercepts, local regression coefficients, significant B-H FDR values, local residuals, local R^2 values, and condition number values, in which the imported incidence of DF fits the GWR models with the explanatory variable of the BI of *Ae. albopictus* during 2009–2011. As presented in Fig. 4, regression coefficients of the incidence rate of *Ae. albopictus* were not significant in all study areas (local $R^2 < 0.09$). The results indicated that local *Ae. albopictus* did not contribute to imported dengue cases in the main island of Taiwan. We used bivariate Moran's I analysis to examine spatial dependence between the imported incidence of DF and BI of *Ae. albopictus*, and the results were negatively significant and demonstrated low correlation (bivariate Moran's index = −0.07; Table 2 and Fig. 3a).

The maps in Fig. 5 are presented as local intercepts, local regression coefficients, significant B-H FDR values, local residuals, local R^2 values, and condition number values, in which the imported incidence of DF fits the GWR models with the explanatory variable of the BI of *Ae. aegypti* during 2009–2011. As presented in Fig. 5, regression coefficients of the incidence rate of *Ae. aegypti* were not significant in all study areas (local $R^2 < 0.08$). The results indicated that local *Ae. aegypti* did not contribute to imported dengue cases in the main island of Taiwan. We used bivariate Moran's I analysis to examine spatial dependence between the imported incidence of DF and BI of *Ae. aegypti*, and the results exhibited no correlation (bivariate Moran's index = 0.03; Table 2 and Fig. 3b).

The maps in Fig. 6 are presented as local intercepts, local regression coefficients, significant B-H FDR values,

Table 2 Spatial dependence tests between the original variables and spatial lag as the second variables, which were calculated using global bivariate Moran's I analysis in Taiwan during 2009–2011

Original variable	Spatial lag (second variable)	Bivariate Moran's I	Pseudo *p*-value	Spatial dependence
Aedes albopictus (Breteau Index)	Imported dengue incidence rate	−0.07	0.0019	Negative
Aedes aegypti (Breteau Index)	Imported dengue incidence rate	0.03	0.0985	No correlation
Aedes albopictus (Breteau Index)	Autochthonous dengue incidence rate	0.06	0.0122	Positive
Aedes aegypti (Breteau Index)	Autochthonous dengue incidence rate	0.51	0.0001	Positive
Aedes albopictus (Breteau Index)	Dengue fever incidence rate	0.06	0.0139	Positive
Aedes aegypti (Breteau Index)	Dengue fever incidence rate	0.51	0.0001	Positive
Human population density	*Aedes albopictus* (Breteau Index)	−0.12	0.0001	Negative
Human population density	*Aedes aegypti* (Breteau Index)	0.21	0.0001	Positive

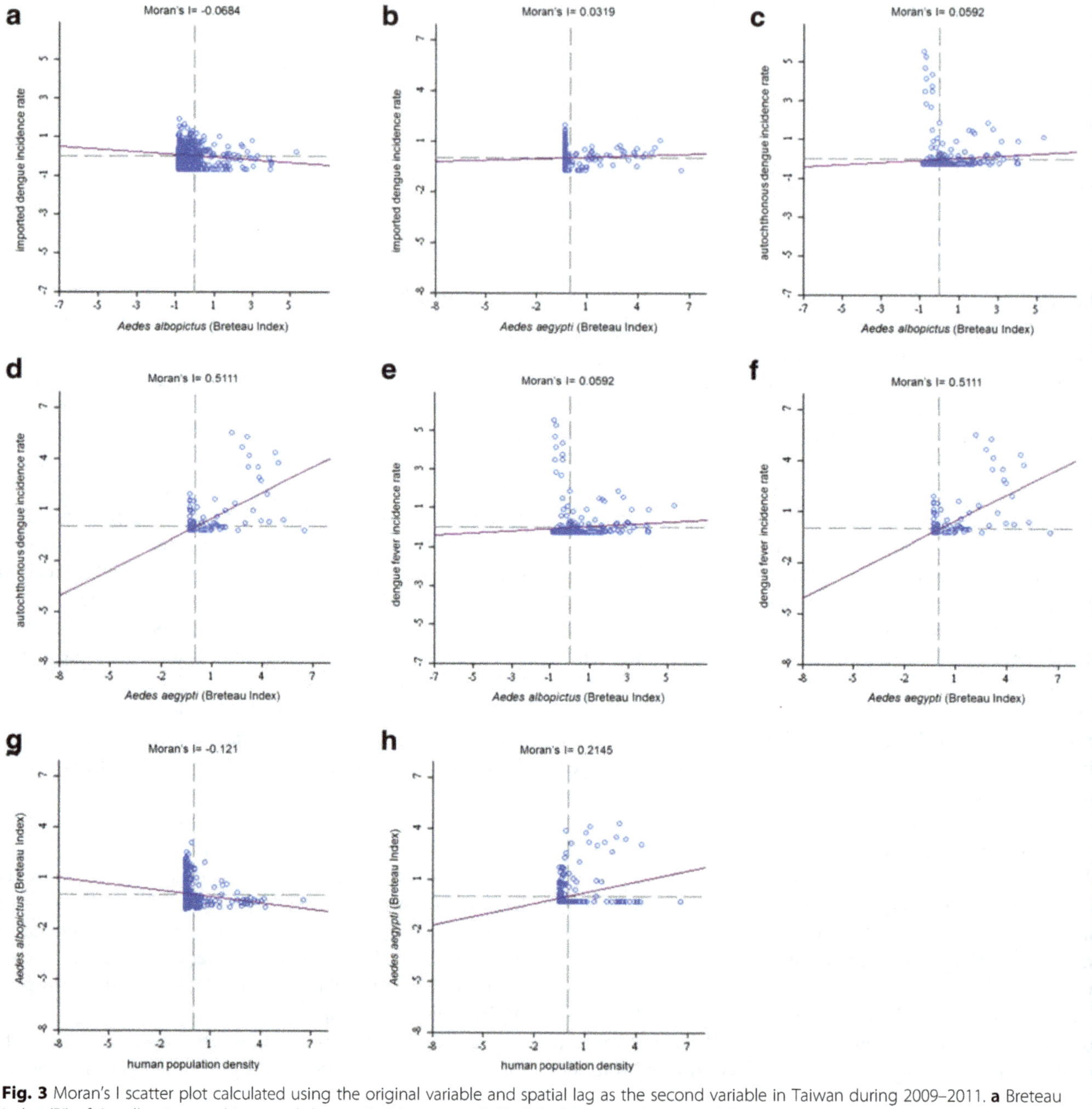

Fig. 3 Moran's I scatter plot calculated using the original variable and spatial lag as the second variable in Taiwan during 2009–2011. **a** Breteau index (BI) of *Ae. albopictus* and imported dengue incidence rate. **b** BI of *Ae. aegypti* and imported dengue incidence rate. **c** BI of *Ae. albopictus* and autochthonous dengue incidence rate. **d** BI of *Ae. aegypti* and autochthonous dengue incidence rate. **e** BI of *Ae. albopictus* and dengue fever incidence rate. **f** BI of *Ae. aegypti* and dengue fever incidence rate. **g** Human population density and BI of *Ae. albopictus*. **h** Human population density and BI of *Ae. aegypti*

local residuals, local R^2 values, and condition number values, in which the autochthonous incidence of DF fits the GWR models with the explanatory variable of the BIs of *Ae. albopictus* during 2009–2011. As presented in Fig. 6, regression coefficients of the incidence rate of *Ae. albopictus* were negatively significant, with clusters covering most areas in the western area of southern Taiwan (local $R^2 < 0.45$). The results indicated that *Ae. albopictus* did not positively contribute to autochthonous dengue cases on the main island of Taiwan. We used bivariate Moran's I analysis to examine spatial dependence between the autochthonous incidence of DF and BI of *Ae. albopictus*, and the results were positively significant but exhibited low correlation (bivariate Moran's index = 0.06; Table 2 and Fig. 3c).

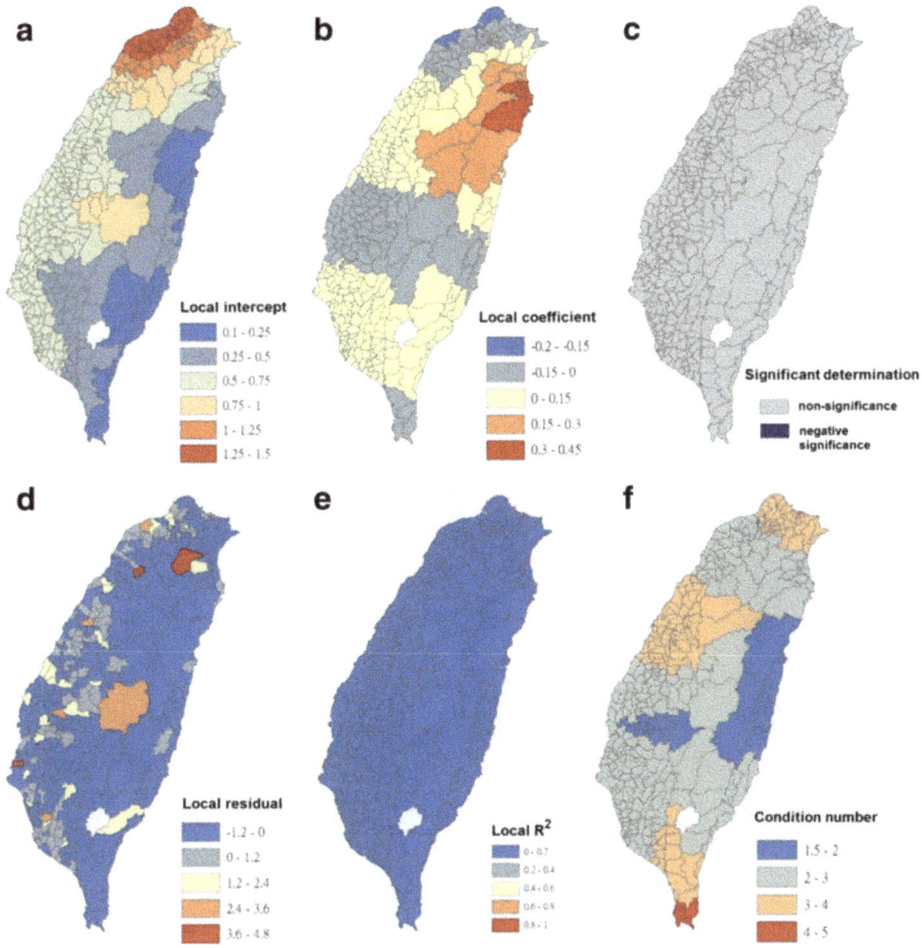

Fig. 4 Results of the GWR model for Breteau indices of *Ae. albopictus* (as the explanatory variable) and imported incidence of dengue fever (as the response variable) in 348 townships in Taiwan during 2009–2011. **a** Local intercepts during 2009–2011. **b** Local regression coefficients during 2009–2011. **c** Significant determination of coefficients according to the Benjamini–Hochberg false discovery rate during 2009–2011. **d** Local residuals during 2009–2011. **e** Local R^2 values during 2009–2011. **f** Local condition number values during 2009–2011

The maps in Fig. 7 are presented as local intercepts, local regression coefficients, significant B-H FDR values, local residuals, local R^2 values, and condition number values, in which the autochthonous incidence of DF fits the GWR models with the explanatory variable of the BIs of *Ae. aegypti* during 2009–2011. As presented in Fig. 7, regression coefficients of the incidence rate of *Ae. aegypti* were positively significant, with clusters covering most areas of Taiwan. A total of 290 townships correlated with local autochthonous dengue incidence (local R^2 < 0.35). The results indicated that autochthonous DF in Taiwan was transmitted by *Ae. aegypti*. Furthermore, the results of bivariate Moran's I analysis revealed that spatial dependence between the autochthonous incidence of DF and BI of *Ae. aegypti* was positively significant (bivariate Moran's index = 0.51; Table 2 and Fig. 3d).

The maps in Fig. 8 are presented as local intercepts, local regression coefficients, significant B-H FDR values, local residuals, local R^2 values, and condition number values, in which the DF incidence fits the GWR models with the explanatory variable of the BI of *Ae. albopictus* during 2009–2011. As presented in Fig. 8, regression coefficients of the incidence rate of *Ae. albopictus* were negatively significant, with clusters covering most areas in the western area of southern Taiwan (local R^2 < 0.45). The results indicated that *Ae. albopictus* did not positively contribute to dengue cases in the main island of Taiwan. We used bivariate Moran's I analysis to examine spatial dependence between the incidence of DF and BI of *Ae. albopictus*, and the results were positively significant but had very low correlation (bivariate Moran's index = 0.06; Table 2 and Fig. 3e).

The maps in Fig. 9 are presented as local intercepts, local regression coefficients, significant B-H FDR values, local residuals, local R^2 values, and condition number values, in which the incidence of DF fits the GWR models with the explanatory variable of the BI of

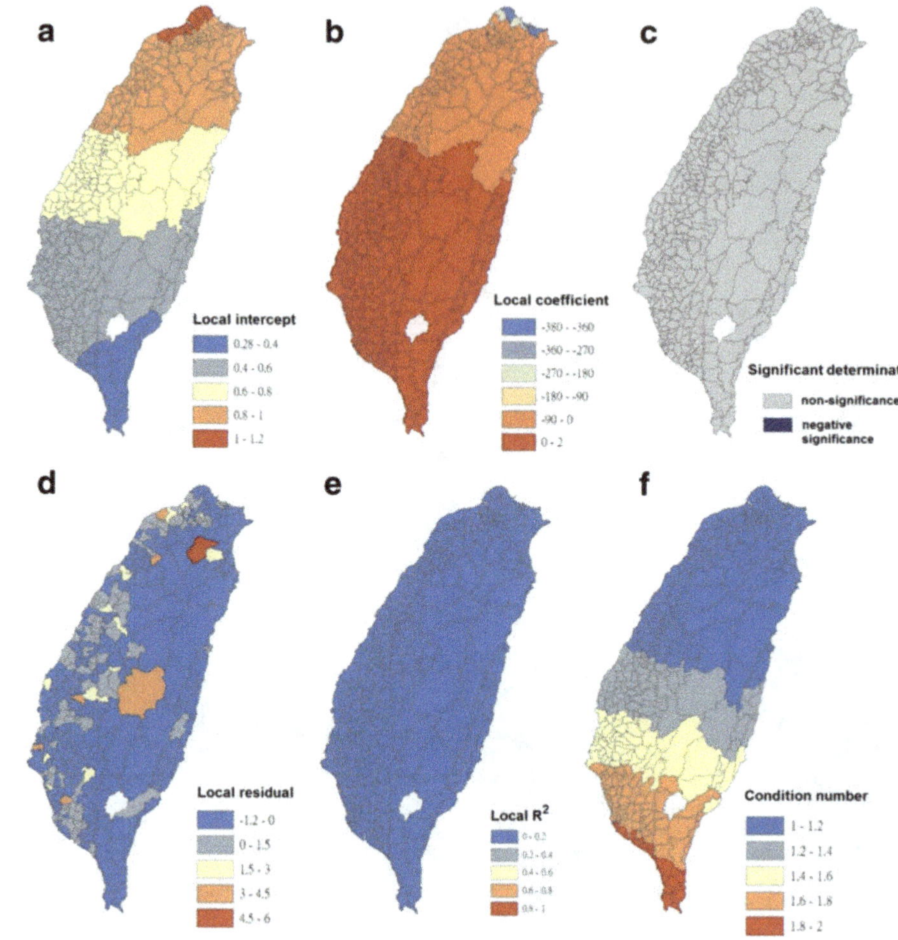

Fig. 5 Results of the GWR model for Breteau indices of *Ae. aegypti* (as the explanatory variable) and the imported incidence of dengue fever (as the response variable) in 348 townships in Taiwan during 2009–2011. **a** Local intercepts during 2009–2011. **a** Local regression coefficients during 2009–2011. **c** Significant determination of coefficients according to the Benjamini-Hochberg false discovery rate during 2009–2011. **d** Local residuals during 2009–2011. **e** Local R^2 values during 2009–2011. **f** Local condition number values during 2009–2011

Ae. aegypti during 2009–2011. As illustrated in Fig. 9, regression coefficients of the incidence rate of *Ae. aegypti* were positively significant, with clusters covering most areas of Taiwan. A total of 290 townships were correlated with DF incidence (local $R^2 < 0.35$). The results indicated that DF incidence in Taiwan was transmitted by *Ae. aegypti*. We used bivariate Moran's I analysis to examine spatial dependence between the incidence of DF and BI of *Ae. aegypti*, and the results were positively significant (bivariate Moran's index = 0.51; Table 2 and Fig. 3f).

The maps in Fig. 10 are presented as local intercepts, local regression coefficients, significant B-H FDR values, local residuals, local R^2 values, and condition number values, in which the BI of *Ae. albopictus* fit the GWR models with the explanatory variable of human population density during 2009–2011. As presented in Fig. 10, regression coefficients of the human population density were negatively significant, with clusters covering most areas of plain and mountainous townships in the south part of Taiwan (local $R^2 < 0.5$). The results indicated that a high density of human population did not positively contribute to the prevalence of *Ae. albopictus*; however, it reduced the mosquito density in the south part of Taiwan. We used bivariate Moran's I analysis to examine spatial dependence between the BI of *Ae. albopictus* and density of human population, and the results were negatively significant (bivariate Moran's index = −0.12; Table 2 and Fig. 3g).

The maps in Fig. 11 are presented as local intercepts, local regression coefficients, significant B-H FDR values, local residuals, local R^2 values, and condition number values, in which the BI of *Ae. aegypti* fits the GWR models with the explanatory variable of the human population density during 2009–2011. As illustrated in Fig. 11, regression coefficients of the human population density were positively significant, with clusters covering most areas of Taiwan's townships in the south of the

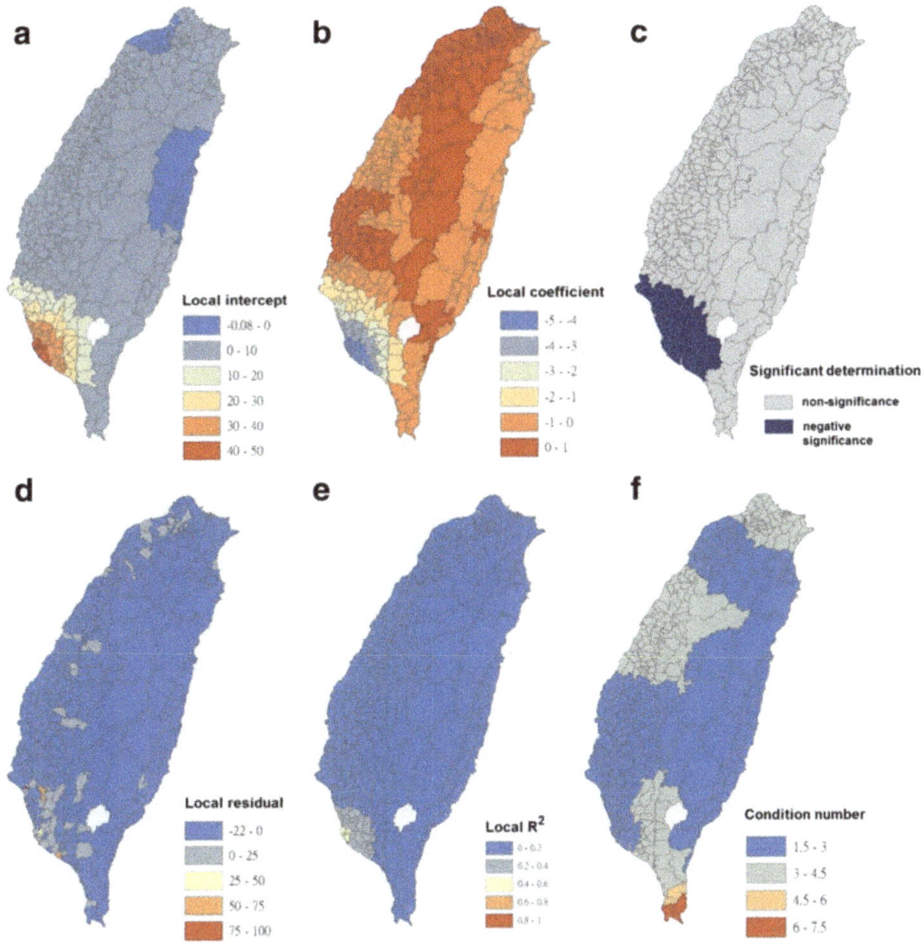

Fig. 6 Results of the GWR model for Breteau indices of *Ae. albopictus* (as the explanatory variable) and autochthonous incidence of dengue fever (as the response variable) in 348 townships in Taiwan during 2009–2011. **a** Local intercepts during 2009–2011. **b** Local regression coefficients during 2009–2011. **c** Significant determination of coefficients according to the Benjamini–Hochberg false discovery rate during 2009–2011. **d** Local residuals during 2009–2011. **e** Local R^2 values during 2009–2011. **f** Local condition number values during 2009–2011

Tropic of Cancer (i.e., 23.5°N; local $R^2 < 0.33$). The results indicated that the human population density contributed to the incidence of *Ae. aegypti* in southern Taiwan. We used bivariate Moran's I analysis to examine spatial dependence between the BI of *Ae. aegypti* and density of human population, and the results were positively significant (bivariate Moran's index = 0.21; Table 2 and Fig. 3h).

We used Yates' chi-square test to examine the patterns of confirmed dengue cases (imported or autochthonous) among 9 dengue outbreak years (i.e., 2002, 2006, 2007, 2009, 2010, 2011, 2012, 2014, and 2015); dengue outbreak years are defined as those having >1000 confirmed dengue cases. The two-sided test had a significance level of 0.05. The results indicated that most of the years had dissimilar incidence patterns. However, few tests did not reject the null hypothesis, and the years with similar incidence patterns were classified into three groups: "2006, 2007, and 2011"; "2010 and 2012"; and "2002 and 2015," as shown in Table 3.

Discussion

Extensive and rapid urbanization without appropriate planning may have directly resulted in large numbers of artificial containers that are suitable for breeding *Aedes* mosquitoes around households. The rapidly developing air transportation has accelerated virus translocation, enabling it to easily migrate from endemic to non-endemic areas [54]. Therefore, the probability of virus introduction through imported cases has considerably increased, even in countries where dengue has never been reported. Moreover, travelers infected with DENV serve as vehicles for its potential transmission [55]. Other environmental factors, such as global warming, have been associated with the occurrence of dengue epidemics [56, 57], causing this disease to be more complicated and thus more difficult to manage. Socioeconomic

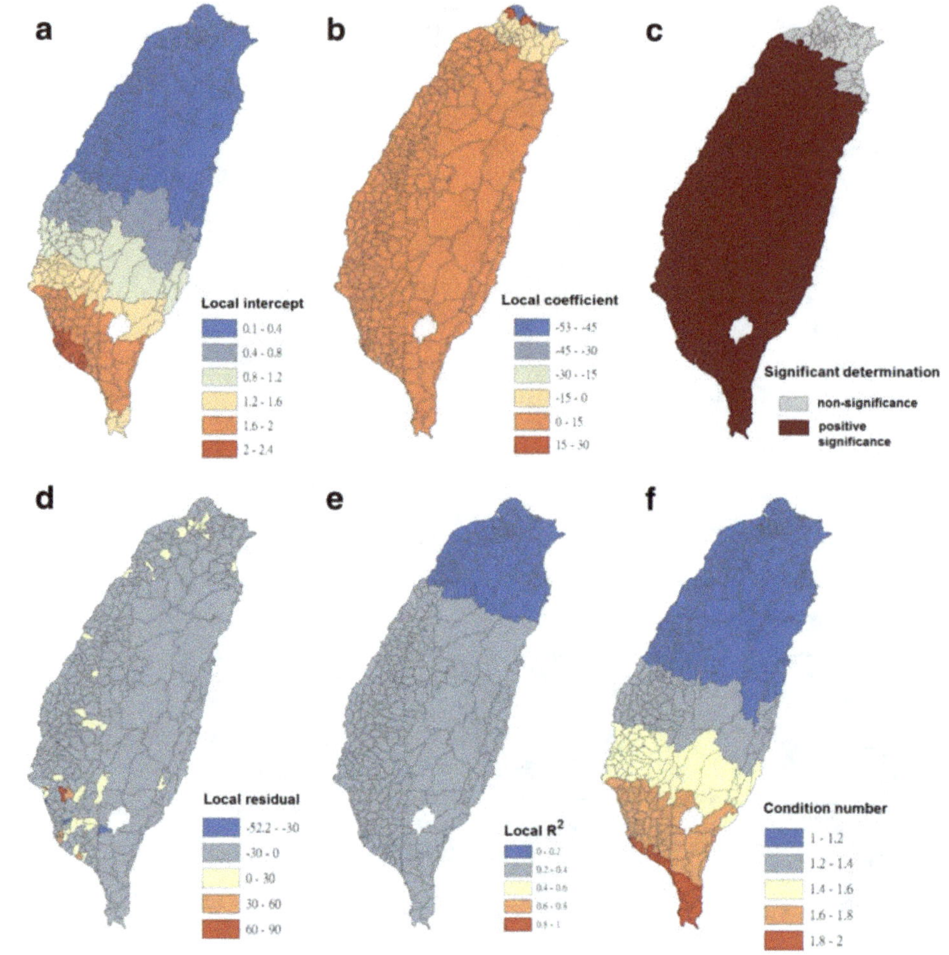

Fig. 7 Results of the GWR model for Breteau indices of *Ae. aegypti* (as the explanatory variable) and autochthonous incidence of dengue fever (as the response variable) in 348 townships in Taiwan during 2009–2011. **a** Local intercepts during 2009–2011. **b** Local regression coefficients during 2009–2011. **c** Significant determination of coefficients according to the Benjamini–Hochberg false discovery rate during 2009–2011. **d** Local residuals during 2009–2011. **e** Local R^2 values during 2009–2011. **f** Local condition number values during 2009–2011

factors affecting the distribution of *Aedes* mosquitoes, other than the use of containers to store water, include air conditioner use, housing quality, and urbanization rate [58, 59]. *Ae. aegypti* and *Ae. albopictus* are found in both urban and rural areas. *Ae. aegypti* tends to breed in urbanized ecological niches, whereas *Ae. albopictus* is more frequently found in rural areas; however, mixed breeding has been reported [60]. In addition, *Ae. aegypti* prefers living indoors, whereas *Ae. albopictus* frequently breeds outdoors [61–63]. Dengue outbreaks have occurred nearly every year in Taiwan since 1987, first appearing in the southern part of Taiwan, which has a high human population density. Dengue outbreaks usually increase during rapid urbanization, and a high human population density has been associated with dengue transmission because of its potential impact on human-mosquito contact [64, 65]. Our study results revealed that the clusters of *Ae. aegypti* were associated with a high density of human population in the southern part of Taiwan, where the risk of dengue outbreaks is high (Figs. 2, 10, and 11). *Ae. aegypti* has more opportunities to increase human-mosquito contact and thus increase the probability of dengue outbreaks. However, the opposite results were observed for *Ae. albopictus*.

Studies on the spatial coexistence of *Ae. aegypti* and *Ae. albopictus* have reported that the two species are sympatric [66, 67]. In North America [68] and Brazil [66], the two species have similar larval ecological niches and often share the same larval habitat. Likewise, in Mayotte, *Ae. albopictus* coexists with *Ae. aegypti* in 40 % of larval habitats [69]. However, as suggested by Paupy et al. [70], the apparent coexistence of the two species could be a transient situation, followed by a reduction [71–73] or displacement [74, 75] of the resident species; interspecific larval competition for resources is the most

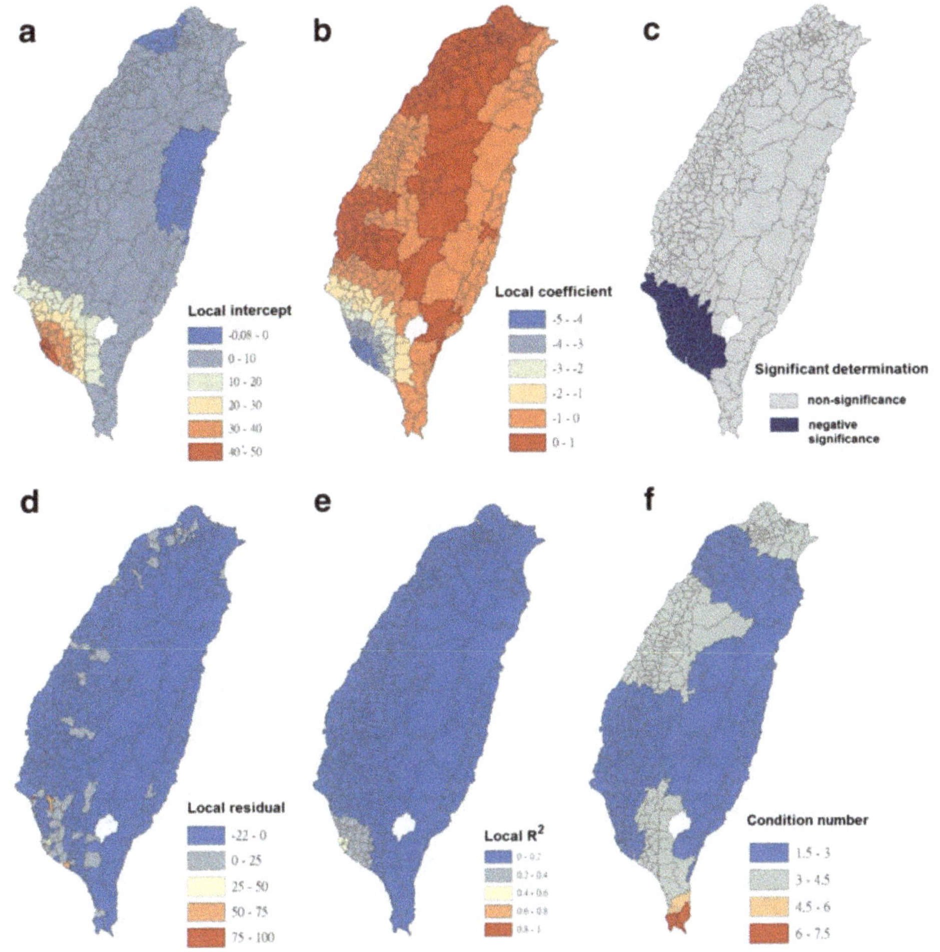

Fig. 8 Results of the GWR model for Breteau indices of *Ae. albopictus* (as the explanatory variable) and dengue fever incidence rates (as the response variable) in 348 townships in Taiwan during 2009–2011. **a** Local intercepts during 2009–2011. **b** Local regression coefficients during 2009–2011. **c** Significant determination of coefficients according to the Benjamini–Hochberg false discovery rate during 2009–2011. **d** Local residuals during 2009–2011. **e** Local R^2 values during 2009–2011. **f** Local condition number values during 2009–2011

ikely reason for this process. Moreover, a few local studies have reported that the local spread of *Ae. albopictus* and decline in *Ae. aegypti* populations might be linked to interspecies competition [68, 76, 77] or non-reciprocal cross-species inseminations [78].

Ae. aegypti almost exclusively feeds on humans in daylight hours and typically rests indoors [79]. By contrast, *Ae. albopictus* is usually exophagic and bites humans and animals opportunistically [70]; however, *Ae. albopictus* has been reported to exhibit strongly anthropophilic behavior similar to that of *Ae. aegypti* in specific contexts [63, 80]. Both species inhabit containers but differ in their behavior and biology; thus, they occupy different niches [81]. Studies have reported that compared with *Ae. aegypti*, which is usually endophagic, *Ae. albopictus* tends to be exophagic and thus prefers to feed on blood indoors [62, 80]. Multiple blood feedings occur frequently in *Ae. albopictus* and *Ae. Aegypti*, which usually becomes engorged after two or three blood meals [80, 82–84]. However, multiple blood feedings in a single gonotrophic cycle are more frequent in *Ae. aegypti* [63, 82, 85]. Such behavioral differences may provide fewer opportunities for *Ae. albopictus* to contact humans infected by DENV. Thus, *Ae. albopictus* has a lower probability of transmitting the virus through the intake of a blood meal [86]. Mosquito behaviors are crucial in determining the occurrence and scale of many arthropod-borne diseases and diseases caused by nematodes, protozoans, and viruses [87].

Both *Ae. albopictus* and *Ae. aegypti* are susceptible to DENV. However, rates of salivary gland infection and transmission are higher in *Ae. aegypti*-fed blood meals than in *Ae. albopictus*-fed blood meals containing DENV, either in mosquitoes from Taiwan or Southeast Asian countries [86, 88]. A study on field-caught mosquitoes conducted in Singapore reported that 6.9 % of

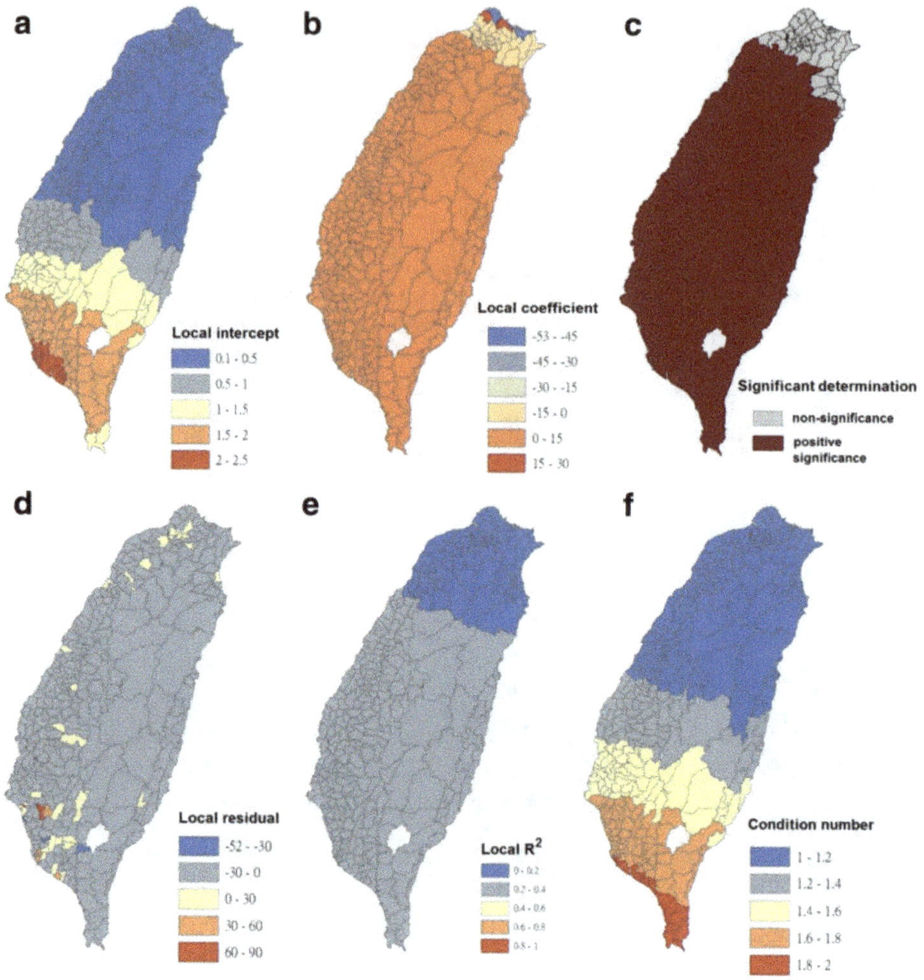

Fig. 9 Results of the GWR model for Breteau indices of *Ae. aegypti* (as the explanatory variable) and dengue fever incidence rates (as the response variable) in 348 townships in Taiwan during 2009–2011. **a** Local intercepts during 2009–2011. **b** Local regression coefficients during 2009–2011. **c** Significant determination of coefficients according to the Benjamini-Hochberg false discovery rate during 2009–2011. **d** Local residuals during 2009–2011. **e** Local R^2 values during 2009–2011. **f** Local condition number values during 2009–2011

Ae. aegypti, but only 2.9 % of *Ae. albopictus* was positive for DENVs [89]. Another study conducted in Singapore reported that infected *Ae. aegypti* were detected as early as six weeks before the start of a dengue outbreak, whereas infected *Ae. albopictus* did not appear until the number of cases was increasing [21]. Furthermore, a study conducted in southern Taiwan demonstrated that DENV was detected in low levels only from 0.2 % positive signs for field-caught *Ae. aegypti*, but not for *Ae. albopictus* [90]. Large outbreaks such as those in 2006 and 2007 occurred one year after the detection of virus-infected *Ae. aegypti* [90]. These results prompt the possibility that *Ae. aegypti* can efficiently establish a preliminary dengue case cluster. Because of frequent subclinical or cryptic infections, dengue outbreaks may be delayed or not reported, resulting in silent transmission [91]. In addition, competition for resources by other intracellular organisms is crucial for mosquitoes to support viral replication [92]. In Taiwan, the endosymbiont Wolbachia has been identified in nearly all *Ae. albopictus* populations; however, it is completely absent from *Ae. aegypti* populations breeding in the field [93]. The artificial introduction of an exogenous strain of Wolbachia, leading to competition for cellular resources, interfered with replication of DENV in *Ae. aegypti*. Wolbachia-mediated pathogen interference may synergistically work with the life-shortening strategy [92]. This suggests that this maternally inherited endosymbiont acts as a factor determining viral infection and its dissemination to other tissues; that is, from the midgut to the salivary glands of the mosquito [94, 95]. In addition, the study results in Malaysia revealed transovarial transmission of dengue virus in the larvae of *Ae. aegypti* and *Ae. albopictus* in the field, with 6.3 % positive results [96]. However, according to a study of virological

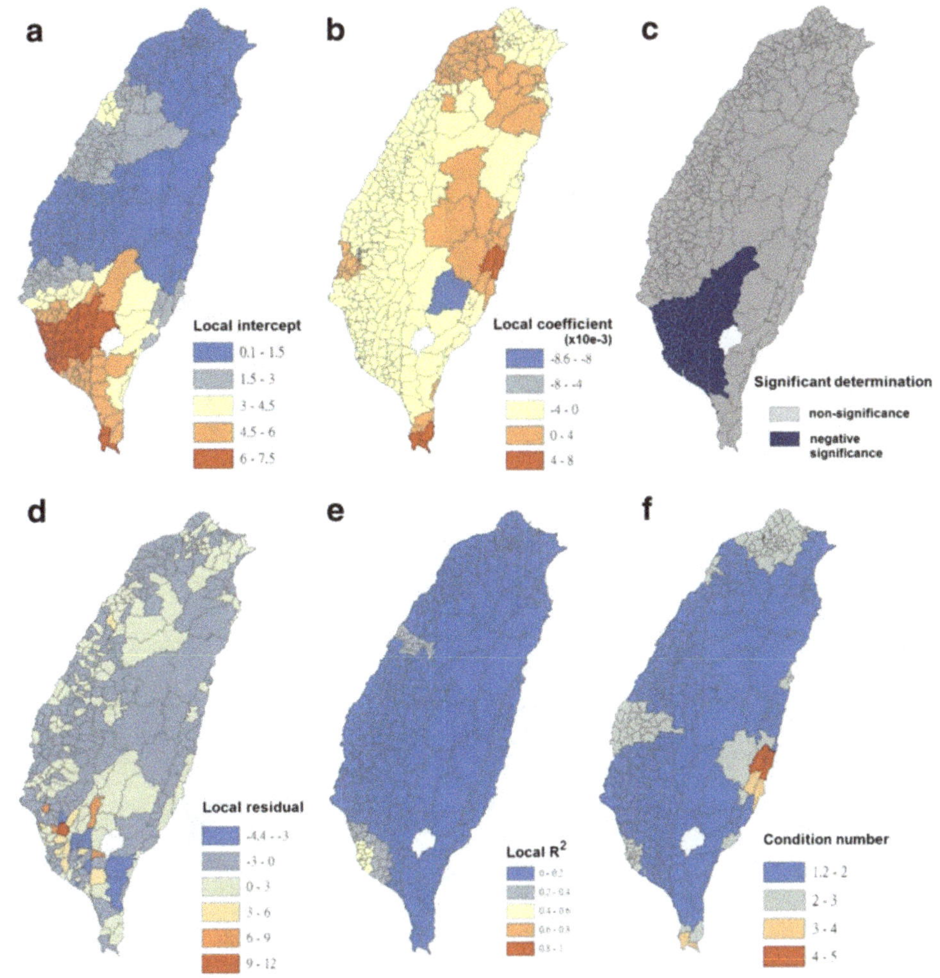

Fig. 10 Results of the GWR model for human population densities (as the explanatory variable) and Breteau indices of *Ae. albopictus* (as the response variable) in 348 townships in Taiwan during 2009–2011. **a** Local intercepts during 2009–2011. **b** Local regression coefficients during 2009–2011. **c** Significant determination of coefficients according to the Benjamini-Hochberg false discovery rate during 2009–2011. **d** Local residuals during 2009–2011. **e** Local R^2 values during 2009–2011. **f** Local condition number values during 2009–2011

surveillance in Taiwan, transovarial transmission in local *Aedes* mosquitos may not occur, or occur at lower rates [90].

Since the epidemic in 1987, few small outbreaks have been reported in north of the Tropic of Cancer, such as those in Chungho (i.e., Jhonghe City) in Taipei County in 1995 (162 cases), Tunghai University in Taichung City in 1995 (8 cases), and Taipei City in 1996 (14 cases); these outbreaks occurred in areas without *Ae. aegypti* [97, 98]. Because *Ae. albopictus* is also susceptible to DENV [86, 99], it may also cause sporadic cases, and occasionally, small outbreaks. In turn, only a few autochthonous cases can occur and thus the scales of outbreaks are limited in northern Taiwan, although more imported cases are reported every year in that area. Despite similarities between *Ae. aegypti* and *Ae. albopictus*, they differ in crucial characteristics, including behaviors and vector competence to the dengue virus. Such differences may cause discrepancies in their roles in dengue outbreaks. Considering the occurrence of DF in past decades in Taiwan, only limited or no outbreaks can be established in which *Ae. aegypti* is absent (northern and central parts of Taiwan where *Ae. albopictus* is prevalent). Yang et al. (2014) [100] hypothesized that the existence of *Ae. aegypti* is a prerequisite for the initiation and establishment of a dengue outbreak, which may be expanded or maintained through participation of *Ae. albopictus*. The outbreak may be terminated when herd immunity in the resident population reaches a level sufficiently high to block the spread of infections. However, this hypothesis is inconsistent with our results presented in Figs. 6 and 7. The clusters in dengue-endemic areas of southern Taiwan were located where the incidence of autochthonous cases was negatively correlated with *Ae. albopictus* and positively correlated with *Ae. aegypti*. Our findings revealed that *Ae. aegypti* in endemic areas

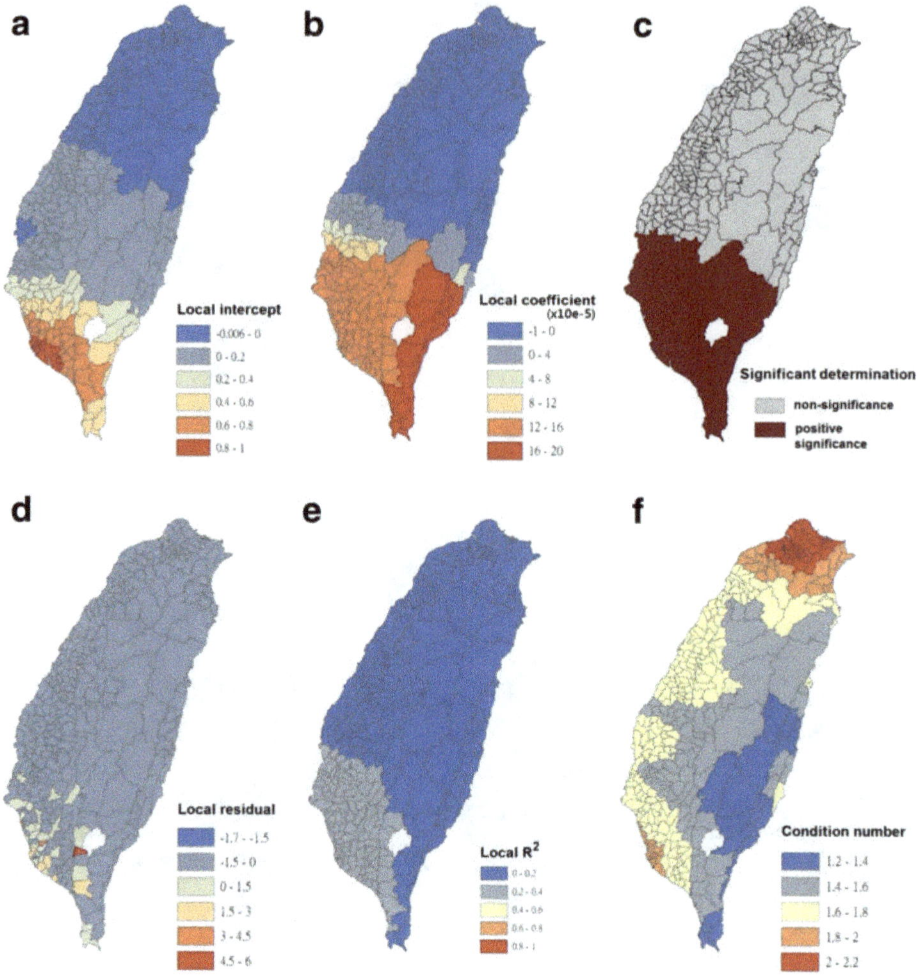

Fig. 11 Results of the GWR model for human population densities (as the explanatory variable) and Breteau indices of *Ae. aegypti* (as the response variable) in 348 townships in Taiwan during 2009–2011. **a** Local intercepts during 2009–2011. **b** Local regression coefficients during 2009–2011. **c** Significant determination of coefficients according to the Benjamini–Hochberg false discovery rate during 2009–2011. **d** Local residuals during 2009–2011. **e** Local R^2 values during 2009–2011. **f** Local condition number values during 2009–2011

Table 3 Yates' chi-square test and matric comparisons of nine dengue outbreak years[a]

Year	2002 (Im/Au)	2006 (Im/Au)	2007 (Im/Au)	2009 (Im/Au)	2010 (Im/Au)	2011 (Im/Au)	2012 (Im/Au)	2014 (Im/Au)	Year	Imported case (Im)	autochthonous case (Au)
									2002	52	5336
2006 (Im/Au)	*307.13								2006	109	965
2007 (Im/Au)	*273.09	3.1							2007	179	2000
2009 (Im/Au)	*778.08	*35.43	*83.76						2009	204	848
2010 (Im/Au)	*681.82	*19.34	*58.58	*5.12					2010	304	1592
2011 (Im/Au)	*305.53	0.55	1.11	*58.12	*36.62				2011	157	1545
2012 (Im/Au)	*539.76	*8.17	*30.67	*12.71	2.5	*17.37			2012	207	1271
2014 (Im/Au)	*8.84	*363.42	*371.93	*1215.21	*1186.02	*405.63	*335.02		2014	240	15492
2015 (Im/Au)	0.84	*861.18	*960.62	*2808.97	*2899.05	*1009.39	*1242.15	*54.38	2015	365	43419

Im imported case, *Au* autochthonous case
Significance (*) is a chi-square value > 3.84 (p value = 0.05)
[a]indicates the number of confirmed dengue > 1000 cases
Data extracted from Taiwan CDC [37]

played a critical role in establishing most scales of dengue outbreaks during 2009–2011. However, *Ae. albopictus* may have a supporting role or cause sporadic cases and occasionally small outbreaks in the absence of *Ae. aegypti.*

Conclusions

Ae. aegypti is a key vector for dengue epidemics in Taiwan. According to the BIs of *Ae. aegypti*, but not of *Ae. albopictus*, high-density clusters of human populations are highly associated with the emergence of dengue epidemics in southern Taiwan. *Ae. albopictus* may have a supporting role during small-scale dengue outbreaks or cause sporadic cases and occasionally small outbreaks in the absence of *Ae. aegypti*. This observation may provide broader considerations for health authorities responsible for dengue prevention, hopefully leading to a more efficient allocation of resources, particularly in the control of mosquito vectors.

Acknowledgments
The authors thank the CDC for providing access to the database on notifiable infectious diseases and related statistics on infectious diseases. The authors also thank the Ministry of the Interior for providing access to the demographic data.

Funding
No funding was obtained for this study.

Authors' contributions
PJ was responsible for the study design, epidemiological enquiry, data collection, statistical calculations, and drafting of the manuscript. HJ assisted with the collection of *Aedes* mosquito data. Both authors read and approved the final manuscript.

Competing interests
The authors declare that they have no competing interests.

Consent for publication
Not applicable.

Author details
[1]Center for General Education, Aletheia University, New Taipei City 25103, Taiwan, ROC. [2]Center for Diagnostics and Vaccine Development, Centers for Disease Control, Taipei, Taiwan, ROC.

References

1. Bhatt S, Gething PW, Brady OJ, Messina JP, Farlow AW, Moyes CL, et al. The global distribution and burden of dengue. Nature. 2013;496(7446):504–7.
2. Armstrong C. Dengue fever. Pub Health Rep. 1923;38:1750–84.
3. Rigau-Pérez JG, Clark GG, Gubler DJ, Reiter P, Sanders EJ, Vorndam AV. Dengue and dengue haemorrhagic fever. Lancet. 1998;352:971–7.
4. Goh KT, Ng SK, Chan YC, Lim SJ, Chua EC. Epidemiological aspects of an outbreak of dengue fever/dengue haemorrhagic fever in Singapore. Southeast Asian J Trop Med Pub Health. 1987;18:291–4.
5. Schaffner F, Mathis A. Dengue and dengue vectors in the WHO European region: past, present, and scenarios for the future. Lancet Infect Dis. 2014; 14(12):1271–80.
6. Brady OJ, Gething PW, Bhatt S, Messina JP, Brownstein JS, Hoen AG, et al. Refining the global spatial limits of dengue virus transmission by evidence-based consensus. PLoS Negl Trop Dis. 2012;6(8):e1760.
7. Simmons CP, Farrar JJ. Nguyen vV, Wills B. Current concept: dengue. N Engl J Med. 2012;366:1423–32.
8. Noisakran S, Perng GC. Alternate hypothesis on the pathogenesis of dengue hemorrhagic fever (DHF)/dengue shock syndrome (DSS) in dengue virus infection. Exp Biol Med (Maywood). 2008;233:401–8.
9. Sam SS, Omar SF, Teoh BT, Abd-Jamil J, AbuBakar S. Review of dengue hemorrhagic fever fatal cases seen among adults: a retrospective study. PLoS Negl Trop Dis. 2013;7(5):e2194.
10. Rudnick A, Marchette NJ, Garcia R. Possible jungle dengue – recent studies and hypotheses. Jpn J Med Sci Biol. 1967;20:69–74.
11. Teoh BT, Sam SS, Abd-Jamil J, AbuBakar S. Isolation of ancestral sylvatic dengue virus type 1, Malaysia. Emerg Infect Dis. 2010;16:1783–85.
12. Calisher CH, Karabatsos N, Dalrymple JM, Shope RE, Porterfield JS, Westaway EG, et al. Antigenic relationships between flaviviruses as determined by cross-neutralization tests with polyclonal antisera. J Gen Virol. 1989;70:37–43.
13 Salazar MI, Richardson JH, Sánchez-Vargas I, Olson KE, Beaty BJ. Dengue virus type 2: replication and tropisms in orally infected *Aedes aegypti* mosquitoes. BMC Microbiol. 2007;7:9.
14 Reinert JF, Harbach RE, Kitching IJ. Phylogeny and classification of tribe Aedini (Diptera: Culicidae). Zool J Linn Soc. 2009. doi:10.1111/j.1096-3642.2009.00570.x.
15 Simmons CP, Farrar JJ, Chau NVV, Wills B. Dengue. N Engl J Med. 2012. doi: 10.1056/NEJMra1110265.
16 Jentes ES, Poumerol G, Gershman MD, Hill DR, Lemarchand J, Lewis RF, et al. The revised global yellow fever risk map and recommendations for vaccination, 2010: consensus of the informal WHO Working Group on Geographic Risk for Yellow Fever. Lancet Infect Dis. 2011;11(8):622–32.
17 Leparc-Goffart I, Nougairede A, Cassadou S, Prat C, de Lamballerie X. Chikungunya in the Americas. Lancet. 2014;383(9916):514.
18 Rodriguez-Morales AJ, Bandeira AC, Franco-Paredes C. The expanding spectrum of modes of transmission of Zika virus: a global concern. Ann Clin Microbiol Antimicrob. 2016;15:13.
19 Brown JE, Evans BR, Zheng W, Obas V, Barrera-Martinez L, Egizi A, et al. Human impacts have shaped historical and recent evolution in *Aedes aegypti*, the dengue and yellow fever mosquito. Evolution. 2014;68(2):514–25.
20 Brown JE, McBride CS, Johnson P, Ritchie S, Paupy C, Bossin H, et al. Worldwide patterns of genetic differentiation imply multiple 'domestications' of *Aedes aegypti*, a major vector of human diseases. Proc Biol Sci. 2011;278(1717):2446–54.
21 Chow VTK, Chan YC, Yong R, Lee KM, Lim LK, Chung YK, et al. Monitoring of dengue viruses in field-caught Aedes aegypti and Aedes albopictus mosquitoes by a type-specific polymerase chain reaction and cycle sequencing. Am J Trop Med Hyg. 1998;58(5):578–86.
22 Delatte AH, Gimonneau G, Triboire A, Fontenille D, Delatte H. Influence of temperature on immature development, survival, longevity, fecundity, and gonotrophic cycles of *Aedes albopictus*, vector of chikungunya and dengue in the Indian Ocean. J Med Entomol. 2009;46(1):33–41.
23 Medlock JM, Hansford KM, Schaffner F, Versteirt V, Hendrickx G, Zeller H, et al. A review of the invasive mosquitoes in Europe: ecology, public health risks, and control options. Vector Borne Zoonotic Dis. 2012;12(6):435–47.
24 Carvalho RG, Lourenc¸o-de-Oliveira R, Braga IA. Updating the geographical distribution and frequency of *Aedes albopictus* in Brazil with remarks regarding its range in the Americas. Mem Inst Oswaldo Cruz. 2014;109(6):787–96.
25 Ngoagouni C, Kamgang B, Nakouné E, Paupy C, Kazanji M. Invasion of *Aedes albopictus* (Diptera: Culicidae) into central Africa: what consequences for emerging diseases? Parasit Vectors. 2015;8:191.
26 Lin TH. Surveillance and control of *Aedes aegypti* in epidemic areas of Taiwan. Kaohsiung J Med Sci. 1994;10(Suppl):S88–93.
27 Lin C, Wang CY, Teng HJ. The study of dengue vector distribution in Taiwan from 2009 to 2011. Taiwan Epidemiol Bull. 2014;30(15):304–10 (in Chinese).
28 Chang LH, Hsu EL, Teng HJ, Ho CM. *Aedes albopictus* (Diptera: Culicidae) larvae exposed to low temperatures in Taiwan. J Med Entomol. 2007;44(2): 205–10.
29 Giménez JO, Fischer S, Zalazar L, Stein M. Cold season mortality under natural conditions and subsequent hatching response of *Aedes (Stegomyia)*

aegypti (Diptera: Culicidae) eggs in a subtropical city of Argentina. J Med Entomol. 2015;52(5):879–85.
30 Lin CC, Huang YH, Shu PY, Wu HS, Lin YS, Yeh TM, et al. Characteristic of dengue disease in Taiwan: 2002–2007. Am J Trop Med Hyg. 2010;82(4):731–9.
31 Shu PY, Su CL, Liao TL, Yang CF, Chang SF, Lin CC, et al. Molecular characterization of dengue viruses imported into Taiwan during 2003–2007: geographic distribution and genotype shift. Am J Trop Med Hyg. 2009;80(6): 1039–46.
32 Huang JH, Su CL, Yang CF, Liao TL, Hsu TC, Chang SF, et al. Molecular characterization and phylogenetic analysis of dengue viruses imported into Taiwan during 2008–2010. Am J Trop Med Hyg. 2012;87(2):349–58.
33 van Panhuis WG, Choisy M, Xiong X, Chok NS, Akarasewi P, Iamsirithaworn S, et al. Region-wide synchrony and traveling waves of dengue across eight countries in Southeast Asia. Proc Natl Acad Sci U S A. 2015;112(42):13069–74.
34 Bureau of Communicable Disease Control. Preliminary investigation report of an outbreak of dengue fever in Kaohsiung and Pingtung, southern Taiwan. Epidemiol Bull. 1987;1987(Dec):93–5.
35 Wu YC. Epidemic dengue 2 on Liouchyou Shaing, Pingtung County in l981. Chinese J Microbiol Immunol. 1986;19:203–11.
36 King CC, Wu YC, Chao DY, Lin TH, Chow L, Wang HT, et al. Major epidemics of dengue in Taiwan in 1981–2000: related to intensive virus activities in Asia. Dengue Bulletin. 2000;24:1–10.
37 Taiwan National Infectious Disease Statistics System. http://nidss.cdc.gov.tw/en/?treeid=00ED75D6C887BB27&nowtreeid=D39475C2DB7CD87B. 2016. Accessed 22 Jan 2016.
38 Dengue Control, World Health Organization (WHO). http://www.who.int/denguecontrol/monitoring/vector_surveillance/en/. 2016. Accessed 4 Sep 2016.
39 Centers for Disease Control, R.O.C. (Taiwan). Guidelines for dengue/chikungunya control. 7th ed. Taipei: Centers for Disease Control, R.O.C. (Taiwan); 2014.
40 Monthly Bulletin of Interior Statistics. http://sowf.moi.gov.tw/stat/month/list.htm. 2015. Accessed 13 Oct 2015.
41 Boots BN, Getis A. Point pattern analysis. Newbury Park: Sage Publications; 1998.
42 Cliff AC, Ord JK. Spatial autocorrelation. London: Pion Limited; 1973.
43 Legendre P, Legendre L. Numerical ecology. 2nd ed. Amsterdam: Elsevier; 1998.
44 Grubesic TH. Zip codes and spatial analysis: problems and prospects. Socio Econ Plan Sci. 2008;42:129–49.
45 Cliff AD, Ord JK. Spatial processes: models and applications. London: Pion Limited; 1981.
46 Anselin L, Syabri I, Smirnov O. Visualizing multivariate spatial correlation with dynamically linked windows. Santa Barbara: University of California; 2002. CD-ROM. http://citeseerx.ist.psu.edu/viewdoc/summary?doi=10.1.1.118.7163. Accessed 5 Sep 2016.
47 Wartenberg D. Multivariate spatial correlation: a method for exploratory geographical analysis. Geogr Anal. 1985;17:263–83.
48 GeoDa 1.4.6. https://spatial.uchicago.edu/software (2016). Accessed 5 Sep 2016.
49 Fotheringham AS, Brunsdon C, Charlton M. Geographically weighted regression: the analysis of spatially varying relationships. Wiley: Chichester; 2002.
50 Fotheringham AS, Brunsdon C, Charlton M. Geographically weighted regression: a natural evolution of the expansion method for spatial data analysis. Environ Planning A. 1998;30:1905–27.
51 Charlton M, Fotheringham AS. Geographically weighted regression (White Paper). National Centre for Geocomputation National University of Ireland, Maynooth. http://www.geos.ed.ac.uk/~gisteac/fspat/gwr/gwr_arcgis/GWR_WhitePaper.pdf. 2009. Accessed 17 Sep 2016.
52 Thissen D, Steinberg L, Kuang D. Quick and easy implementation of the Benjamini-Hochberg procedure for controlling the false positive rate in multiple comparisons. J Educ Behav Stat. 2002;27:77–83.
53 Rosner B. Hypothesis testing: on sample inference. In: Fundamentals of biostatistics. 7th ed. Boston: Brooks/Cole, Cengage Learning; 2011. p. 204–57.
54 Gubler DJ. Epidemic dengue/dengue hemorrhagic fever as a public health, social and economic problem in the 21st century. Trends Microbiol. 2002;10:100–3.
55 Jelinek T. Dengue fever in international travelers. Clin Infect Dis. 2000; 31(1):144–7.
56 Herrera-Martinez AD, Rodríguez-Morales AJ. Potential influence of climate variability on dengue incidence registered in a western pediatric hospital of Venezuela. Trop Biomed. 2010;27(2):280–6.
57 Liu-Helmersson J, Stenlund H, Wilder-Smith A, Rocklöv J. Vectorial capacity of *Aedes aegypti*: effects of temperature and implications for global dengue epidemicpotential. PLoS One. 2014;9(3):e89783.
58 Ramos MM, Mohammed H, Zielinski-Gutierrez E, Hayden MH, Lopez JLR, Fournier M, et al. Epidemic dengue and dengue hemorrhagic fever at the Texas-Mexico border: results of a household-based seroepidemiologic survey, December 2005. Am J Trop Med Hyg. 2008;78(3):364–9.
59 Aström C, Rocklöv J, Hales S, Béguin A, Louis V, Sauerborn R. Potential distribution of dengue fever under scenarios of climate change and economic development. Ecohealth. 2012;9(4):448–54.
60 Calderón-Arguedas O, Troyo A, Solano ME, Avendano A, Beier JC. Urban mosquito species (Diptera: Culicidae) of dengue endemic communities in the Greater Puntarenas area. Rev Biol Trop. 2009;57(4):1223–34.
61 Hwang JS, Hsu EL, Chen YR. Investigations on the density and breeding habitats of *Aedes* mosquitoes in dengue epidemic areas in Taiwan. Chin J Pub Health (Taiwan). 1995;14:228–36.
62 Thavara U, Tawatsin A, Chansang C. Larval occurrence, oviposition behavior and biting activity of potential mosquito vectors of dengue on Samui Island. Thailand J Vector Ecol. 2001;26(2):172–80.
63 Ponlawat A, Harrington LC. Blood feeding patterns of *Aedes aegypti* and *Aedes albopictus* in Thailand. J Med Entomol. 2005;42(5):844–9.
64 Padmanabha H, Durham D, Correa F, Diuk-Wasser M, Galvani A. The interactive roles of *Aedes aegypti* super-production and human density in dengue transmission. PLoS Negl Trop Dis. 2012;6(8):e1799.
65 Rodrigues Mde M, Marques GR, Serpa LL, Arduino Mde B, Voltolini JC, Barbosa GL, et al. Density of *Aedes aegypti* and *Aedes albopictus* and its association with number of residents and meteorological variables in the home environment of dengue endemic area, São Paulo, Brazil. Parasit Vectors. 2015;8:115.
66 Braks MA, Honorio NA, Lourencqo-De-Oliveira R, Juliano SA, Lounibos LP. Convergent habitat segregation of *Aedes aegypti* and *Aedes albopictus* (Diptera: Culicidae) in southeastern Brazil and Florida. J Med Entomol. 2003; 40(6):785–94.
67 Chen CD, Nazni WA, Lee HL, Seleena B, Mohd Masri S, Chiang YF, et al. Mixed breeding of *Aedes aegypti* (L.) and *Aedes albopictus* Skuse in four dengue endemic areas in Kuala Lumpur and Selangor, Malaysia. Trop Biomed. 2006;23(2):224–7.
68 Juliano SA, Lounibos LP, O'Meara GF. A field test for competitive effects of *Aedes albopictus* on *A. aegypti* in South Florida: differences between sites of coexistence and exclusion? Oecologia. 2004;139(4):583–93.
69 Bagny L, Freulon M, Delatte H. First record of *Aedes albopictus*, vector of arboviruses in the Eparse Islands of the Mozambique Channel and updating of the inventory of Culicidae. Bull Soc Pathol Exot. 2009;102(3):193–8.
70 Paupy C, Delatte H, Bagny L, Corbel V, Fontenille D. *Aedes albopictus*, an arbovirus vector: from the darkness to the light. Microbes Infect. 2009; 11(14–15):1177–85.
71 Bagny L, Delatte H, Quilici S, Fontenille D. Progressive decrease in *Aedes aegypti* distribution in Reunion Island since the 1900s. J Med Entomol. 2009; 46(6):1541–5.
72 Bagny L, Delatte H, Elissa N, Quilici S, Fontenille D. *Aedes* (Diptera: Culicidae) vectors of arboviruses in Mayotte (Indian Ocean): distribution area and larval habitats. J Med Entomol. 2009;46(2):198–207.
73 Raharimalala FN, Ravaomanarivo LH, Ravelonandro P, Rafarasoa LS, Zouache K, Tran-Van V, et al. Biogeography of the two major arbovirus mosquito vectors, *Aedes aegypti* and *Aedes albopictus* (Diptera, Culicidae), in Madagascar. Parasit Vectors. 2012;5:56.
74 Lounibos LP. Invasions by insect vectors of human disease. Annu Rev Entomol. 2002;47:233–66.
75 Juliano SA, Lounibos LP. Ecology of invasive mosquitoes: effects on resident species and on human health. Ecol Lett. 2005;8(5):558–74.
76 O'Meara GF, Evans LF, Gettman AD, Cuda JP. Spread of *Aedes albopictus* and decline of *Ae. aegypti* (Diptera: Culicidae) in Florida. J Med Entomol. 1995; 32(4):554–62.
77 Daugherty MP, Alto BW, Juliano SA. Invertebrate carcasses as a resource for competing *Aedes albopictus* and *Aedes aegypti* (Diptera: Culicidae). J Med Entomol. 2000;37(3):364–72.
78 Bargielowski IE, Lounibos LP, Carrasquilla MC. Evolution of resistance to satyrization through reproductive character displacement in populations of invasive dengue vectors. Proc Natl Acad Sci U S A. 2013;110(8):2888–92.
79 Scott TW, Takken W. Feeding strategies of anthropophilic mosquitoes result in increased risk of pathogen transmission. Trends Parasitol. 2012;28(3):114–21.

80 Delatte H, Desvars A, Bou'etard A, Bord S, Gimonneau G, Vourc'h G, et al. Blood-feeding behavior of *Aedes albopictus*, a vector of chikungunya on La Reunion. Vector Borne Zoonotic Dis. 2010;10(3):249–58.

81 Eisen L, Moore CG. *Aedes (Stegomyia) aegypti* in the continental United States: a vector at the cool margin of its geographic range. J Med Entomol. 2013;50(3):467–78.

82 Scott TW, Clark GG, Lorenz LH, Amerasinghe PH, Reiter P, Edman JD. Detection of multiple blood feeding in *Aedes aegypti* (Diptera: Culicidae) during a single gonotrophic cycle using a histologic technique. J Med Entomol. 1993;30(1):94–9.

83 Xue RD, Edman JD, Scott TW. Age and body size effects on blood meal size and multiple blood feeding by *Aedes aegypti* (Diptera: Culicidae). J Med Entomol. 1995;32(4):471–4.

84 Xue RD, Barnard DR, Ali A. Influence of multiple blood meals on gonotrophic dissociation and fecundity in Aedes Albopictus. J Am Mosq Control Assoc. 2009;25(4):504–7.

85 Canyon DV, Hii JL, Muller R. The frequency of host biting and its effect on oviposition and survival in *Aedes aegypti* (Diptera: Culicida). J Med Entomol. 1999;36(3):301–8.

86 Chen WJ, Wei HL, Hsu EL, Chen ER. Vector competence of *Aedes albopictus* and *Ae. aegypti* (Diptera: Culicidae) to dengue 1 virus in Taiwan: development of the virus in the orally and parenterally infected mosquitoes. J Med Entomol. 1993;30(3):524–30.

87 Day JF. Host-seeking strategies of mosquito disease vectors. J Am Mosq Control Assoc. 2005;21(4 Suppl):17–22.

88 Vazeille M, Rosen L, Mousson L, Failloux AB. Low oral receptivity for dengue type 2 viruses of *Aedes albopictus* from Southeast Asia compared with that of *Aedes aegypti*. Am J Trop Med Hyg. 2003;68(2):203–8.

89 Chung YK, Pang FY. Dengue virus infection rate in field populations of female Aedes aegypti and Aedes albopictus in Singapore. Trop Med Int Health. 2002;7(4):322–30.

90 Chen CF, Shu PY, Teng HJ, Su CL, Wu JW, Wang JH, et al. Screening of dengue virus in field-caught *Aedes aegypti* and *Aedes albopictus* (Diptera: Culicidae) by one-step SYBR green-based reverse transcriptase-polymerase chain reaction assay during 2004-2007 in Southern Taiwan. Vector Borne Zoonotic Dis. 2010;10(10):1017–25.

91 Chen WJ, Chen SL, Chien LJ, Chen CC, King CC, Harn MR, et al. Silent transmission of the dengue virus in southern Taiwan. Am J Trop Med Hyg. 1996;55(1):12–6.

92 Moreira LA, Iturbe-Ormaetxe I, Jeffery JA, Lu G, Pyke AT, Hedges LM, et al. A Wolbachia symbiont in *Aedes aegypti* limits infection with dengue, Chikungunya, and Plasmodium. Cell. 2009;139(7):1268–78.

93 Tsai KH, Huang CG, Lien JC, Wu WJ, Chen WJ. Molecular (sub) grouping of the endosymbiont Wolbachia infection among mosquitoes of Taiwan. J Med Entomol. 2004;41(4):677–83.

94 Lu P, Bian G, Pan X, Xi Z. Wolbachia induces density-dependent inhibition to dengue virus in mosquito cells. PLoS Negl Trop Dis. 2012;6(7):e1754.

95 Mousson L, Zouache K, Arias-Goeta C, Raquin V, Mavingui P, Failloux AB. The native Wolbachia symbionts limit transmission of dengue virus in *Aedes albopictus*. PLoS Negl Trop Dis. 2012;6(12):e1989.

96 Rohani A, Aidil Azahary AR, Malinda M, Zurainee MN, Rozilawati H, Wan Najdah WM, et al. Eco-virological survey of *Aedes* mosquito larvae in selected dengue outbreak areas in Malaysia. J Vector Borne Dis. 2014;51(4): 327–32.

97 Department of Health (DOH). Report cases of infectious diseases in Taiwan. Health Rep. 1996;13:1–406 (in Chinese).

98 Wu YC. Recent outbreaks in Taiwan area. Health Rep. 1996;6:2–6 (in Chinese).

99 Gratz NG. Critical review of the vector status of *Aedes albopictus*. Med Vet Entomol. 2004;18(3):215–27.

100 Yang CF, Hou JN, Chen TH, Chen WJ. Discriminable roles of *Aedes aegypti* and *Aedes albopictus* in establishment of dengue outbreaks in Taiwan. Acta Trop. 2014;130:17–23.

Seasonal patterns of dengue fever and associated climate factors in 4 provinces in Vietnam from 1994 to 2013

Hu Suk Lee[1*], Hung Nguyen-Viet[1], Vu Sinh Nam[2], Mihye Lee[3], Sungho Won[4,5,6], Phuc Pham Duc[7] and Delia Grace[8]

Abstract

Background: In Vietnam, dengue fever (DF) is still a leading cause of hospitalization. The main objective of this study was to evaluate the seasonality and association with climate factors (temperature and precipitation) on the incidences of DF in four provinces where the highest incidence rates were observed from 1994 to 2013 in Vietnam.

Methods: Incidence rates (per 100,000) were calculated on a monthly basis from during the study period. The seasonal-decomposition procedure based on loess (STL) was used in order to assess the trend and seasonality of DF. In addition, a seasonal cycle subseries (SCS) plot and univariate negative binomial regression (NBR) model were used to evaluate the monthly variability with statistical analysis. Lastly, a generalized estimating equation (GEE) was used to assess the relationship between monthly incidence rates and weather factors (temperature and precipitation).

Results: We found that increased incidence rates were observed in the second half of each year (from May through December) which is the rainy season in each province. In Hanoi, the final model showed that 1 °C rise of temperature corresponded to an increase of 13% in the monthly incidence rate of DF. In Khanh Hoa, the final model displayed that 1 °C increase in temperature corresponded to an increase of 17% while 100 mm increase in precipitation corresponded to an increase of 11% of DF incidence rate. For Ho Chi Minh City, none of variables were significant in the model. In An Giang, the final model showed that 100 mm increase of precipitation in the preceding and same months corresponded to an increase of 30% and 22% of DF incidence rate.

Conclusion: Our findings provide insight into understanding the seasonal pattern and associated climate risk factors.

Keywords: Vietnam, Dengue fever, Monthly incidence rate, Seasonality, Climate factors, Temperature and precipitation

Background

Dengue fever (DF) is a mosquito-borne viral disease which is a leading cause of illness and death in tropical and subtropical countries [1, 2]. Currently, four dengue virus serotypes (DEN-1, DEN-2, DEN-3 and DEN-4) are circulating in Asia, Africa and the America [1–3]. Infection with one of those serotypes does not have cross-protective immunity, so people in endemic areas can have four serotypically different dengue infections during their lifetimes [4]. It was estimated that 3.5 billion people are living in areas at risk for infection with approximately 390 million dengue infections annually (95% credible interval 284–528 million), of which 96 million (67-136 million) clinically manifest [5, 6]. It becomes a major public health problem due to expanding geographical distribution with climate change and an evolution from epidemic cycle with long term intervals to endemic with seasonal patterns [7–11]. Climate variability/changes have a significant impact on vector populations. Factors, such as temperature, precipitation and humidity can influence vector development/survival rates, behavior and habitats [12–14]. Previous studies

* Correspondence: H.S.Lee@cgiar.org
[1]International Livestock Research Institute, Regional Office for East and Southeast Asia, Room 301-302, B1 Building, Van Phuc Diplomatic Compound, 298 Kim Ma Street, Ba Dinh District, Hanoi, Vietnam
Full list of author information is available at the end of the article

have suggested that temperature and precipitation were associated with the occurrence of DF, but relationships have not been consistently described [15–19]. For instance, in Thailand, temperature and precipitation were positively associated with dengue transmission [20]. In a Taiwanese study, the incidence rate was negatively associated with monthly temperature and relative humidity [18]. These discrepancies may be attributed to different climate/environmental conditions and different data analysis methods.

In Vietnam, a National Dengue Control Programme (NDCP) was established in 1999, which relies mainly on vector control to decrease the transmission from vectors to humans. However, dengue is still a leading causes of hospitalization, and Vietnam has the highest number of cases in the Western Pacific region [21]. To our knowledge, few studies have been conducted to assess the seasonal pattern of DF and its associated climate factors in Vietnam. The main objective of this study was to evaluate the seasonality and association with climate factors (temperature and precipitation) on the incidences of DF in Hanoi, Khanh Hoa, Ho Chi Minh City and An Giang provinces where the highest incidence rates were observed from 1994 to 2013 in Vietnam.

Methods

Study locations and data

Hanoi (population: 6.7 million), Khanh Hoa (population: 1.2 million), Ho Chi Min City (population: 7.5 million) and An Giang (population: 2.2 million) provinces with the highest incidence rates were selected for this study, which are located in North, Central and Southern part of Vietnam, respectively (Fig. 1). The annual temperature ranges from 16 °C to 29 °C in Hanoi whereas other three provinces are relatively higher between 24 °C and 29 °C (Table 1). Generally, there are two seasons: the rainy (from May to October) and dry seasons (from November to April) in Vietnam.

According to the national surveillance system of infectious diseases in Vietnam, DF is one of the 28 pathogens which are reported on a monthly basis by the preventive medicine networks. A case of dengue is determined as a suspected case who meets the WHO (World Health Organization) case definition: acute febrile illness (≥38 °C) of 2-7 days duration with two of the following symptoms: severe headache, retro-orbital pain, nausea, vomiting, myalgia, arthralgia, hemorrhagic manifestations and leucopenia [22]. Most of cases are clinically diagnosed and only 10-20% of cases are serologically confirmed. The numbers of cases and deaths are collected at provincial preventive medicine centers which are reported to the regional preventive medicine institutes, and then to the National Institute of Hygiene and Epidemiology (NIHE). Annually, the NIHE and then Ministry of Health (MOH) publish books of reported dengue fever cases. We obtained the data from the annual book of communicable diseases published from 1994 and 2013 of DF cases, these were entered in Excel sheets by our research team. In addition, monthly meteorological data [total precipitation (100 mm) and average temperature (°C)] were obtained from four provinces (source: Institute of Meteorology and Hydrology and Climate Change).

Data analysis

Incidence rates (per 100,000) were calculated on a monthly basis during the study period. The seasonal-decomposition procedure based on loess (STL) was used in order to assess the trend and seasonality of DF. This is a statistical technique to decompose a time series dataset into trend, seasonal and remainder on a yearly basis (12 months) [23]. In addition, a seasonal cycle sub-series (SCS) plot and univariate negative binomial regression (NBR) model were used to evaluate the monthly variability with statistical analysis [24]. The SCS displays a horizontal line for the average incidence rate of each month over the total period, and each vertical line above and below the horizontal line indicates the specific incidence rate for that month in each year of the data. In order to evaluate the monthly differences, univariate NBR models were constructed for each province while February was used as reference.

A generalized estimating equation (GEE) was used to assess the relationship between monthly incidence rates and weather factors (temperature and precipitation), because serial correlations were detected between observations. We employed the GEE with Autoregressive (AR)(1) as working correlation matrix and sandwich estimators were used to adjust the residual correlations. It should be noted that sandwich estimator in GEE guarantees the robustness against the misspecified correlation structure [25]. A negative binomial distribution (NBD) was selected for the GEE model which includes a Poisson distribution with an extra-dispersion term (alpha (α)). Generally, a Poisson regression distribution should be considered for count data but the Poisson distribution model is not able to take into account the overdispersed count outcomes [26, 27]. A likelihood ratio was implemented in order to confirm the presence of overdispersion, and the test showed the presence of overdispersion in the model.

For the variable screening, we conducted the correlations between monthly temperature and precipitation while the correlations between the original monthly variables and their one lag (preceding month) counterparts were investigated in order to evaluate the possible lagged effect in the model. The linearity of effect of temperature and precipitation on DF incidence was explored using loess smoothing curves. If there was evidence of non-linearity, a quadratic function of the predictor was considered in the model if $P < 0.05$. For the model building,

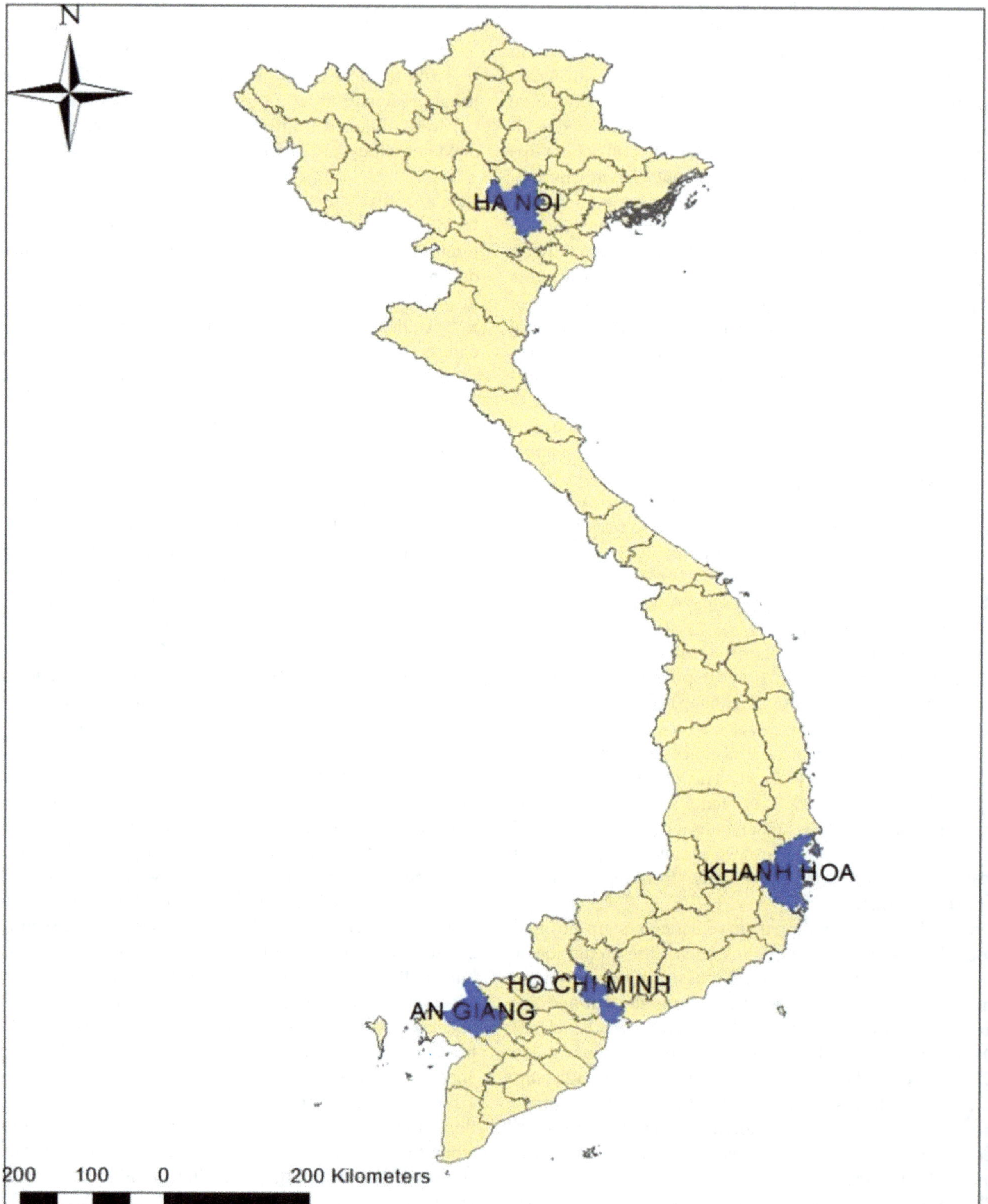

Fig. 1 Map of the area in Hanoi, Khanh Hoa, Ho Chi Minh City, An Giang provinces

Table 1 Monthly weather conditions in Hanoi, Khanh Hoa, Ho Chi Minh City and An Giang from 1994 to 2013

Month	Hanoi		Khanh Hoa		Ho Chi Minh City		An Giang	
	Temperature (° C)	Precipitation (mm)	Temperature (° C)	Precipitation (mm)	Temperature (° C)	Precipitation (mm)	Temperature (° C)	Precipitation (mm)
Jan	16.67	19.59	24.17	49.74	27.18	104.39	25.79	8.97
Feb	18.36	21.9	24.81	13.87	26.77	156.74	26.32	4.97
Mar	20.62	47.98	26.04	33.02	27.59	147.74	27.58	15.04
Apr	24.44	68.95	27.70	52.95	27.06	138.36	28.78	84.02
May	27.34	205.05	28.55	101.34	27.15	124.34	28.43	147.42
Jun	29.34	246.82	28.97	56.61	27.45	136.61	27.95	114.16
Jul	29.25	307.14	28.74	53.57	27.19	110.26	27.41	175.45
Aug	28.51	316.37	28.69	52.94	27.23	131.81	27.73	215.41
Sep	27.43	203.24	27.96	201.51	27.09	161.86	27.62	160.4
Oct	25.52	160.29	26.89	359.30	27.46	118.08	27.52	252.95
Nov	22.18	80.54	25.98	429.06	27.20	145.00	27.36	155.66
Dec	18.38	39.13	24.76	198.70	27.61	142.75	26.22	48.96
Summary[a]	24.0 ± 4.6	143.08 ± 131.07	26.94 ± 1.76	133.55 ± 175.69	27.24 ± 0.96	134.82 ± 116.32	27.39 ± 1.17	115.28 ± 113.58

[a]mean and standard deviation

the strong correlation (r = 0.72, P < 0.001) was observed between temperature and precipitation for Hanoi, therefore we developed two multivariable models – a model had the temperature without precipitation and vice versa. For other provinces, both variables (temperature and precipitation) with one lag were screened in the models.

Variables with P-values <0.05 were considered to be significant in the final models. In addition, the Bonferroni-adjusted significance level obtained by dividing the significance level α, by the number of P-values was used for multiple comparison problems. The accuracy of the proposed model was evaluated with the root-mean-square error (RMSE). To minimize the overfitting problem, our data were split into train and test data. Train data consist of observations from January 1995 to December 2012, and were used to provide the linear model. The remaining data (from January 2013 to December 2013) were assigned as test data, and used to calculate RMSE. The results for the NBR were demonstrated as incidence rate ratio (IRR) and 95% confidence interval (CI). All data were created in Microsoft Excel 2010 and analyzed using R (version 3.2.2) and STATA (version 14.0, Stata Corp, College Station, TX, USA). ArcGIS version 10.3 ArcMap (ESRI, Redlands, CA, USA) was used to generate the map. This study was approved by the Hanoi Medical University Institutional Review Board (HMU IRB: no. 00003121), Vietnam.

Results

STL analysis and seasonal cycle subseries by province

In Hanoi, a total of 46,043 cases (average 3.436 per 100,000; 95% CI: 3.432-3.439) were reported from 1994 to 2013. The trend plot showed the mild fluctuations (apart from dramatically increase and decrease incidence in 1998) (Fig. 2-a: first plot). The STL plot exhibited the seasonal patterns with a strong peak during the last half of the calendar year and a smaller peak in July (Fig. 2-a: second plot). The remainder component showed varying residuals with intermittently large values. The seasonal cycle subseries plot demonstrated that the highest incidence rate was noted in October whereas the lowest was in February (Fig. 3-a). An univariate NBR model showed that all months (except for March and April) were at increased risk for DF incidence rates compared to February at an alpha level of 0.05 while January was not statistically significant with Bonferroni adjustment (P < 0.05/11) (Table 2). In particular, incidence rates of disease were highly increased in October followed by November and September.

In Khanh Hoa, a total of 61,404 cases (average 23.473 per 100,000; 95% CI: 23.468-23.479) were recorded during the study period. The trend plot showed the large fluctuations with an apparent overall increase and decrease in 1995, 1998, 2005, 2010 and 2012 (Fig. 2-b: first plot) while the STL plot had two peaks with seasonal pattern in the second half of each year (Fig. 2-b: second plot). In the remainder component, large residuals were observed in 1996, 2005 and 2010. The seasonal cycle subseries showed that incidence rates were relatively higher in the second half (Fig. 3-b). In an univariate NRB analysis, there were significantly increased incidences of disease from May to December compared to February (α = 0.05) while May, June and December were not statistically at an increased risk of acquiring the disease when Bonferroni correction was applied (Table 2).

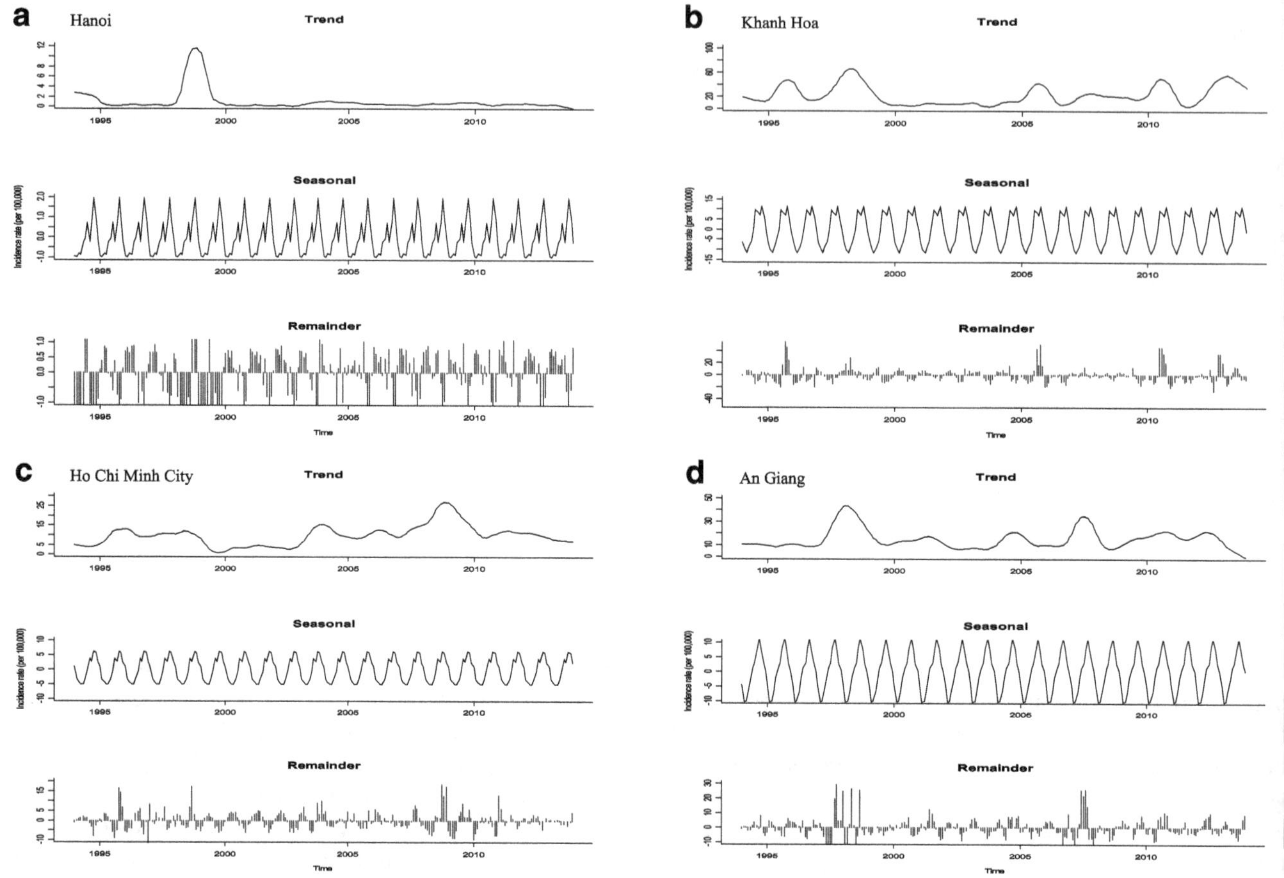

Fig. 2 Seasonal-trend decomposition (Trend, Seasonal and Remainder) of the monthly incidence rates of DF in four provinces from 1994 to 2013 (Each plot has different Y-axis scales)

For Ho Chi Minh City, a total of 61,404 cases (average 10.349 per 100,000; 95% CI: 10.348-10.351) were reported during the study period. The STL trend plot presented the largest fluctuations with its peaks in 1997, 2003 and 2008 (Fig. 2-c: first plot). The seasonal plot had primary and secondary peaks at the end of year (Fig. 2-c: first plot). In the remainder plot, large values were observed in 1995, 1998, 2008 and 2011. The highest rates on the seasonal cycle subseries plot were in October, November and August whereas the lowest rates were in May, April and March (Fig. 3-b). There were significantly increased incidence rates of disease in January and from August to December compared to February whereas the risk was significantly reduced between March and June at an alpha level of 0.05. For the Bonferroni adjustment, September was not statistically at an increased risk.

In An Giang, a total of 61,404 cases (average 15.391 per 100,000; 95% CI: 15.381-15.402) were reported during the study period. The STL plot showed the largest fluctuations with its peaks in 1997, 2004, 2009 and 2012 (Fig. 2-d: first plot). The seasonal plot showed a single peak in the early second half of each year (Fig. 2-d: second plot). The remainder plot appeared to have random variations although large values were noted in 1998 and 2007. The highest rates on seasonal cycle subseries plot were in September, October and August whereas the lowest rates were observed in March, April and March (Fig. 3-d). In an univariate NBR analysis, there were significantly increased risks of disease in all months (except for March) with $\alpha = 0.05$ while March and April were statistically not at an increased risk with Bonferroni correction.

GEE model by each province

In Hanoi, the final model showed that 1 °C rise of temperature corresponded to an increase of 13% in the monthly incidence rate of DF (Table 3) while the precipitation was not significant in the model. The preceding month for temperature was not significant in the final model while linearity was observed between temperature and DF incidence rate with RMSE = 14.92.

In Khanh Hoa, the final model displayed that 1 °C increase in temperature corresponded to an increase of 17% while 100 mm increase in precipitation corresponded to an increase of 11% of DF incidence rate with

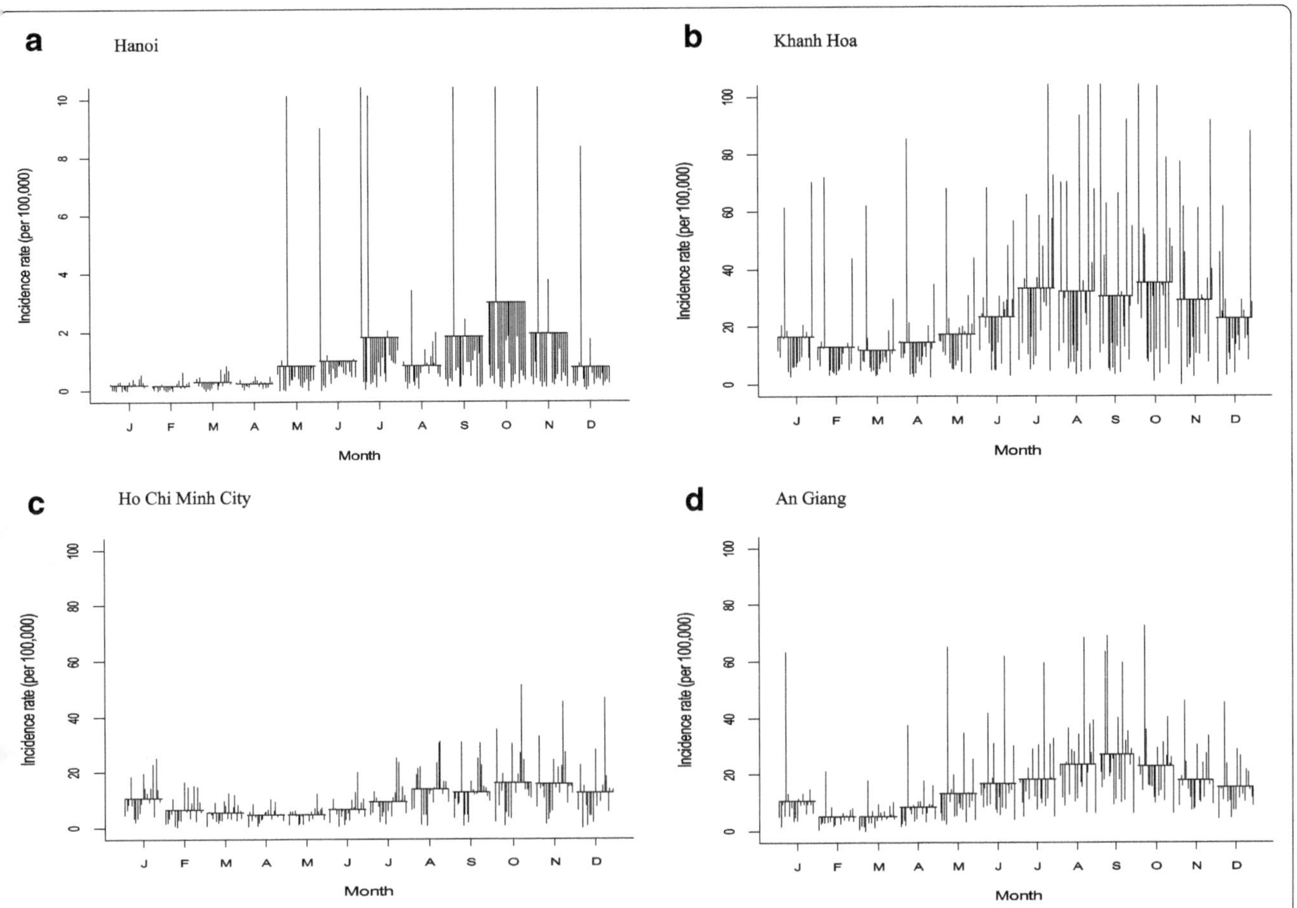

Fig. 3 Seasonal cycle subseries plot of the monthly incidence rates of DF in four provinces from 1994 to 2013 (only Hanoi has different Y-axis scales)

Table 2 Univariate negative binomial regression (NBR) models for the DF incidence rates by month with incidence rate ratio (IRR) and 95% confidence interval (CI)

Month	Hanoi	Khanh Hoa	Ho Chi Minh City	An Giang
January	2.73 (1.19-6.26)*	1.26 (0.73-2.18)	1.61 (1.03-2.53)*	2.12 (1.39-3.22)*†
February	Reference: 1	Reference: 1	Reference: 1	Reference: 1
March	1.36 (0.59-3.14)	0.90 (0.52-1.56)	0.84 (0.54-1.32)	1.04 (0.68-1.59)
April	1.43 (0.62-3.30)	1.12 (0.65-1.92)	0.71 (0.45-1.11)	1.69 (1.11-2.56)*
May	5.14 (2.24-11.77)*†	1.34 (0.78-2.30)*	0.71 (0.45-0.11)	2.58 (1.70-3.92)*†
June	6.63 (2.90-15.19)*†	1.79 (1.04-3.09)*	0.99 (0.63-1.54)	3.28 (2.16-4.98)*†
July	14.94 (6.52-34.17)*†	2.55 (1.43-4.39)*†	1.40 (0.89-2.19)	3.58 (2.36-5.45)*†
August	22.02 (9.63-50.34)*†	2.46 (1.43-4.24)*†	2.06 (1.31-3.22)*†	4.57 (3.01-6.94)*†
September	38.47 (16.83-87.94)*†	2.35 (1.36-4.04)*†	1.91 (1.22-2.99)*	5.26 (3.46-8.00)*†
October	55.07 (23.65-123.59)*†	2.69 (1.56-4.63)*†	2.40 (1.53-3.76)*†	4.49 (2.95-6.83)*†
November	46.69 (20.43-106.73)*†	2.22 (1.29-3.83)*†	2.35 (1.50-3.67)*†	3.49 (2.30-5.31)*†
December	13.44 (5.88-30.74)*†	1.75 (1.02-3.01)*	1.84 (1.18-2.89)*†	3.01 (1.98-4.58)*†

* = statistically significant ($P < 0.05$)
† = Bonferroni adjustment ($P < 0.05/11$)

Table 3 Final NBR models of DF incidence rates in Hanoi, Khanh Hoa, Ho Chi Minh City and An Giang

Province/Variable	Adjusted incidence rate ratios (IRRs)	95% CI	*P* value	RMSE
Hanoi (0.717, <0.001)				
Monthly average temperature (°C)	1.13	1.09-1.17	<0.001[a]	14.92
Khanh Hoa (−0.140)				
Monthly average temperature (°C)	1.17	1.09-1.26	<0.001[a]	22.40
Monthly total precipitation (100 mm)	1.11	1.03-1.20	0.004[a]	
Ho Chi Minh City (0.232)				
Null	Null	Null	Null	Null
An Giang (0.1672)				
Monthly total precipitation (100 mm) in the preceding month	1.30	1.13-1.50	<0.001[a]	44.06
Monthly total precipitation (100 mm) in the same month	1.22	1.06-1.40	0.006[a]	

[a] = Bonferroni adjustment ($P < 0.05/4$)

RMSE = 22.40. The preceding months for both variables were not statistically significant in the models. In addition, linearities were observed. For Ho Chi Minh City, none of the variables were significant in the model. In An Giang, the final model showed that 100 mm increase of precipitation in the preceding and the same months corresponded to an increase of 30% and 22% in the monthly incidence rate of DF with RMSE = 44.06, respectively while linearity was observed (apart from 1 outlier). All variables in the final modes were statistically significant with Bonferroni adjustment (*P*-value < 0.05/4).

Discussion

The aim of this study was to evaluate the seasonal pattern and association between incidence rates and weather risk factors in four provinces during last 20 years (1994-2013). We found that increased incidence rates were observed in the second half of each year (from May through December) which is the rainy season ("called dengue season") in Vietnam [28, 29]. The big outbreaks appear to be occurring every 10 years (in 1987, 1998 and 2010). We were able to identify a number of some peaks associated with sudden increase in each province which were assumed to be related to emergence of new serotypes or drop in herd immunity.

Dengue fever occurs across the country, with the highest number of cases in the southern part of the country. In Hanoi (capital city), average incidence rates were lower (3-7 times lower) than other three provinces. However, dramatically high IRRs for the rainy season were observed compared to other provinces. This may be attributed to the more active surveillance, easy access to the healthcare system and increased public awareness (including clinicians and general public). However, an absolute number of suspected cases are high during the rainy season across the country, so that increased awareness is less likely to influence on our results. The National surveillance system for DF has been consistently collecting cases from local authorities in collaboration with well-trained clinicians so that surveillance dataset may be representative of all regions of Vietnam. In terms of clinical diagnosis, results of hematocrit and thrombocyte counts could be used to help to differentiate between dengue and malaria or JE/meningitis. In addition, distributions of malaria, JE or meningitis are different compared to dengue (dengue in urban, sub-urban and populated areas; mostly malaria in mountainous areas and JE in rural areas with rice field). Therefore, doctors also can utilize geographical areas to aid diagnosing patients. We found that temperature and precipitation were positively associated with the occurrence of disease which were consistent with findings from the previous studies [20, 28, 30, 31]. For stance, a positive correlation was observed between rainfall and vector population in Malaysia [32]. In an Indonesian study, it was suggested that higher temperatures had led to shorter incubation periods and increased virus replication [33].

Vietnam has one of the highest rates of urbanization in the world, both spatially and demographically and this is likely to affect the ecology of mosquitoes [34]. One study found that urbanization was positively correlated with density, larval development rate and adult survival rate of vectors, which can potentially increase the transmission of disease [35]. This study highlights the highly dynamic nature of DF epidemiology and the need to base disease surveillance and control on timely and representative data. Moreover, in Vietnam, people have a tendency to store water near to their houses due to a lack of reliable water supply in peri-urban/rural areas. A significant portion of people also live in poorly sanitized areas. The stagnant water and substandard sanitary and hygiene practices can lead to creation of good breeding sites for the vectors. In Ho Chi Minh City, we did not find the association between climate factors and DF. It could be possible that DF incidence is more likely to be influenced by other potential risk factors (such as lifestyle and man-made water containers). Actually, because of various water storage behaviors in different regions, vector population in southern regions is 5-10 times higher than northern regions (unpublished data). For An Giang, DF incidence rate had a significant association with the precipitation in the preceding and current months that may be useful to develop the predictive early warning indicators in that region. Overall, our models have the relatively large RMSEs, therefore in order to improve performance of models, other unmeasured environmental factors (such as control measures, herd immunity demographic/socioeconomic changes and urbanizations) should be considered which may be attributed to dengue transmission.

Several limitations should be addressed as follows. It is possible that DF cases were under reported, especially in rural areas due to lack of healthcare and diagnostic facilities. A retrospective study showed that among acute undifferentiated fever cases, 33.6% of cases were caused by dengue fever, which may suggest the possibility of substantial underestimation in local areas [36]. In addition, there was a possibility of misdiagnosis with other diseases as most of cases were reported based on clinical manifestation and hematocrit/platelet counts. It could be possible that more cases were likely to be diagnosed by clinicians during the rainy season. We were not able to identify the proportions of the 4 different serotypes, or the age and gender of respondents, which could be associated with the likelihood of exposure to the vectors. All four serotypes have been identified in Southern Vietnam [3]. One study found that 18.4% and 2.4% of the patients from Khanh Hoa and Binh Thuan provinces were confirmed with DF virus serotype 4 and 2, respectively [37]. In addition, male cases with ≥15 years of age were predominately reported from 6 Asian countries [38]. This study has suggested that this may be related to gender and age differences due to exposure differences among older adolescents and adults. Further study is necessary in order to identify circulating serotypes and more vulnerable groups depending on the provinces. We assumed that human population was the same on a yearly basis which is not realistic, however, the effect of this was limited because the relatively large denominators could not have an impact on a monthly incidence rate.

The STL and SCS methods have been commonly used in the economic and environmental areas, but have not been commonly used in the epidemiology/medical fields [24, 39, 40]. There are several advantages of the STL and SCS method [23]. Firstly, it is a straightforward procedure to decompose a time series with missing data. Secondly, it has flexibility in specifying the amount of deviation in seasonal and trend components of time series data. In addition, trend and seasonal components are very robust, so that these are not easily distorted by outliers in the data. Lastly, the STL method is a valuable tool for understanding the complexity of time series data. For SCS plot, it helps visualize patterns both between and within groups during the study period. However, it must be interpreted cautiously because the horizontal lines (average for vertical lines) are highly influenced by large values.

Conclusions

We found that each province showed slightly different seasonal patterns. Overall, increased incidence rates were observed between July and December during the study period. Our findings provide insight into understanding the seasonal pattern and associated climate risk factors in each province. This study may be another way of providing evidence to aid clinicians when making a diagnosis and foresee the timing of outbreaks, therefore may be utilized to raise public awareness during the high peak seasons in order to prevent or reduce further potential outbreaks or onwards transmission during an outbreak.

Abbreviations

AR: Autoregressive; CI: Confidence interval; DF: Dengue fever; GEE: Generalized estimating equation; IRR: Incidence rate ratio; MOH: Ministry of health; NBD: Negative binomial distribution; NBR: Negative binomial regression; NDCP: National dengue control programme; NIHE: National institute of hygiene and epidemiology; RMSE: Root-mean-square error; SCS: Seasonal cycle subseries; STL: Seasonal-decomposition procedure based on loess; WHO: World health organization

Acknowledgments

The authors thank National Dengue Control Programme (NDCP) under the Ministry of Health and Institute of Meteorology and Hydrology and Climate Change, Ministry of Natural Resources and Environment (IMHEN) for providing information on DF cases and metrological data.

Funding

We acknowledge the CGIAR Fund Council, Australia (ACIAR), Irish Aid, European Union, International Fund for Agricultural Development (IFAD), Netherlands, New Zealand, Switzerland, UK, USAID and Thailand for funding to the CGIAR Research Program on Climate Change, Agriculture and Food Security (CCAFS).

Authors' contributions

Conceived and designed the experiments: HSL. Performed the experiments: HSL, Analyzed the data: HSL and SHW Wrote the paper: HSL, VSN, MHL, SHW, HNV, PPD and DG gave inputs and revised the paper. All co-authors approved the content of the paper.

Competing interests

The authors declare that they have no competing interests.

Consent for publication

Not applicable.

Author details
[1]International Livestock Research Institute, Regional Office for East and Southeast Asia, Room 301-302, B1 Building, Van Phuc Diplomatic Compound, 298 Kim Ma Street, Ba Dinh District, Hanoi, Vietnam. [2]Vector Borne Diseases and Training, National Institute of Hygiene and Epidemiology, Hanoi, Vietnam. [3]Medical microbiology Department, The Royal Bournemouth Hospital, Bournemouth, UK. [4]Graduate School of Public Health, Seoul National University, Seoul, Korea. [5]Interdisciplinary Program of Bioinformatics, Seoul National University, Seoul, Korea. [6]Institute of Health and Environment, Seoul National University, Seoul, Korea. [7]Center for Public Health and Ecosystem Research (CENPHER), Hanoi School of Public Health, Hanoi, Vietnam. [8]International Livestock Research Institute, Nairobi, Kenya.

References

1. WHO. Comprehensive Guidelines for Prevention and Control of Dengue and Dengue Haemorrhagic Fever (2011) Available: http://apps.searo.who.int/pds_docs/B4751.pdf. Accessed 20 Mar 2016.
2. Gubler DJ. Dengue and dengue hemorrhagic fever. Clin Microbiol Rev. 1998;11:480–96.
3. Ha DQ, Tien N, Huong V, Loan H, Thang C. Dengue epidemic in southern Vietnam, 1998. Emerg Infect Dis. 2000;6:422–5.
4. Gubler DJ, Clark GG. Dengue/dengue hemorrhagic fever: the emergence of a global health problem. Emerg Infect Dis. 1995;1:55–7.
5. Beatty M, Letson W, Edgil D, Margolis H. Estimating the total world population at risk for locally acquired dengue infection. Abstract presented at the 56th Annual Meeting of the American Society of Tropical Medicine and Hygiene. AmJTrop Med Hyg. 2007;77:Suppl 5170–257.
6. Bhatt S, Gething PW, Brady OJ, Messina JP, Farlow AW, Moyes CL, Drake JM, Brownstein JS, Hoen AG, Sankoh O, Myers MF, George DB, Jaenisch T, Wint GRW, Simmons CP, Scott TW, Farrar JJ, Hay SI. The global distribution and burden of dengue. Nature. 2013;496:504–7.
7. CDC. Dengue Available at: https://www.cdc.gov/dengue/ Accessed 25 Mar 2016
8. Gibbons RV, Vaughn DW. Dengue: an escalating problem. Brit Med J. 2002; 324:1563–6.
9. Guzmán MG, Kouri G. Dengue: an update. Lancet Infect Dis. 2002;2:33–42.
10. Morin CW, Comrie AC, Ernst K. Climate and dengue transmission: evidence and implications. Environ Health Perspect. 2013;121:1264–72.
11. Colón-González FJ, Fezzi C, Lake IR, Hunter PR. The effects of weather and climate change on dengue. PLoS Negl Trop Dis. 2013;7:e2503.
12. Reiter P. Climate change and mosquito-borne disease. Environ Health Perspect. 2001;109(suppl 1):141–61.
13. Tun-Lin W, Burkot T, Kay B. Effects of temperature and larval diet on development rates and survival of the dengue vector *Aedes aegypti* in north Queensland. Australia Med Vet Entomol. 2000;14:31–7.
14. Halstead SB. Dengue virus-mosquito interactions. Annu Rev Entomol. 2008; 53:273–91.
15. Li C, Lim T, Han L, Fang R. Rainfall, abundance of *Aedes aegypti* and dengue infection in Selangor, Malaysia. Southeast Asian J Trop Med Public Health. 1985;16:560–8.
16. Depradine C, Lovell E. Climatological variables and the incidence of Dengue fever in Barbados. Int J Environ Health Res. 2004;14:429–41.
17. Chowell G, Sanchez F. Climate-based descriptive models of dengue fever: the 2002 epidemic in Colima, Mexico. J Environ Health. 2006;68:40–4.
18. Wu P-C, Guo H-R, Lung S-C, Lin C-Y, Su H-J. Weather as an effective predictor for occurrence of dengue fever in Taiwan. Acta Trop. 2007;103:50–7.
19. Rosa-Freitas MG, Schreiber KV, Tsouris P, ETdS W, Luitgards-Moura JF. Associations between dengue and combinations of weather factors in a city in the Brazilian Amazon. Rev Panam Salud Publica. 2006;20:256–67.
20. Promprou S, Jaroensutasinee M, Jaroensutasinee K. Climatic Factors Affecting Dengue Haemorrhagic Fever Incidence in Southern Thailand. Avilable at: http://apps.who.int/iris/bitstream/10665/164135/1/dbv29p41.pdf%20/. Accessed 30 Mar 2016.
21. WPRO. Dengue in the Western Pacific Region. Available at: http://www.wpro.who.int/emerging_diseases/Dengue/en/. Accessed 31 Mar 2016.
22. WHO. Dengue: Guidelines for Diagnosis, Treatment, Prevention and Control. Available at: http://www.who.int/tdr/publications/documents/dengue-diagnosis.pdf. Accessed 1 Apr 2016.
23. Cleveland RB, Cleveland WS, McRae JE, Terpenning I. STL: A seasonal-trend decomposition procedure based on loess. J Off Stat. 1990;6:3–73.
24. Lee H, Levine M, Guptill-Yoran C, Johnson A, Kamecke P, Moore GE. Regional and temporal variations of Leptospira seropositivity in dogs in the United States, 2000–2010. J Vet Intern Med. 2014;28:779–88.
25. Liang K-Y, Zeger SL. Longitudinal data analysis using generalized linear models. Biometrika. 1986;73:13–22.
26. Calvin JA, Long JS. Regression models for categorical and limited dependent variables. Technometrics. 1998;40:80–1.
27. Gardner W, Mulvey EP, Shaw EC. Regression analyses of counts and rates: Poisson, overdispersed Poisson, and negative binomial models. Psychol Bull. 1995;118:392.
28. Wiwanitkit V. An observation on correlation between rainfall and the prevalence of clinical cases of dengue in Thailand. J Vector Borne Dis. 2006;43:73–6.
29. Hopp J, Foley JA. Worldwide fluctuations in dengue fever case related to climate variability. Clim Res. 2003;25:85–94.
30. Pham HV, Doan HT, Phan TT, Minh NN. Ecological factors associated with dengue fever in a Central Highlands province, Vietnam. BMC Infect Dis. 2011;11:172.
31. Hurtado-Daz M, Riojas-Rodrguez H, Rothenberg S, Gomez-Dantes H, Cifuentes E. Impact of climate variability on the incidence of dengue in Mexico. Tropical Med Int Health. 2007;12:1327–237.
32. Rozilawati H, Zairi J, Adanan C. Seasonal abundance of *Aedes albopictus* in selected urban and suburban areas in Penang, Malaysia. Trop Biomed. 2007;24:83–94.
33. Bangs MJ, Larasati RP, Corwin AL, Wuryadi S, Jakarta I. Climatic factors associated with epidemic dengue in Palembang, Indonesia: implications of short-term meteorological events on virus transmission. Southeast Asian J Trop Med Public Health. 2006;37:1103–16.
34. Vietnam urbanization reivew: techinical assistance report. Available at: http://documents.worldbank.org/curated/en/225041468177548577/pdf/669160ESW0P1130Review000Full0report.pdf. Accessed 15 June 2016.
35. Li Y, Kamara F, Zhou G, Puthiyakunnon S, Li C, Liu Y, Zhou Y, Yao L, Yan G, Chen XG. Urbanization increases *Aedes albopictus* larval habitats and accelerates mosquito development and survivorship. PLoS Negl Trop Dis. 2014;8:e3301.
36. Phuong H, de Vries PJ, Nga TT, Giao PT, Hung LQ, Binh TQ, Nam NV, Nagelkerke N, Kager PA. Dengue as a cause of acute undifferentiated fever in Vietnam. BMC Infect Dis. 2006;6:123.
37. Buchy P, Vo VL, Bui KT, Trinh TX, Glaziou P, Le TT, Le VL, Bui TC. Secondary dengue virus type 4 infections in Vietnam. Southeast Asian J Trop Med Public Health. 2005;36:178–85.
38. Anker M, Arima Y. Male-female differences in the number of reported incident dengue fever cases in six Asian countries. Western Pac Surveil Response J. 2011;2:17–23.
39. Sun L, Klein EY, Laxminarayan R. Seasonality and temporal correlation between community antibiotic use and resistance in the United States. Clin Infect Dis. 2012;55:687–69.
40. Li L, Qian J, Ou C-Q, Zhou Y-X, Guo C, Guo Y. Spatial and temporal analysis of Air Pollution Index and its timescale-dependent relationship with meteorological factors in Guangzhou, China, 2001–2011. Environ Pollut. 2014;190:75–81.

10

High frequency of pre-existing neutralizing antibody responses in patients with dengue during an outbreak in Central Brazil

Angela Ferreira Lopes de Teive e Argolo[1,2*], Valéria Christina de Rezende Féres[3], Marli Tenório Cordeiro[4], Lucimeire Antonelli da Silveira[1], Adriana Oliveira Guilarde[1], Ernesto Torres de Azevedo Marques Jr.[4,5], Wayner Vieira de Souza[4] and Celina Maria Turchi Martelli[1,4]

Abstract

Background: This study aims to identify dengue neutralizing antibody response in patients with dengue from a well-characterized cohort during an outbreak in central Brazil, 2012–2013.

Methods: We analyzed paired samples from 40 patients with severe dengue and 20 patients with dengue. Eligibility criteria were: IgM, NS1Ag and/or RT-PCR positivity and positive IgG result. Plaque reduction neutralization test ($PRNT_{50}$) from DENV-1 to DENV-4 was performed to identify serotype-specific NAbs response. An infecting serotype was defined as ≥4-fold increase in DENV NAbs in paired samples. Monotypic response was classified as $PRNT_{50} \geq 1/20$ to only one DENV serotype, and multitypic response was considered to be $PRNT_{50} \geq 1/20$ to two or more serotypes simultaneously.

Results: Patients were mainly adults. Virological dengue infection was confirmed by RT-PCR: DENV-4($n = 14$) and DENV-1($n = 10$). Forty-four out of 60(73.3 %) patients had NAbs to DENV-4, DENV-1(68.3 %), DENV-2(68.3 %) and DENV-3(61.6 %) respectively. Fifteen percent of the cases presented monotypic response, whereas 85 % had multitypic response. DENV-4 infected-patients presented the greatest difference in $PRNT_{50}$ titers compared with other serotypes. Pre-existing DENV NAbs was not correlated with disease severity. This was the first time that DENV-4 was implicated in an epidemic in the region.

Conclusion: Our data indicates high exposure of multiple DENV serotypes in all age groups in the pre-dengue vaccine era and also previous to Zika virus introduction in Brazil.

Keywords: Dengue virus, Neutralizing antibody, Dengue fever, Brazil

Background

Dengue is one of the most relevant arboviruses in the world, endemic in more than 120 countries in tropical and subtropical areas [1]. Dengue virus is a mosquito-borne flavivirus with four characterized antigenically distinct serotypes (DENV-1, DENV-2, DENV-3 and DENV-4). Approximately 390 million dengue infections occur every year with ~100 million symptomatic illnesses according to a recent modeling estimation [2]. In the American region, nearly 61 % of the 2.38 million dengue cases were reported in Brazil in 2013 [3]. Nationwide there was evidence of an upward trend in the number of reported dengue cases, hospitalization and deaths in the last decade [4–6]. In central Brazil the first dengue outbreak was registered in 1994 with the detection of DENV-1, followed by DENV-2 (1998), DENV-3 (2002) and DENV-4 (2011) [7, 8]. Over the last two decades the peak of dengue transmission occurred

* Correspondence: angelafarmaceutica@hotmail.com
[1] Institute of Tropical Pathology and Public Health of Federal University of Goiás, Rua 235, St Universitário, Goiânia 74.605-050, GO, Brazil
[2] Public Health Laboratory of Secretaria Estadual de Saúde de Goiás (LACEN-GO), Av. Contorno, 3.556, Jd. Bela Vista, 74.853-120 Goiânia, GO, Brazil
Full list of author information is available at the end of the article

in 2013 with ~55 thousand cases registered with an incidence rate of 4411 per 100,000 inhabitants [9].

Dengue may develop as an unapparent infection with the majority of cases presenting mild disease, but life-threatening conditions, death may occur [1]. Susceptible individuals mount a specific immune response when they are infected by one of the four DENV serotypes. Sequential infections also occur after exposure to different serotypes [10, 11]. DENV infection is believed to induce a long-lasting protective immunity to homologous serotypes. In addition, due to cross-protection, a transient immunity to heterologous serotypes may play a beneficial role in clinical outcomes [12]. By contrast, the viral infection mediated by antibodies (ADE) may be amplified during a secondary infection with a heterologous serotype, leading to deleterious immune response and disease severity [13–15].

The plaque reduction neutralization test (PRNT) is currently the gold standard to identify dengue serotype-specific neutralizing antibodies. This assay allows the detection of pre-existing and/or current DENV infection and seems to be correlated with protection [16]. In the current study, we aimed to identify the DENV neutralizing antibody response in paired samples collected from patients with dengue enrolled in hospital and ambulatory settings in central Brazil. The objective was also to assess the correlation of pre-existing DENV neutralizing antibodies by PRNT with dengue outcomes during the 2012–2013 outbreak. The study was conducted alongside the first DENV-4 outbreak, examining simultaneous co-circulation of the four serotypes in the region. The antibody profile is crucial to understanding the risk factors for disease severity and the protective role of the forthcoming dengue vaccines.

Methods

Study population

A clinical cohort of 452 laboratory-confirmed dengue cases was assembled in the city of Goiania in central Brazil (1.3 million inhabitants) [17] during the dengue outbreak of 2012–2013. The study area also has endemic yellow fever with high vaccination coverage (17DD yellow fever) in the population [18]. We recruited cases in eight public health clinics and in one public and two private hospitals. Briefly, patients were clinically and epidemiologically evaluated at baseline alongside with collection of blood samples at acute phase of disease (≤7 days of onset of symptoms) (t0). The follow-up consisted of a clinical evaluation and blood collection during a recent convalescence at 8–15 days (t1) and late convalescence at 20–30 (t2) days after the onset of symptoms. The patients were clinically classified as dengue, dengue with warning signs (DWS) or severe dengue (SD) according to the World Health Organization criteria [1].

For the current study, dengue cases were defined by at least one of the following tests: IgM, NS1Ag and/or RT-PCR. At least one positive IgG result in paired sera was required to perform PRNT.

Out of the entire cohort, we selected the first 40 patients who were diagnosed with either DWS (dengue with warning signs) or SD (severe dengue), considering the previously defined eligibility criteria. As a comparison group, we also selected the first 20 enrolled dengue eligible patients.

Laboratory procedures

Blood samples collected during the clinical evaluation (t0, t1 and t2) were processed, and sera were cryopreserved according to biosafety guidelines at the Laboratory of Molecular Biology and Immunology of Infectious Diseases of Federal University of Goias in Goiania, Brazil.

We performed the following tests at baseline and follow-up: hematocrit, platelet, aspartate aminotransferase (16-50U/L), alanine aminotransferase (19–41 U/L) and albumin (3.5–5.0 g/dL); normal ranges reported in parentheses. For hematocrit 10 % increase in paired samples was defined hemoconcentration. The platelet count nadir was defined as the lowest platelet value obtained.

Specific dengue tests

Acute (t0) and convalescent (t1 or t2) paired sera were tested by enzyme-linked immunosorbent assay (ELISA) using Dengue IgM-capture (PanBio, Ltd, Brisbane, Australia) and Dengue IgG Indirect (PanBio, Ltd, Brisbane, Australia) commercial kits. The NS1Ag test (Biorad Platelia™) and RT-PCR (Lanciotti et al., 1992) [19] were performed in acute serum samples. All of the tests were conducted according to the manufacturers' instructions.

Reverse Transcriptase – Polymerase Chain Reaction (RT-PCR)

Viral RNA was extracted from serum samples using a purification column from the PureLink™ Viral RNA/DNA Kit (Invitrogen, Carlsbad, CA). In one-step reverse transcription, cDNA was obtained and amplified using consensus primers to viral genome region (Capsid/prM). The nested PCR was performed to amplify the products of DNA using specific-serotypes primers to identify DENV-1 to 4 [19]. The amplicon were visualized on 1.2 % agarose gel electrophoresis according molecular size specific to each of the serotypes and stained with Gel Red (Biotium, BRA).

Plaque reduction neutralization test ($PRNT_{50}$)

Dengue serotype-specific neutralizing antibodies (NAbs) were determined in paired samples by a $PRNT_{50}$

following a modified protocol by Morens et al. (1985) [20] and according to WHO guidelines [16]. In brief, the $PRNT_{50}$ were conducted on Vero cells seeded at the density of 3 x 10^5 cells/mL in MEM (Invitrogen, USA) with 10 % Fetal Bovine Serum (FBS) (GIBCO) in 24-well plates (0.5 mL/well) 24 h before assay. Serum samples were heat inactivated at 56 °C for 30 min than were diluted with MEM (1/20 to 1/2560) onto 96-well microtiter plates and incubation of 100 PFU of challenge virus. The assay was carried out using the DENV strains Brazil: DENV-1 (PE/97-42735), DENV-2 (PE/95-3808), DENV-3 (PE/02-95016) isolated in the State of Pernambuco, and DENV-4 isolated in the State of Roraima in 1982. After incubation for 1 h at 37 °C, 5 % CO_2, the medium was discharged and 50 µl of each dilution of the mixture serum/virus was inoculated in triplicate. The plates were then incubated at the same conditions to allow virus adsorption. The cells were covered with 500 µl of semi-solid medium and incubated for 7 days at 37 °C, 5 % CO_2. After discarding the semi-solid medium, the cell monolayer was fixed with formalin, stained with crystal violet and plaques counted. We considered a sample as positive when NAbs levels were ≥1:20 against at least one serotype. The reciprocal of dilution of PRNT positivity was defined based on a 50 % reduction in plaque counts ($PRNT_{50}$). To ensure accuracy and avoid inter-test variations, all of the procedures were performed by the same technician at a Public Health Laboratory Dr. Giovanni Cysneiros (LACEN-GO) in Goias state with technical supervision at the LaViTE, Centro de Pesquisas Aggeu Magalhães/FIOCRUZ in Recife, Pernambuco. The Brazilian institutions are part of the National Dengue Diagnosis Network.

Definitions

The infecting serotype/current infection was defined as follows: a) ≥ 4-fold increase in serotype-specific NAbs titers among paired sera, or b) positive serotype-specific NAbs ($PRNT_{50} \geq 1/20$) in a convalescent sample but as a negative result in acute sample. Moreover, the infecting serotype was also defined by RT-PCR in acute samples.

A monotypic response was defined by the presence of NAbs against only one of the four DENV serotypes. A multitypic response was defined as a concomitant detection of NAbs against two (dual), three or more serotypes.

A primary infection was defined by detecting NAbs against the infecting serotype in the absence of pre-existing NAbs in paired sera. A secondary infection was defined by detecting the infecting serotype and the presence of preexistent heterologous NAbs.

A sequential DENV infection was identified when there was seroconversion of NAbs for the infecting serotype and a detection of similar titers of heterologous NAbs in paired sera. It was not possible to determine the sequence of infections in the presence of NAbs against three or more serotypes.

Statistical analyses

The main characteristics of the study population were described. The percentage of increase in hematocrit and the platelet count nadirs were stratified by severe and dengue cases. Albumin, AST and ALT values were categorized according to reference levels and compared among the dengue groups. The X^2 test was applied for categorical variables, t-test to detect difference between means, 2-tailed $p < 0.05$ was considered statistically significant.

The reciprocal of dilution of $PRNT_{50}$ values were log-transformed (log base 10) after adding one (setting PRNT <1/20 to a value of 1). The geometric mean titers (GMT) and 95 % CIs were calculated. The median values of the PRNT titers (log base 10) difference among paired samples was compared using a non-parametric test of Friedman.

Statistical analyses was performed using SPSS v.18.0 (Inc., Chicago, IL, USA) and GraphPad Prism v.6.04 (GraphPad Software, USA)

Results

Sixty subjects with paired samples of dengue confirmed cases were selected for the $PRNT_{50}$ to all four DENV serotypes. The age range of severe dengue and dengue patients varied from 3 to 81 years old and from 11 to 79 years old, respectively, with a statistical significant difference in the mean ages between the groups (*t-test* = 5.26). There was a significant association between severity of dengue and hospitalization $X^2 = 6.91$; $p = 0.02$). Six patients had positive tourniquet test as the only hemorrhagic manifestation and were classified as dengue cases. Hemorrhagic manifestation was predominant among the severe dengue cases, a statistical significant association when compared to dengue cases ($X^2 = 22.85$; $p < 0.01$). When considering the platelet count nadir, the severe dengue cases had a higher frequency of low platelets levels (57.5 % ≤ 100 platelets/mm^3) compared with 25 % in the dengue group, yielding a statistically significant association between the groups. An increase of 10 % or more in the hematocrit levels was not significantly different between the groups ($X^2 = 1.60$; $p = 0.34$). Higher frequencies of low albumin levels (<3.5 g/dL) were detected among the severe dengue cases (47.5 %) compared with the control group (20.0 %) ($X^2 = 4.19$; $p = 0.04$). Severe dengue cases presented higher values of AST compared with the control group ($X^2 = 4.07$; $p = 0.04$) (Table 1).

In total all patients presented NAbs for one or more DENV serotypes. Overall, 44 out of the 60 dengue

Table 1 Characteristics of dengue patients by disease severity during outbreak in central Brazil

Characteristics	Severe dengue[a] $n = 40$	Dengue $n = 20$	p[b]
Age, mean SD, years	33.6 ± 18.5	47.05 ± 20.5	<0.001
Sex, ratio of females to males	2.1:1.0	0.8:1.0	
Educational level, years[c](%)			
≤ 8	17(51.5)	7(41.2)	0.49
> 8	16(48.5)	10(58.8)	
Race[d], (%)			
White	18(48.7)	7(36.8)	0.46
Mixed/Black	19(51.3)	12(63.2)	
Hospitalization, (%)	20(50.0)	3(15.0)	<0.01
Hemorrhagic manifestation, (%)	36(90.0)	6[e](30.0)	<0.01
Platelet count nadir, platelets/mm[3f]			
> 100	16(40.0)	15(75.0)	0.02
> 50 to ≤ 100	18(45.0)	5(25.0)	
≤ 50	6(15.0)	-	
Hematocrit increase, (%)			
< 10	32(80.0)	13(65.0)	0.35
≥ 10	8(20.0)	7(35.0)	
Albumin, (%)			
< 3.5 – low values	19(47.5)	4(20.0)	0.04
3.5–5.5 – normal values	21(52.5)	16(80.0)	
AST, (%)			
< 50 – normal values	13(32.5)	12(60.0)	0.04
≥ 50 – high values	27(67.5)	8(40.0)	
ALT, (%)			
< 41 – normal values	18(45.0)	11(55.0)	0.46
≥ 41 – high values	22(55.0)	9(45.0)	

Data are the no. (%) of subjects, unless otherwise indicated; *AST* aspartate aminotransferase, *ALT* alanine aminotransferase. Platelet count nadir was defined as the lowest platelet value obtained
[a]Clinically classified as dengue with warning signs or severe dengue
[b]X^2 test was used for categorical variables
[c]Data were missing for seven severe dengue cases and three dengue cases
[d]Data were missing for three severe dengue cases and one dengue case
[e]Positive tourniquet test as the only hemorrhagic manifestation
[f]The platelet count nadir was defined as the lowest platelet value obtained

patients (73.3 %) had NAbs to DENV-4, followed by DENV-1 (68.3 %), DENV-2 (68.3 %) and DENV-3 (61.6 %), considering each serotype per se. The majority of dengue cases independent of severity had multitypic infection (85 %). Nine out of the 40 severe dengue cases (22.5 %) had NAbs against all four DENV serotypes while seven out of 20 dengue cases (35.0 %) also had this multitypic response. There is no association between antibody response (monotypic, dual or multitypic) and severity of disease ($X^2 = 0.43$; $p = 0.81$) (Table 2).

All of the patients had positive IgG results in acute or in convalescent serum samples according to inclusion criteria.

Table 2 Characteristics of serotype-specific neutralizing antibody response by $PRNT_{50}$ of the dengue patients stratified by dengue severity

Characteristics	Severe dengue[a] $n = 40$	Dengue $n = 20$
Antibody response		
Monotypic, (%)	6(15.0)	3(15.0)
DENV-1	2	1
DENV-2	-	2
DENV-3	-	-
DENV-4	4	-
Multitypic dual, (%)	11(27.5)	4(20.0)
DENV-1/DENV-2	4	-
DENV-1/DENV-3	-	1
DENV-1/DENV-4	1	-
DENV-2/DENV-4	1	3
DENV-3/DENV-4	5	-
Multitypic three or more, (%)	23(57.5)	13(65.0)
DENV-1/DENV-2/DENV-3	3	3
DENV-1/DENV-2/DENV-4	4	1
DENV-1/DENV-3/DENV-4	5	-
DENV-2/DENV-3/DENV-4	2	2
DENV-1/DENV-2/DENV-3/DENV-4	9	7

43 out of 60 subjects were IgM positive (71.6 %); 34 were NS1Ag positive (56.6 %). Twenty-four out of the 60 patients had a virological dengue infection confirmed by RT-PCR with the following results: DENV-4 ($n = 14$) and DENV-1 ($n = 10$) with negative virological results in 36 patients. At baseline, all of the patients had serum collected within 1–7 days, except one patient whose serum was collected at 9 days (median = 4.5 days). The range in the number of days for the serum collection in the follow-up period varied from 8 to 30 days with extreme values (7 days in 1 patient and 7 patients with a range of 31–44 days) (median = 21 days). The difference of the collection dates between convalescent and acute sera varied from 2 to 42 days (median = 16 days). Fifty-two out of 60 patients (86.6 %) had at least a four-fold increase in neutralizing antibodies in paired samples. Seroconversion by $PRNT_{50}$ was not detected in the following eight patients: two DENV-1 infected cases (subjects 5 and 7) by RT-PCR and six (subjects 4, 30, 36, 39, 42, and 56) serologically-confirmed dengue cases (IgM and/or NS1Ag) presented with NAbs titers compatible with previous exposure without recognizing the infecting serotype. One patient who was 43 years old (subject 34) had DENV-1 and DENV-2 concurrent infections by NAbs seroconversion with type 1 confirmed by RT-PCR (Additional file 1: Table S1).

Older age groups presented with higher frequencies of NAbs to three or more dengue serotypes compared with

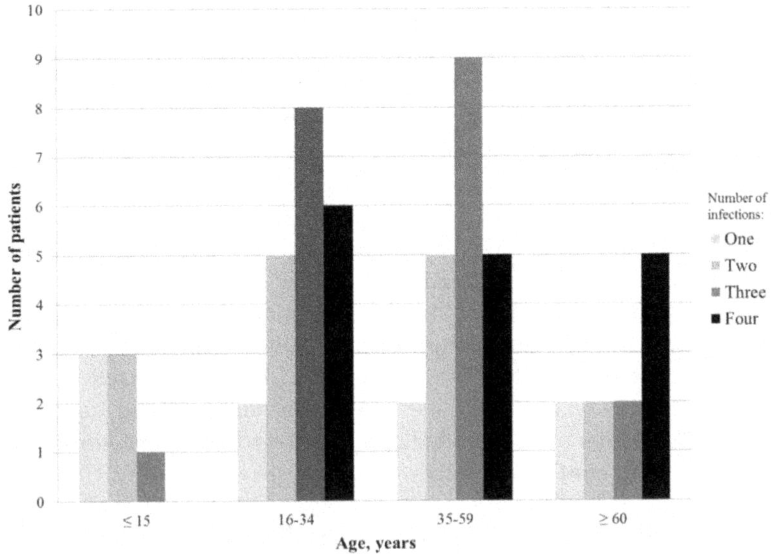

Fig. 1 Neutralizing antibody response defined by $PRNT_{50}$ to DENV-1 to 4 by age groups

patients who were ≤ 15 years old. Serological evidence for exposure to all four dengue serotypes occurred in 16 out of 60 (26.6 %) participants. All of them were sixteen years old or more (Fig. 1). The youngest patient (3 years old) presented with a monotypic response with a seroconversion to serotype 4 by $PRNT_{50}$ and had a confirmed DENV-4 infection by RT-PCR. A nine year old patient presenting with a DENV-4 infection by seroconversion had also pre-existing NAbs against serotype 3. Five dengue patients aged 10–15 years old had the following: monotypic response to DENV-4 (10 years old, subject 3); to DENV-2 (11 years old, subject 5); multitypic response to DENV-3/DENV-4 (11 years old, subject 4); DENV-2/DENV-4 (15 years old, subject 7) and response to DENV-2/DENV-3/DENV-4 (13 years old, subject 6) (Additional file 1: Table S1).

The geometric mean titers (GMT) values varied slightly from acute to convalescent sera with overlapping

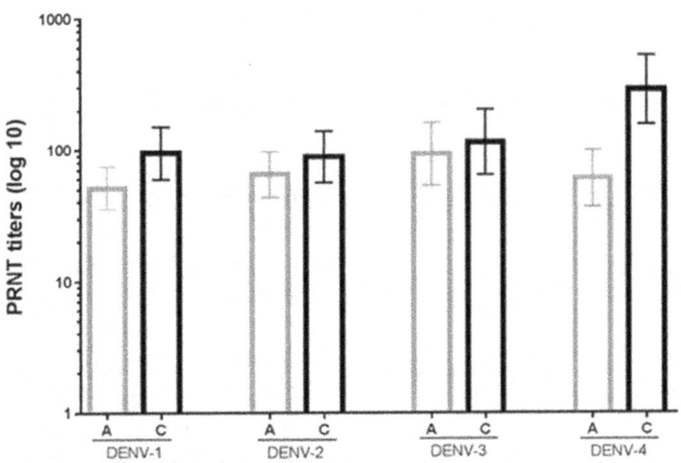

Sample collection	DENV-1(n=41) GMT (95%C.I.)	DENV-2 (n=41) GMT (95%C.I.)	DENV-3(n=37) GMT (95%C.I.)	DENV-4(n=44) GMT (95%C.I.)
Acute	51.57 (35.48-74.13)	64.98 (42.65-95.49)	92.96 (52.48-158.48)	60.63 (36.30-97.72)
Convalescent	95.12 (58.88-151.35)	87.09 (56.23-138.03)	112.20 (63.09-199.52)	281.83 (154.88-512.86)

Fig. 2 Representation of reciprocal $PRNT_{50}$ titers in acute (A) and convalescent (C) sera. Neutralizing Abs titers to DENV-4 among paired samples (*t test* $p < 0,001$)

confidence intervals for DENV-1, 2 and 3. Neutralizing Abs titers to DENV-4 were higher in the convalescent sera (GMT = 281.83; IC95% 154.88-512.86) compared with the acute sera (GMT = 60.63; IC95% 36.30–97.72) ($p < 0{,}001$) (Fig. 2). We presented the box-plot distribution of the difference between the NAbs titers ($\log_{10}$) measured in convalescent and acute samples for all DENV serotypes (Friedman Test $X^2 = 31.76$; $p < 0.001$). The difference in the DENV-4 NAbs titers ($\log_{10}$) in paired samples varied from zero to 2.41; IQR (0.0–1.2) and median value of 0.60. Our results showed that the DENV-4 infected patients presented with the highest difference in $PRNT_{50}$titers compared with the other serotypes (Additional file 2: Figure S1).

Figure 3 presents with individual NAbs titers stratified by DENV-1 or DENV-4 infected cases confirmed by RT-PCR. Seroconversion to serotype 4 by $PRNT_{50}$ was detected among all DENV-4 virologically-confirmed patients. Among the 10 DENV-1 infected patients, eight also showed seroconversion to serotype 1. Two patients did not present with seroconversion in NAbs titers to serotype 1 probably due to the small lag time (≤7 days) between sample collections.

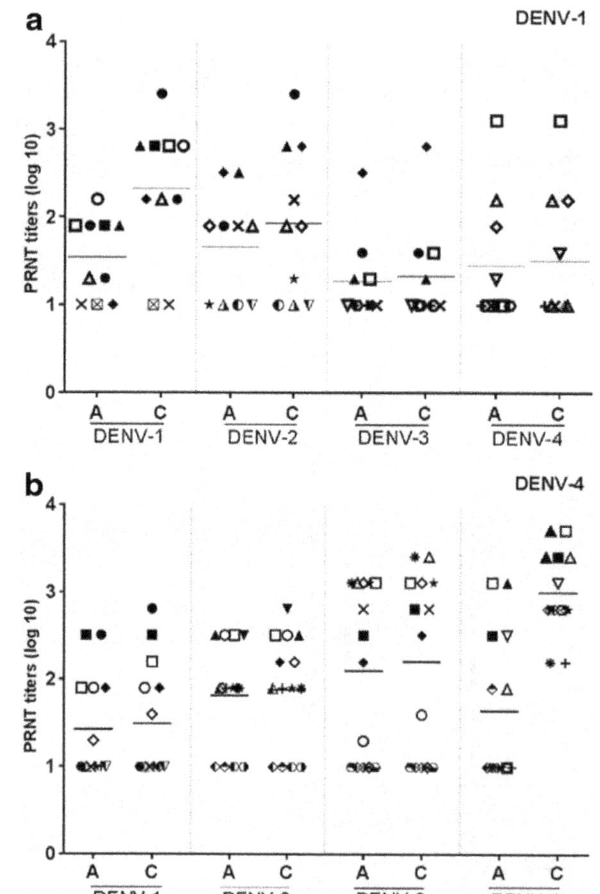

Fig. 3 Graphical representation $PRNT_{50}$ titers paired sera among patients infected by DENV-1 or DENV-4. Legend: $PRNT_{50}$ titers (log10) in paired sera stratified for acute (A) or convalescent (C) phase of disease among patients infected by DENV-1 or DENV-4 determined by RT-PCR. (A) 10 patients infected by DENV-1; (B) 14 patients infected by DENV-4. Line represents mean

Discussion

Our study showed evidence of the simultaneous circulation of all four DENV serotypes during the major outbreak in the year 2013 in central Brazil. The dengue patients presented with a high seroprevalence of neutralizing antibodies against DENV-1, DENV-2, DENV-3 and/or DENV-4 detected by $PRNT_{50}$ mainly as a multitypic response. These results may reflect cumulative exposure to the circulating dengue virus in the study setting. In our study, DENV-4 was the predominant serotype during the outbreak in consonance with the main dengue virus isolated in the same period by surveillance data [8].

Most dengue patients presented with pre-existing NAbs levels for at least two DENV serotypes simultaneously. A multitypic response was predominant among children and adults suggesting early and continuous transmission of DENV serotypes in the study setting. Our results of a high frequency of multitypic response are in line with a previous population-based study in the northeast area of Brazil (2005–2006) [21].

In the present study, there was a high frequency of multitypic responses independently of the severity of the dengue cases. Tertiary or quaternary immune responses were similarly distributed between the severe dengue and control group.

One female adult (43 years old) recruited in the hospital was classified as a severe dengue case and had concurrent infections by DENV-1 and DENV-2 according to the $PRNT_{50}$ results. DENV-1 was detected by RT-PCR, but DENV-2 was not, probably due to lower viral load of this serotype. The regional epidemiological scenario seems to be compatible with other studies that have also described the occurrence of concurrent dengue infections mainly during dengue outbreaks in hyperendemic areas with co-circulation of all four DENV serotypes in Asia [22–25] and in the Americas [26–28]. To our knowledge, this is the first concurrent dengue infection reported in Goias state, central Brazil.

Several recent studies have noted potential variations in $PRNT_{50}$ assay such as virus strains, cell linage and other test components that may influence detection, quantification of NAbs titers with possible effects in $PRNT_{50}$ results and comparability among studies [29–31] In our study, we analyzed serotype-specific NAbs titers for the subset of patients with virological confirmation (RT-PCR). Subjects with the infecting DENV-1 or DENV-4 serotypes defined by $PRNT_{50}$ had the same virological marker (DENV-1 or DENV-4) by RT-PCR suggesting the consistency of the assays performed. Our data also suggested a booster of pre-existing NAbs during a heterologous DENV infection as described in other studies [32, 33]. The need of paired samples to diagnose dengue infections by $PRNT_{50}$ limits its application in clinical settings [1, 34, 35].

One of the constraints of the present study is the small sample size. PRNT consists of a laborious technique that requires a long time to run and technical skilled personnel, which limits its use in large-scale studies [16]. Our results represent a NAbs response in symptomatic dengue patients recruited in ambulatory and hospital settings, showing a point-of care situation. We are aware that our results should be interpreted with caution and may not be extrapolated to other Brazilian regions. However, this is a timely study that characterized the dengue specific-serotype immune response during a large dengue outbreak. It highlights the high frequency of multitypic response pattern in all age groups.

This paper adds knowledge about serotype-specific antibody profile in dengue patients during a DENV-4 outbreak in central Brazil. To our knowledge this is the first evidence of multiple dengue infections in a clinical cohort of severe and non-severe dengue cases in this setting.

Conclusions

Our data indicates high exposure of multiple DENV serotypes in all age groups in the pre-dengue vaccine era and also previous to Zika virus introduction in Brazil. This is essential information for future dengue vaccines programs.

Acknowledgments

We thank all of the staff of virology laboratory of LACEN-GO, State Secretariat of Health, Goias, Brazil, including Carmen Ramos, Vinícius Lemes, Lucileis Fernandes e Marlene Camargo. We also thank all of the members of dengue study group from the Institute of Tropical Pathology and Public Health-UFG, Brazil: Mônica da Guarda, Isabela Cinquini, Priscila Teixeira and Benigno Rocha. We are thankful to all of the research staff of the Laboratory of Virology and Experimental Therapy (LaViTE), Centro de Pesquisas Aggeu Magalhães/FIOCRUZ in Recife, Pernambuco particularly Dr. Ernesto Marques, Dr. Laura Gil and Msc. Priscila Castanha. Martelli CMT and Souza WV received research scholarship [CNPq #306489/2010-4] and [307484/2007-6], respectively. We thank Prof. João Bosco Siqueira for helpful comments and all staff of Rômulo Rocha Laboratory, Pharmacy College of Federal University of Goiás.

Funding

This work was supported by the Fundação de Amparo a Pesquisa em Goias [FAPEG] and Conselho Nacional de Desenvolvimento Científico e Tecnológico [CNPq] [PRONEX-REDE DENGUE 73/2009 # 201210267000729]. C.M.T.M. and W.V.S. received research scholarships [CNPq numbers 306489/2010-4, 305281/2010-0].

Authors' contributions

AFLTA, VCRF, LAS, MTC and CMTM were in charge for the study design, data analyses, interpretation of the results and writing the manuscript. AFLTA carried out the immunoassays. AOG was in charge of clinical evaluation. WVS participated in the design of the study and performed the statistical analysis. ETMJ have been involved in drafting the manuscript and revising it critically. All authors have read and approved the final manuscript.

Authors' information

Not applicable.

Competing interests

The authors declare that they have no competing interests.

Consent for publication

Not Applicable.

Author details

[1]Institute of Tropical Pathology and Public Health of Federal University of Goiás, Rua 235, St Universitário, Goiânia 74.605-050, GO, Brazil. [2]Public Health Laboratory of Secretaria Estadual de Saúde de Goiás (LACEN-GO), Av. Contorno, 3.556, Jd. Bela Vista, 74.853-120 Goiânia, GO, Brazil. [3]Pharmacy College of Federal University of Goiás, Av. Universitaria, St. Universitario, 74.605-220 Goiânia, GO, Brazil. [4]Centro de Pesquisas Aggeu Magalhães da Fundação Oswaldo, Av. Prof. Moraes Rego, 1235, Cidade Universitária, 50.670-901 Recife, PE, Brazil. [5]Center for Vaccine Research, Department of Infectious Diseases and Microbiology, University of Pittsburgh, Pittsburgh, PA, USA.

References

1. World Health Organization. Dengue: guidelines for diagnosis, treatment, prevention, and control, new ed. Geneva: World Health Organization; 2009.
2. Bhatt S, Gething PW, Brady OJ, Messina JP, Farlow AW, Moyes CL, et al. The global distribution and burden of dengue. Nature. 2013;496:504–7.
3. Pan American Health Organization. World Health Organization. Communicable Diseases and Health Analysis. Health Information and Analysis. Health Situation in the Americas: Basic Indicators 2013. Washington, D.C., United States of America, 2014. http://www.paho.org/hq/index.php?option=com_docman&task=cat_view&gid=1784&Itemid=2518&lang=pt.
4. Siqueira JB, Martelli CMT, Coelho GE, Simplicio ACR, Hatch DL. Dengue and dengue hemorrhagic fever, Brazil, 1981–2002. Emerg Infect Dis. 2005;11:48–53.
5. Teixeira MG, Siqueira JB, Ferreira GLC, Bricks L, Joint G. Epidemiological trends of dengue disease in Brazil (2000–2010): a systematic literature search and analysis. PLoS Negl Trop Dis. 2013;7:e2520.
6. Brazilian Ministry of Health. Health Brazil 2010: Health analysis and selected evidences on impact of health surveillance actions. [in portuguese]. 2011: 157–171. Available at: http://bvsms.saude.gov.br/bvs/publicacoes/saude_brasil_2010.pdf. Accessed 23 Oct 2014.
7. Feres VCR, Martelli CMT, Turchi MD, Junior JBS, Nogueira RMR, Rocha BAM, et al. Laboratory surveillance of dengue virus in Central Brazil, 1994–2003. J Clin Virol. 2006;37:179–83.
8. Secretariat of Health of Goias. Dengue buletin - Goiás 2013 [in portuguese]. 2013. Available at: www.sgc.goias.gov.br/upload/links/arq_850_RelatorioABoletimASemanalA-ASEA21.pdf. Accessed 19 Dec 2014.
9. Brazilian Ministry of Health. Dengue cases. Brazil, major regions and federative units, 1990–2013. [in portuguese]. 2014. Available at: http://portalsaude.saude.gov.br/images/pdf/2014/julho/31/Dengue-classica-at—2013.pdf. Accessed 05 Jan 2015.

10. Roehrig JT, Hombach J, Barrett ADT. Guidelines for plaque-reduction neutralization testing of human antibodies to dengue viruses. Viral Immunol. 2008;21:123–32.
11. Simmons CP, Farrar JJ, van Nguyen VC, Wills B. Dengue. N Engl J Med. 2012;366:1423–32.
12. Wahala MPB, De Silva AM. The human antibody response to dengue virus infection. Viruses. 2011;3:2374–95.
13. Halstead SB, Rojanasuphot S, Sangkawibha N. Original antigenic sin in dengue. Am J Trop Med Hyg. 1983;32:154–6.
14. Guzman MG, Alvarez M, Halstead SB. Secondary infection as a risk factor for dengue hemorrhagic fever/dengue shock syndrome: An historical perspective and role of antibody-dependent enhancement of infection. Arch Virol. 2013;158:1445–59.
15. Rothman AL. Immunity to dengue virus: a tale of original antigenic sin and tropical cytokine storms. Nat Rev Immunol. 2011;11:532–43.
16. World Health Organization. Guidelines for plaque reduction neutralizing testing of human antibodies to dengue viruses. Geneva: World Health Organization; 2007. Available at: http://whqlibdoc.who.int/hq/2007/who_ivb_07.07_eng.pdf. Accessed 12 Oct 2014.
17. Brazilian Institute of Geography and Statistics (IBGE). Statistical series [in portuguese]. Available at: http://seriesestatisticas.ibge.gov.br/series.aspx?vcodigo=CD90&t=populacao-recenseada-residente-e-presente. Accessed 07 Jan 2015.
18. Barreto ML, Teixeira MG. Dengue no Brasil: situação epidemiológica e contribuições para uma agenda de pesquisa. Estud av. 2008;22(64):53–72.
19. Lanciotti RS, Calisher CH, GUBLER DJ, Chang GJ, Vorndam AV. Rapid detection and typing of dengue viruses from clinical samples by using reverse transcriptase-polymerase chain reaction. J Clin Microbiol. 1992;30(3):545–51.
20. Morens DM, Halstead SB, Repik PM, Putvatana R, Raybourne N. Simplified plaque reduction neutralization assay for dengue viruses by semimicro methods in BHK-21 cells: comparison of the BHK suspension test with standard plaque reduction neutralization. J Clin Microbiol. 1985;22:250–4.
21. Castanha PMS, Cordeiro MT, Martelli CMT, Souza WV, Marques ETA, Braga C. Force of infection of dengue serotypes in a population-based study in the northeast of Brazil. Epidemiol Infect. 2012;141:1080–8.
22. Laille M, Deubel V, Sainte-Marie FF. Demonstration of concurrent dengue 1 and dengue 3 infection in six patients by the polymerase chain reaction. J Med Virol. 1991;34:51–4.
23. Gubler DJ, Kuno G, Sather GE, Waterman SH. A case of natural concurrent human infection with two dengue viruses. Am J Trop Med Hyg. 1985;34:170–3.
24. Loroño-Pino MA, Cropp CB, Farfán JA, Vorndam AV, Rodríguez-Angulo EM, Rosado-Paredes EP, et al. Common occurrence of concurrent infections by multiple dengue virus serotypes. Am J Trop Med Hyg. 1999;61:725–30.
25. VinodKumar CS, Kalapannavar NK, Basavarajappa KG, Sanjay D, Gowli C, Nadig NG, et al. Episode of coexisting infections with multiple dengue virus serotypes in central Karnataka, India. J Infect Public Health. 2013;6:302–6.
26. Santos CSL, Bastos MAA, Sallum MAM, Rocco IM. Molecular characterization of dengue viruses type 1 and 2 isolated from a concurrent human infection. Rev Inst Med Trop Sao Paulo. 2003;45:11–6.
27. Araújo FMDC, Nogueira RMR, Araújo JMG, Ramalho ILC, Roriz MLFDS, De Melo MEL, et al. Concurrent infection with dengue virus type-2 and DENV-3 in a patient from Ceará Brazil. Mem Inst Oswaldo Cruz. 2006;101:925–8.
28. de Figueiredo RMP, Naveca FG, Oliveira CM, Bastos Mde S, Mourão MPG, Viana Sde S, et al. Co-infection of Dengue virus by serotypes 3 and 4 in patients from Amazonas, Brazil. Rev Inst Med Trop Sao Paulo. 2011;53:321–3.
29. Salje H, Rodríguez-Barraquer I, Rainwater-Lovett K, Nisalak A, Thaisomboonsuk B, Thomas SJ, et al. Variability in dengue titer estimates from plaque reduction neutralization tests poses a challenge to epidemiological studies and vaccine development. PLoS Negl Trop Dis. 2014;8:e2952.
30. Thomas SJ, Nisalak A, Anderson KB, Libraty DH, Kalayanarooj S, Vaughn DW, et al. Dengue plaque reduction neutralization test (PRNT) in primary and secondary dengue virus infections: How alterations in assay conditions impact performance. Am J Trop Med Hyg. 2009;81:825–33.
31. Rainwater Lovett K, Rodriguez-Barraquer I, Cummings DA, Lessler J. Variation in dengue virus plaque reduction neutralization testing: systematic review and pooled analysis. BMC Infect Dis. 2012;12:233.
32. Corbett KS, Katzelnick L, Tissera H, Amerasinghe A, Silva AD, Silva AM. Preexisting neutralizing antibody responses distinguish clinically inapparent and apparent dengue virus infections in a Sri Lankan pediatric cohort. J Infect Dis. 2015;211:590–9.
33. van Panhuis WG, Gibbons RV, Endy TP, Rothman AL, Srikiatkhachorn A, Nisalak A, et al. Inferring the serotype associated with dengue virus infections on the basis of pre- and postinfection neutralizing antibody titers. J Infect Dis. 2010;202:1002–10.
34. Guzmán MG, Kourí G. Dengue diagnosis, advances and challenges. Int J Infect Dis. 2004;8:69–80.
35. World Health Organization. Dengue haemorrhagic fever: diagnosis, treatment, prevention, and control. 2nd ed. Genev: World Health Organization; 1997. p. 1–58. Available at: http://www.who.int/csr/resources/publications/dengue/Denguepublication/en/. Accessed 15 Nov 2014.

11

Clinical and epidemiological features of the 2014 large-scale dengue outbreak in Guangzhou city, China

Yong Ping Lin[1,2†], Yasha Luo[3,5†], Yuan Chen[1†], Mart Matthias Lamers[4], Qiang Zhou[3], Xiao Han Yang[3], Sumana Sanyal[4], Chris Ka Pun Mok[4*] and Zhong Min Liu[1*]

Abstract

Background: Dengue virus is transmitted by mosquito around the tropical and sub-tropical regions. There was a large-scale dengue epidemic in Guangdong province, China during 2014 and around fifty thousands dengue fever cases, including six deaths, have been reported. In this study, we aimed to understand the clinical characteristics of hospitalized patients with laboratory-confirmed dengue virus (DENV) infection and determined the origin of the virus from the outbreak.

Methods: We have summarized the data from 138 hospitalized patients who were laboratory confirmed for dengue infection in Guangzhou city. Patients were classified as either non-severe dengue fever or severe dengue fever according to the guidelines from the WHO. Viral serotypes were determined by real time RT-PCR. Genetic sequences of the envelope and non-structural genes were amplified and analyzed from the serum samples of eleven patients.

Results: Co-circulation of dengue serotype 1 and 2 were identified from the outbreak. Patients infected by serotype 1 or 2 showed similar clinical features. Patients with severe dengue fever showed prolonged hospitalization and significant impairment of organ functions. Four samples from serotype 1 and five samples from serotype 2 were closely related respectively and clustered with Guangzhou isolates from previous years. The remaining isolates of serotype 1 were related to viruses found in Malaysia, India, Bangladesh and Singapore.

Conclusion: The phylogenetic grouping of Guangdong isolates suggests that dengue is no longer an imported disease in China. Analysis of the isolates obtained in this study together with the size of the outbreak are suggestive of endemic circulation in Guangdong province.

Keywords: Dengue, China, Clinical, Outbreak, Endemic

Background

Dengue virus is a mosquito-borne pathogen and mainly transmits around the tropical and sub-tropical regions. It belongs to the family of *Flaviviridae* and is an enveloped, positive sense single-stranded RNA virus with the size of around 11 kb. Infection of either one of the four serotypes causes mild to severe disease symptoms [1]. It is estimated that around 50 to 100 millions people were infected by the dengue viruses every year and over 100 countries are being affected [2, 3]. In mainland China, outbreaks of dengue fever mainly occurred in the southern area (i.e. Guangdong, Yunnan) [4, 5]. Dengue infection in China was first reported in Guangdong province in 1978. From 1978 to 1989, Guangdong province was suffered from several times of serious dengue outbreaks [6]. Up-to-date, all four serotypes have been identified in Guangdong province but DENV-1 is still the main serotype circulating in the area. It has been suggested that the outbreaks occurred in China were mainly initiated by the import cases from Southeast

* Correspondence: ch02mkp@hku.hk; gylzm08@126.com
†Equal contributors
[1]HKU-Pasteur Research Pole, School of Public Health, HKU Li Ka Shing Faculty of Medicine, The University of Hong Kong, Hong Kong, China
[3]Department of Laboratory Medicine, The First Affiliated Hospital of Guangzhou Medical University, Guangdong, China
Full list of author information is available at the end of the article

Asian countries [7]. Although cases of dengue infection have been identified in every year, China has not experienced any large DENV outbreak (more than 10,000 cases) since 1990 [8]. However, from July to November of 2014, there was an unusual large-scale dengue outbreak in Guangdong province. Around fifty thousands of dengue fever cases have been reported, resulting in six deaths. The objective of the study was to describe the clinical characteristics of hospitalized patients with laboratory-confirmed dengue infection and determine the origin of the virus from the outbreak.

Methods

Patients and sample collection

Hospitalized patients diagnosed as laboratory-confirmed DENV infection at the First Affiliated Hospital of Guangzhou Medical University were included in this study. Dengue fever cases were confirmed either by real time reverse transcription-polymerase chain reaction (DAAN, China), dengue NS1 antigen ELISA detection (WANTAI, China) or the IgM/IgG capture ELISA kits (PanBio) from the serum samples of the suspected cases. At the time of enrolment and hospitalization, the subject's clinical history, physical examination, hematological, biochemical and microbiological investigations were recorded. Presumed day of onset was defined from the first day of presenting fever. Severe dengue cases were classified as those who determined as laboratory-confirmed DENV infection and showed severe bleeding, severe plasma leakage or severe organ involvement according to the guidelines provided by the WHO [2]. We determined further investigation of severe plasma leakage by several criteria: 1) High or progressively rising haematocrit; 2) Pleural effusion or ascites; 3) circulatory compromise or shock (tachycardia, cold and clammy extremities, capillary refill time greater than three seconds, weak or undetectable pulse, narrow pulse pressure or, in late shock, unrecordable blood pressure. This study was approved by the ethics committee of the First Affiliated Hospital of Guangzhou Medical University (2015–8) which waived the need for written consent since virologic testing was a routine diagnostic procedure and patient information saved at the study database was delinked from individual patient identifiers.

DENV serotyping

Dengue virus serotyping was determined by real time PCR kit with in-house designed primers: dengue 1: Forward : 5'-TCAATATGCTGAAACGCGCGAGAAACCG-3', Reverse: 5'-CGTCTCAGTGATCCGGGGG-3'; dengue 2: Forward: 5'-TCAATATGCTGAAACGCGCGAGAAACCG-3', Reverse: 5'-CGCCACAAGGGCCATGAACAG-3' which were targeted to the envelope gene. Reaction conditions were performed by the Bio-Rad CFX96 real-time PCR system.

Genomic analysis

The full genomes of E and NS1 genes of the serotype 1 and 2 viruses were amplified by RT-PCR and the sequences of the PCR products were identified by sanger sequencing method. The sequences have been uploaded to Genebank (accession numbers: KT751340-KT751363).

Phylogenetic analysis

Multiple sequence alignment was performed using ClustalW software. Phylogenetic trees were drawn using the Maximum likelihood method by the TN93 model with gamma-distribution of among-site in MEGA 6.06 (www.megasoftware.net). Bootstrap analyses with 1,000 re-samplings were used to determine confidence values for groupings within the phylogenetic trees (Additional files 1, 2, 3 and 4).

Statistical analysis

Descriptive statistics for the study population characteristics and laboratory findings were performed using SPSS Inc. (Chicago, IL, Version 17.0). Quantitative data are presented as the mean ± standards deviation (SD) and are compared by non-pair student *t* test. The categorical variables are reported as frequencies and percentages following comparison with chi-square test.

Results

Total of 387 hospitalized patients who developed fever higher than 38 °C with unknown origin between the 20th of September and the 20th of November 2014 were suspected as dengue fever, of which 138 (35.7 %) were positive for dengue infection. 130 (94.2 %) of the patients were classified as non-severe dengue fever (NSDF) and 8 (5.8 %) were severe dengue fever (SDF) (4 DENV-1, 1 DENV-2, 3 Unidentified). Two patients with SDF died during hospitalization. Among the 138 cases, 107 (77.5 %) and 17 (12.3 %) were infected by serotype 1 and 2 respectively while 14 were unidentified due to the negative detection of vRNA from the serum samples.

The mean age of the patients with SDF was 62.9 ± 27.7 years which was higher than the age of patients with NSDF (DENV1: 56.1 ± 22.1; DENV2: 57.2 ± 23.6). However, there was no statistical difference between the two groups ($p > 0.05$). Moreover, the mean age of the hospitalized patients with dengue infection was higher than that of non-hospitalized patients (mean age: 40.2 ± 19.5 years, $p < 0.05$). The period of hospitalization of patients with SDF was significantly longer than that of patients with NSDF (SDF:18.6 ± 9.5 vs NSDF: DENV1 8.8 ± 4.0/DENV2 8.9 ± 3.3 days, $p < 0.05$). Patients with dengue infection commonly showed typical clinical symptoms including fever, nausea, vomiting, diarrhea, abdominal pain, rash and aches/pains (Table 1). Among the severe cases, 2 (25 %) developed shock while 6 (75 %) showed impaired consciousness (Table 1).

The laboratory diagnosis showed that the levels of alanine aminotransferase (ALT) and aspartate aminotransferase (AST), lactate dehydrogenase (LDH), D-Dimer, creatine kinase (CK) and urine protein were higher than the normal range in patients either with NSDF or SDF (Table 1). All of the clinical parameters listed above, together with levels of the creatinine (Cr) and blood urea nitrogen (Bun), were 2–3 folds higher in SDF patients compared to NSDF patients (Cr and Bun levels are normal in NSDF group) ($p < 0.05$). Majority of the patients, in both the NSDF and SDF group, showed leukopenia and thrombocytopenia, while the platelet count of SDF patients was significantly lower than that of DF patients (29.5 ± 29.8 vs DENV-1 69.9 ± 35.8/DENV-2 65.9 ± 31.2, $p < 0.05$).

The envelope (E) and non-structural 1 (NS1) genes from the serum samples of 11 patients (6 from serotype 1 and 5 from serotype 2) were amplified and sequenced. Phylogenetic analysis showed that the DENV-1 viruses belonged to two separate groups. Four samples from serotype 1 belonged to genotype 1 and were closely related to viruses from Guangzhou, detected between 2006 and 2013 (99.3–99.9 % nt identity in E) (Figs. 1 and 3a). The closest relatives of these isolates were several strains isolated in Guangzhou in 2013 (accession numbers

Table 1 The clinical features and laboratory tests from the patients with dengue infection

	Non-severe dengue	Severe dengue	*P*
Total numbers	*N* = 130	*N* = 8*	N.D.
Age (years)	55.7(51.8 ~ 59.5)	62.9(35.2 ~ 90.6)	N.S.
Sex(Male) [N(%)]	59(45.4 %)	6(75 %)	N.S.
Number of deaths	0	2(25 %)	N.D.
Days of hospitalization	8.8(8.1 ~ 9.5)	18.6(10.7 ~ 26.6)	<0.001
Clinical symptoms	*N* = 122	*N* = 8	
Fever [N(%)]	122(100 %)	8(100 %)	N.S.
Temperature (°C)	39.1(39.0 ~ 39.2)	39.5(39.1 ~ 40.0)	N.S.
Nausea [N(%)]	32(26.2 %)	2(25 %)	N.S.
Vomiting [N(%)]	21(17.2 %)	2(25 %)	N.S.
Diarrhea [N(%)]	26(21.3 %)	2(25 %)	N.S.
Abdominal pain [N(%)]	23(18.9)	2(25 %)	N.S.
Rash [N(%)]	42(34.4 %)	3(37.5 %)	N.S.
Aches/pains [N(%)]	67(54.9 %)	4(50 %)	N.S.
Shock [N(%)]	0	3(37.5 %)	<0.001
Impaired consciousness [N(%)]	0	6(75 %)	<0.001
Laboratory tests	*N* = 120	*N* = 7	
WBC(4–10 × 109) ※	2.71(2.54 ~ 2.87)	2.47(1.70 ~ 3.24)	N.S.
Leukopenia [N(%)]	108(90 %)	8(100 %)	N.S.
PLT(100–300 × 109) ※	71(65 ~ 77)	30(4 ~ 55)	0.003
Thrombocytopenia [N(%)]	102(85 %)	7(100 %)	N.S.
Hct rising [N(%)]	6(5.0 %)	2(28.6 %)	<0.001
ALT(5-40U/L) ※	47.2(39.5 ~ 55.0)	138.3(0–290.5)	<0.001
AST(5-40U/L) ※	65.8(56.2 ~ 75.5)	179.5(70.8 ~ 288.2)	<0.001
D-Dimer(68–494 ng/ml) ※	1769(1366 ~ 2172)	5114(1449 ~ 8779)	<0.001
LDH(109-255U/L) ※	279(262 ~ 297)	2743(0 ~ 8430)	<0.001
CK(10-190U/L) ※	273(210 ~ 336)	1970(0 ~ 5504)	<0.001
Cr(33-133umol/L) ※	76.9(72.4 ~ 81.3)	276.4(0 ~ 655.1)	<0.001
Bun(2.9–7.2 mmol/L) ※	4.3(3.8 ~ 4.7)	10.0(3.7 ~ 16.4)	<0.001
Urine Protein(<0.3 g/L) ※	0.4(0.3 ~ 0.5)	1.0(0.3 ~ 1.8)	0.007

*: Four, Den1; One, Den2; Three, Undefined; ※: Normal range; N.S.: No significant; N.D.: Not detected

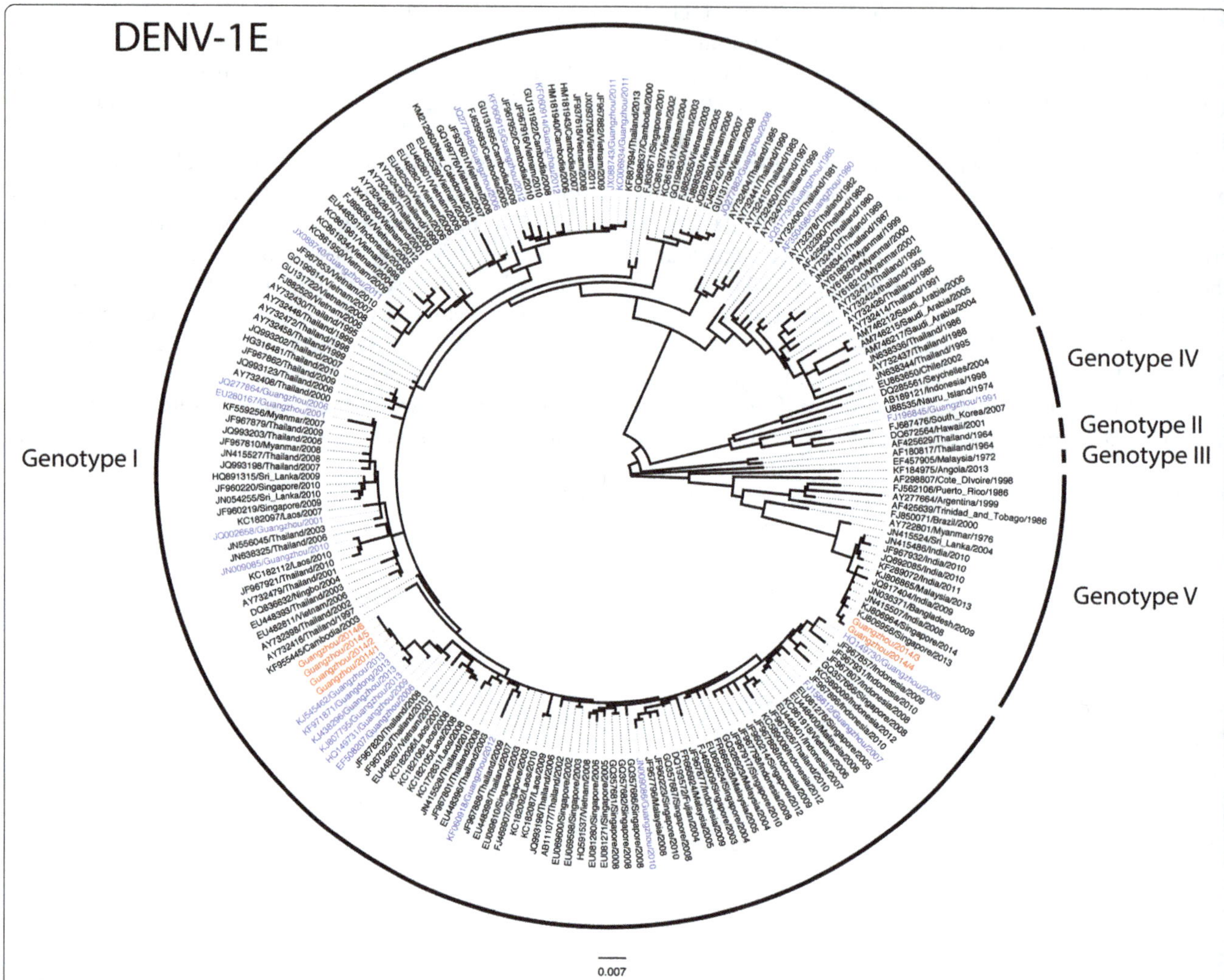

Fig. 1 Phylogenetic tree of the complete E gene of DENV-1 isolates. Maximum likelihood trees were constructed by the TN93 + G model in MEGA 6.06 (http://www.megasoftware.net). Bootstrap values were calculated on 1,000 replicates. The DENV-1 isolates obtained in this study are in red and other isolates from Guangdong province are in blue. Scale bars indicate nucleotide substitutions per site

KJ545462, KJ807795, KJ438296) with E gene nucleotide identities of 99.7–99.9 %. The remaining two DENV-1 isolates belonged to genotype 5 and clustered with isolates from Malaysia (KJ806865), India (JN415507), Bangladesh (JN036371) and Singapore (KJ806964), with nucleotide identities between 99.3 and 99.6 % nt in E.

Phylogenetic analysis of the E gene indicated that the DENV-2 isolates belonged to the Cosmopolitan genotype (Fig. 2). All five isolates clustered monophyletically with DENV-2 sequences from virus strains circulating in Guangzhou in 2001 and 2013 (JQ277886, KJ807797; 98.9–99.5 % nt identity in E) and with Indonesian strains between 2008 and 2010 (Fig. 2) (JF967954, JF968000, JF968031; 98.5–99.3 % nt identity in E).

Phylogenetic analyses of the NS genes of the DENV-1 and DENV-2 isolates supported the clustering patterns of the E genes although for DENV-2 there is no sequences available to show the persistence of the strains in consecutive years in Guangdong (Fig. 3).

Discussion

The dengue outbreak occurred in Guangdong province during 2014 is largest epidemic in China since 1990. Although Guangdong province has the highest rate of dengue virus infection among China and the four serotypes can all be found, the scales of the outbreaks were relatively small and occurred in limited areas throughout the past twenty years [9]. In GuangZhou city, DENV-1 was predominant over the past two decades but other serotypes can be identified in some years. Molecular epidemiological study showed that the DENV-1 isolated in GuangZhou belongs to genotype I, IV and V and the recent isolates are all belongs to I and V

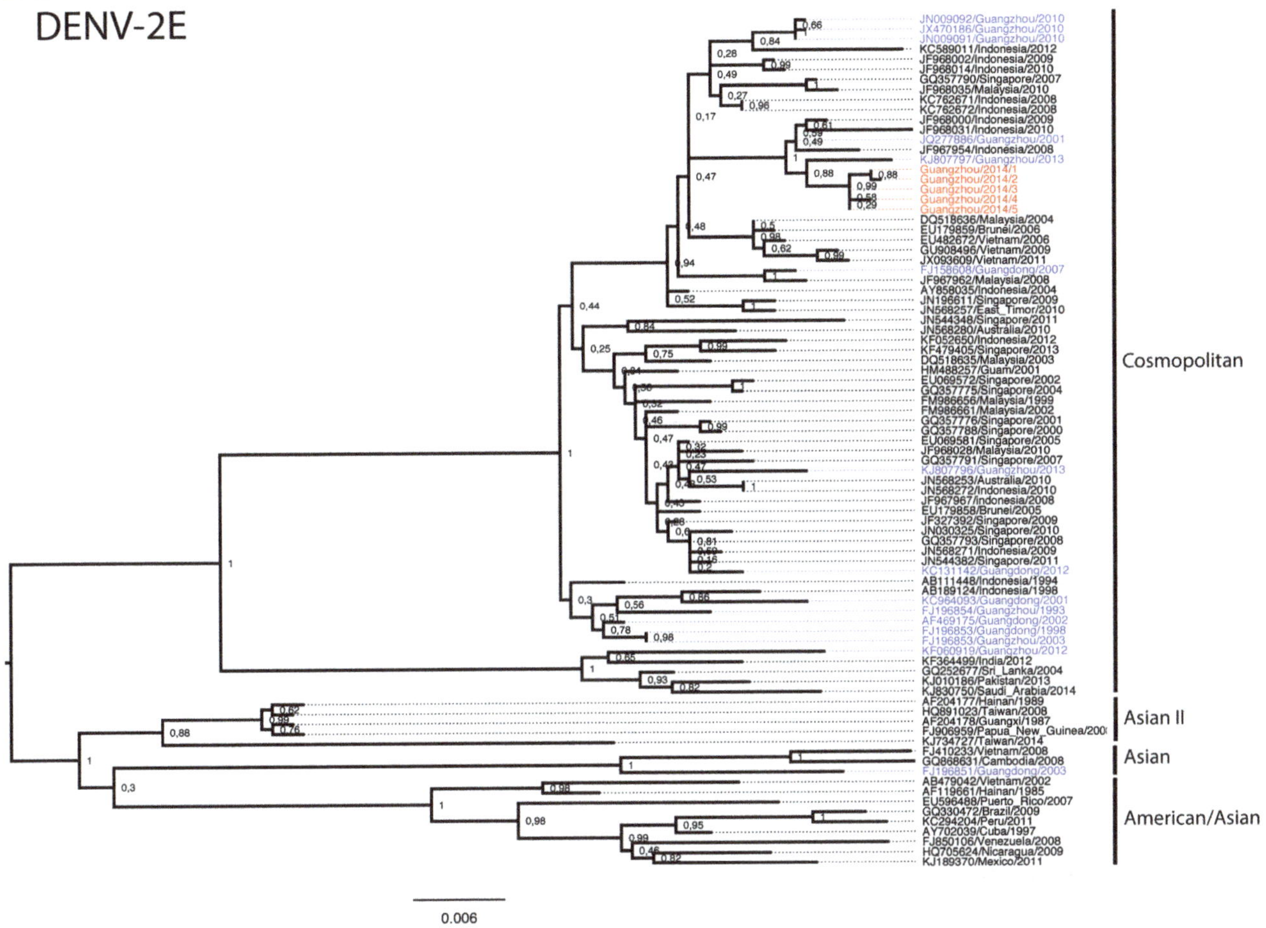

Fig. 2 Phylogenetic tree of the complete E gene of DENV-2 isolates. Maximum likelihood trees were constructed by the TN93 + G model in MEGA 6.06 (http://www.megasoftware.net). Bootstrap values were calculated on 1,000 replicates. The DENV-2 isolates obtained in this study are in red and other isolates from Guangdong province are in blue. Scale bars indicate nucleotide substitutions per site

while almost all the DENV-2 isolated in GuangZhou belongs to Cosmopolitan genotype [10].

The factors that contribute to this epidemic in 2014 are still not very clear. Although *A. aegypti* is known as the most important vector of dengue viruses, *A. albopictus* is predominant in Southern China and found as the major species to carry the dengue virus [9]. Changing of the activity of *A. albopictus* by urbanization and global climate were suggested to associate with the dengue transmission [11]. Recent study using mathematic modeling as analysis approach showed that the mosquito density and temperatures influence the development of this dengue epidemic in Guangzhou city [12]. However, comprehensive studies from epidemiology, virology and surveillance are required to further understand the cause of the outbreak.

Majority of the patients admitted to our hospital showed typical but mild dengue fever. Even in the limited severe cases, development of severe haemorrhagic manifestation, plasma leakage or shock was rarely seen. Our results showed that there was no significant difference on clinical features or laboratory tests between the patients infected with serotype 1 or 2. Several studies suggested that the risk of causing severe dengue infection is lower in serotype 1 compared to other three serotypes [13–16]. While there were only 8 (5.8 %) patients who developed severe dengue fever, most of them were older than the group with mild disease [Mean age: 55.7 vs 62.9 (years old)]. We believe that the reason of the disease progression from the SDF group may mainly due to the older in age instead of the serotypes. Interestingly, among 6 out of 8 (75 %) patients with severe dengue fever showed impairment of consciousness during hospitalization. This is a common presentation of DHF/DSS with prolong and profound shock and organ(s) failure, especially liver failure. Hepatic encephalopathy is likely to be the causes of this impaired consciousness. This was confirmed by higher degree of AST elevation and BUN, Creatinine values of SDF compare to NSDF. Other causes may be electrolyte (hyponatremia) or metabolic (hypoglycemia) disturbance.

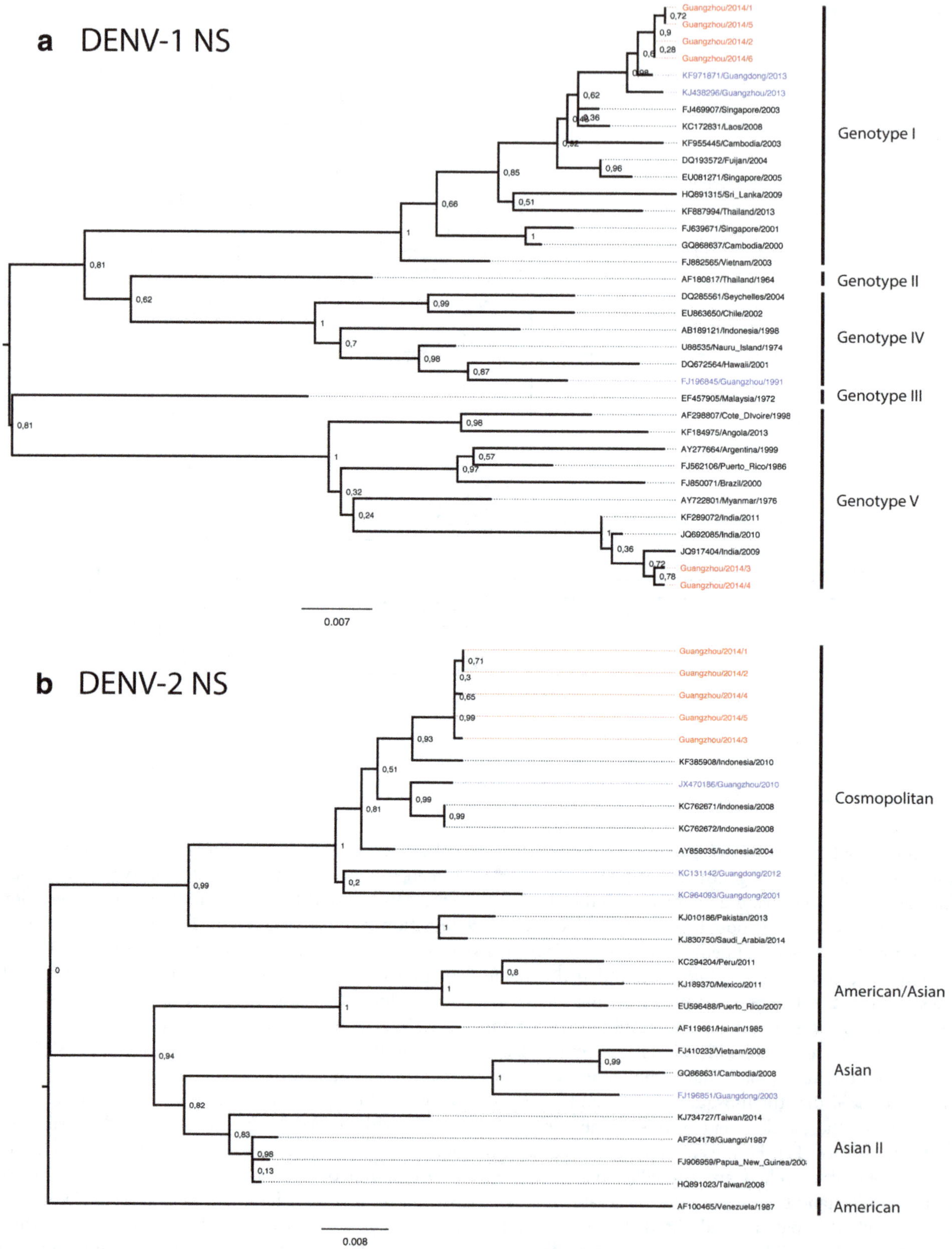

Fig. 3 Phylogenetic tree of the complete NS gene of DENV-1 (**a**) and DENV-2 (**b**) isolates. Maximum likelihood trees were constructed by the TN93 + G model in MEGA 6.06 (http://www.megasoftware.net). Bootstrap values were calculated on 1,000 replicates. The DENV-1 and DENV-2 isolates obtained in this study are in red and other isolates from Guangdong province are in blue. Scale bars indicate nucleotide substitutions per site

Some studies suggested that this clinical sign may associate to the disease progression and mortality during dengue infection [17, 18]. However, the diagnosis of impaired consciousness to predict the progression of dengue infection is needed to further investigated.

While several outbreaks of DENV in China were caused by imported cases from Southeast Asia, the size of this dengue epidemic in Guangzhou may indicate the establishment of endemic DENV transmission [19–21]. Our results support this notion since the majority of the serotype 1 isolates and all serotype 2 isolates we obtained clustered in the same clade and were most related to isolates found in Guangdong in the past successive years. Two serotype 1 isolates were not detected previously in Guangdong and these clustered with isolated found in India, Bangladesh, Singapore and Malaysia. This indicates that part of the epidemic may have been caused by the import of viruses from Southeast Asia and subsequent local transmission. In a recent report, the authors concluded that the dengue is overall still an imported disease in China [7]. The authors came to this conclusion due to the lack of Chinese isolates that clustered together in their phylogenetic analysis. However, in this analysis the authors did not include any isolates from the major epidemic in Guangdong in 2014 and therefore they failed to identify the monophyletic clustering of the Guangdong DENV-1 and DENV-2 isolates with viruses from previous years.

Conclusion

In conclusion, our results showed the general clinical features from the patients infected by the 2014 dengue outbreak in Guangdong, China. The phylogenetic grouping of Guangdong isolates suggests that dengue is no longer an imported disease in China. Analysis of the isolates obtained in this study together with the size of the outbreak are suggestive of endemic circulation in Guangdong province.

Abbreviations

DENV: dengue virus; NS1: non-structural protein 1; SD: standards deviation; E: envelope; NSDF: non-severe dengue fever; SDF: severe dengue fever; ALT: alanine aminotransferase; AST: aspartate aminotransferase; LDH: lactate dehydrogenase; CK: creatine kinase; Cr: creatinine; Bun: blood urea nitrogen; DHF: dengue hemorrhagic fever; DSS: dengue shock syndrome.

Competing interest

The authors declare that they have no competing interests.

Authors' contributions

LY, CY, ZQ and YXH preformed the experiments; MCKP, LYP and LMM analyzed the data; LYP, LY, SS, MCKP and LZM designed the study. All authors read and approved the final manuscript.

Acknowledgement

This study was supported by the science and technology planned projects fund of Guangdong province and the BNP Paribas CIB fund.

Author details

[1]Department of Laboratory Medicine, The First Affiliated Hospital of Guangzhou Medical University, Guangdong, China. [2]Research Centre of Translational Medicine, The First Affiliated Hospital of Guangzhou Medical University, Guangdong, China. [3]Department of Laboratory Medicine, The Second Affiliated Hospital of Guangzhou University of Chinese Medicine, Guangdong, China. [4]HKU-Pasteur Research Pole, School of Public Health, HKU Li Ka Shing Faculty of Medicine, The University of Hong Kong, Hong Kong, China. [5]Department of Laboratory Medicine, Guangdong Women and Children Hospital, Guangzhou, China.

References

1. Heilman JM, De Wolff J, Beards GM, Basden BJ. Dengue fever: a Wikipedia clinical review. Open Medicine. 2014;8:e105–15.
2. World Health Organization. Dengue: guidelines for diagnosis, treatment, prevention and control. http://www.who.int/csr/resources/publications/dengue_9789241547871/en (2009). Accessed 25 July 2015.
3. Bhatt S, Gething PW, Brady OJ, Messina JP, Farlow AW, Moyes CL, et al. The global distribution and burden of dengue. Nature. 2013;496:504–7.
4. Wu JY, Lun ZR, James AA, Chen XG. Dengue fever in mainland China. AmJTrop Med Hyg. 2010;83:664–71.
5. Guo RN, Lin JY, Li LH, Ke CW, He JF, Zhong HJ, et al. The prevalence and endemic nature of dengue infections in Guangdong, South China: an epidemiological, serological, and etiological study from 2005–2011. PLoS One. 2014;9, e85596.
6. Xiong Y, Chen Q. Epidemiology of dengue fever in China since 1978. Nan Fang Yi Ke Da Xue Xue Bao. 2014;2014(34):1822–5.
7. Sang S, Chen B, Wu H, Yang Z, Di B, Wang L, et al. Dengue is still an imported disease in China: a case study in Guangzhou. Infect Genet Evol. 2015;32:178–90.
8. Lai S, Huang Z, Zhou H, Anders KL, Perkins TA, Yin W, et al. The changing epidemiology of dengue in China, 1990–2014: a descriptive analysis of 25 years of nationwide surveillance data. BMC Med. 2015;13:100.
9. Luo L, Liang HY, Hu YS, Liu WJ, Wang YL, Jing QL, et al. Epidemiological, virological, and entomological characteristics of dengue from 1978 to 2009 in Guangzhou, China. J Vector Ecol. 2012;37:230–40.
10. Jiang L, Wu X, Wu Y, Bai Z, Jing Q, Luo L, et al. Molecular epidemiological and virological study of dengue virus infections in Guangzhou, China, during 2001–2010. Virol J. 2013;10:4.
11. Fan WF, Yu SR, Cosgriff TM. The reemergence of dengue in China. Rev Infect Dis. 1989;11 Suppl 4:S847–53.
12. Shen JC, Luo L, Li L, Jing QL, Ou CQ, Yang ZC, et al. The impacts of mosquito density and meteorological factors on dengue fever epidemics in Guangzhou, China, 2006–2014: a time-series analysis. Biomed Environ Sci. 2015;28:321–9.
13. Qiu FX, Gubler DJ, Liu JC, Chen QQ. Dengue in China: a clinical review. Bull World Health Organ. 1993;71:349–59.
14. Ocazionez RE, Cortes FM, Villar LA, Gomez SY. Temporal distribution of dengue virus serotypes in Colombian endemic area and dengue incidence. Re-introduction of dengue-3 associated to mild febrile illness and primary infection. Mem Inst Oswaldo Cruz. 2006;101:725–31.
15. Ocazionez RE, Gomez SY, Cortes FM. Dengue hemorrhagic fever serotype and infection pattern in a Colombian endemic area. Rev Salud Publica (Bogota). 2007;9:262–74.
16. Zhang FC, Zhao H, Li LH, Jiang T, Hong WX, Wang J, et al. Severe dengue outbreak in Yunnan, China, 2013. Int J Infect Dis. 2014;27:4–6.
17. Leo YS, Thein TL, Fisher DA, Low JG, Oh HM, Narayanan RL, et al. Confirmed adult dengue deaths in Singapore: 5-year multi-center retrospective study. BMC Infect Dis. 2011;11:123.

18. Rigau-Pérez JG, Laufer MK. Dengue-related deaths in Puerto Rico, 1992–1996: diagnosis and clinical alarm signals. Clin Infect Dis. 2006;42:1241–6.
19. Jing QL, Yang ZC, Luo L, Xiao XC, Di B, He P, et al. Emergence of dengue virus 4 genotype II in Guangzhou, China, 2010: survey and molecular epidemiology of one community outbreak. BMC Infect Dis. 2012;12:87.
20. Chen S. The origin of dengue viruses caused the DF outbreak in Guangdong province, China, in 2006. Infect Genet Evol. 2011;11:1183–7.
21. Peng HJ, Lai HB, Zhang QL, Xu BY, Zhang H, Liu WH, et al. A local outbreak of dengue caused by an imported case in Dongguan China. BMC Public Health. 2012;12:83.

12

Epidemiological and molecular characteristics of emergent dengue virus in Yunnan Province near the China-Myanmar-Laos border, 2013–2015

Ting-Song Hu[1,6†], Hai-Lin Zhang[1,2†], Yun Feng[2], Jian-Hua Fan[3], Tian Tang[1], Yong-Hua Liu[4], Liu Zhang[1], Xiao-Xiong Yin[4], Gang Chen[1], Hua-Chang Li[5], Jin Zu[3], Hong-Bin Li[3], Yuan-Yuan Li[3], Jing Yu[1], Fu-Qiang Zhang[1*] and Quan-Shui Fan[1*]

Abstract

Background: Yunnan Province is located in southwestern China and neighbors the Southeast Asian countries, all of which are dengue-endemic areas. In 2000–2013, sporadic imported cases of dengue fever (DF) were reported almost annually in Yunnan Province. During 2013–2015, we confirmed that a large-scale indigenous DF outbreak emerged in cities of Yunnan Province near the China-Myanmar-Laos border.

Methods: Epidemiological characteristics of DF in Yunnan Province during 2013–2015 were evaluated by retrospective analysis. A total of 232 dengue virus (DENV)-positive sera were randomly collected for sequence analysis of the capsid/premembrane region of DENV from patients with DF in Yunnan Province. The envelope gene of DENV isolates was also amplified and sequenced. Phylogenetic analyses were performed using the neighbor-joining method with the Tajima-Nei model.

Results: Phylogenetically, all DENV-positive samples could be classified into DENV-1 genotype I and DENV-2 Asian I genotype during 2013–2015 and DENV-4 genotype I in 2015 from Ruili City; and DENV-3 genotype II in 2013 and DENV-2 Cosmopolitan genotype in 2015 from Xishuangbanna Prefecture.

Conclusions: Our results indicated that imported DF from patients from Laos and Myanmar was the primary cause of the DF epidemic in Yunnan Province. Additionally, DENV strains of all four serotypes were identified in indigenous cases in Yunnan Province during the same time period, while the dengue epidemic pattern observed in southwestern Yunnan showed characteristics of a hypoendemic nature: circulation of DENV-1 and DENV-2 over consecutive years.

Keywords: Dengue fever, Dengue virus, Molecular epidemiology, Public health, E gene, Homology, Phylogenetic analysis

* Correspondence: zfq1968@aliyun.com; fqs168@126.com
† Equal contributors
[1] Center for Disease Control and Prevention, Chengdu Military Region, 168 Daguan Road, Kunming 650032, People's Republic of China
Full list of author information is available at the end of the article

Background

Dengue is a mosquito-borne disease caused by the dengue virus (DENV), which is transmitted by *Aedes aegypti* and *Aedes albopictus* mosquitoes that are present in most tropical and sub-tropical regions worldwide [1, 2]. As a member of the family *Flaviviridae* and the genus *Flavivirus*, DENV has four distinct serotypes: DENV-1, DENV-2, DENV-3, and DENV-4 [3]. The disease is prevalent throughout tropical and subtropical regions of the world and is the most rapidly spreading disease, with a 30-fold increase in global incidence over the past 50 years. It is estimated that 390 million dengue infections occur worldwide annually [4, 5]. Complex factors, including climate change, poor vector control, virus evolution, increased population mobility, uncontrolled urbanization, and the lack of effective vaccines, have aggravated the incidence and geographic expansion of dengue [6–8].

Epidemic dengue outbreaks have been reported in Asia and almost all countries in Southeast Asia, including Laos, Myanmar, Indonesia, Cambodia, Malaysia, Philippines, Thailand, and Vietnam [9–18]. Since the first reported dengue outbreak in 1978 in Foshan, Guangdong Province, China, outbreaks have been reported in Hainan, Guangxi, Guangdong, Fujian, Zhejiang, and Yunnan Provinces [19–24]. Moreover, DENV strains of all four serotypes have been identified in southeastern China.

Yunnan Province, which comprises 16 prefectures and 129 counties, is located in Southwest China. It has tropical and subtropical regions and shares a 4060-km border with its neighboring countries Vietnam, Laos, and Myanmar, all of which are dengue-endemic areas. Since 2000, sporadic imported cases of dengue fever (DF) have been reported almost annually in Yunnan Province, China [24]. In 2008, a reported epidemic of DF was imported from Mujie City, Myanmar to Ruili City, Yunnan Province, China [25]. Since 2013, one large-scale dengue outbreak has occurred in Xishuangbanna and Dehong Prefectures of Yunnan Province, which border Laos and Myanmar [23, 26]. From 2013 to 2015, dengue outbreaks have been reported annually in these areas.

In the current study, we analyzed the phylogenetic, molecular, and epidemiological characteristics of DENV outbreaks and their origins in Yunnan Province that occurred from 2013 to 2015.

Methods

DF case data sources

The case information in this study was retrieved in a blinded manner from datasets preserved at the Xishuangbanna Center for Disease Control and Prevention (CDC), Lincang CDC, and Dehong CDC. The patients' acute-phase sera (collected within 1–5 days of illness onset) were also obtained from these CDCs. DF case data were obtained from an infectious diseases database report that was officially compiled by the Yunnan Provincial CDC and Chinese CDC. Detailed information was obtained by epidemiologic investigations. Epidemiological characteristics of DF in Yunnan Province during 2013–2015 were descriptive with a retrospective analysis (including temporal and regional distribution, seasonal distribution of dengue cases, demographic distribution, and occupational distribution of DF patients). These data were analyzed by Graphpad Prism v5.0 (GraphPad Software Inc.). Characteristics of age distribution were compared between different age groups using one-way analysis of variance (one-way ANOVA) and Tukey's multiple comparison test. Results with P values of less than 0.05 were considered statistically significant.

Case definitions and dengue diagnosis

DF was defined according to diagnostic criteria for DF (WS 216–2008) of the Health Department of China. Criteria for clinical-diagnosed DF included a history of mosquito bite and DF symptoms. A laboratory-confirmed case constituted the detection of DENV non-structural protein 1 (NS1) antigen in acute-phase serum. In this study, all DF cases in Xishuangbanna, Dehong, and Lincang Prefectures in 2013–2015 were laboratory-confirmed cases in which DENV NS1 antigen was detected by the Dengue Ag Rapid Test (CTK Biotech, Inc., San Diego, CA, USA).

Serotype identification and amplification of the capsid/premembrane region (*CprM*) and envelope (*E*) gene

A total of 232 DENV-positive sera were randomly collected to amplify and sequence the *CprM* gene of DENV from patients with DF. Nucleic acids were extracted using an AxyPrep Body Fluid Viral DNA/RNA Miniprep Kit (Axygen, Inc., USA). Reverse transcription PCR (RT-PCR) of viral RNA was performed using the SuperScript® III One-Step RT-PCR System with Platinum®Taq Kit (Invitrogen, Inc., USA). Testing for amplification of the *CprM* gene and serotype identification were performed by RT-PCR after RNA extraction using serotype identification primers as previously described by Lanciotti et al. [27]. The *E* gene was amplified with the following primers: DENV1 EF, 5′CAGATACAAAGAG TGGAGACTTGG3′ and DENV1 ER, 5′ATTTGCTTC CACATGATGTTCTC3′; DENV2 EF, 5′TGGATGTCAT CAGAAGGGG3′ and DENV2 ER, 5′GGTGTTATTTGT TTCCACATTAG3′; DENV3 EF, 5′AGCTTGGAGACA AGTCGAGAAG3′ and DENV3 ER, 5′CCACAATAGA TTCTCCATTCTGG3′; DENV4 EF, 5′AACACCACATT CAGGAATGGG3′ and DENV4 ER, 5′CAGTGAGG TCATGTCCTCCTTC3′. *CprM* and *E* genes were amplified and cloned into the pMD18T vector (Takara, Inc., China.) for sequencing. DNA was sequenced using the ABI BigDye Terminator Cycle Sequencing protocol on an

ABI 3730 sequencer (Applied Biosystems, Foster City, CA, USA).

DENV isolation

Virus isolation was carried out in *Ae. albopictus* mosquito C6/36 cells, which were purchased from the ATCC. Acute-phase serum positive for DENV NS1 antigen was diluted 1:20 with Dulbecco's minimum essential medium (DMEM) (Life Technologies, USA) and inoculated into C6/36 cells for 1–2 h. Inoculated cells were maintained in DMEM supplemented with 100,000 U/mL penicillin, 100 μg/mL streptomycin, and 2% fetal bovine serum (Life Technologies) at 28 °C in 5% CO_2. Infected cells were subcultured 3 times and observed daily for the occurrence of cytopathic effects (CPE). Upon CPE in the third subculture, the supernatant was collected and stored at −80 °C until further analysis.

Phylogenetic analysis of isolated DENV

Nucleotide sequences were analyzed using DNAman version 6.0 and compared with sequences available from the BLAST database (http://blast.ncbi.nlm.nih.gov/Blast.cgi). Phylogenetic analyses were performed using the neighbor-joining method with the Tajima-Nei model (MEGA, version 6.0; http://www.megasoftware.net/) [28]. Bootstrap values ≥70%, calculated from 1000 replicates, are shown at the tree branches. DENV genotype was analyzed by including related reference sequences with known genotypes in the phylogenetic tree [19, 21–23, 26, 29].

Ethics statement

All participants were informed of the aims of the study and the procedures involved in study participation at enrollment; written informed consent was obtained before sample collection. The study was approved by the Institutional Ethical Committee of the Center for Disease Control and Prevention, Chengdu Military Region, the People's Republic of China.

Results

Epidemiological characteristics

Temporal and regional distribution

From 2013 to 2015, 4019 dengue cases were reported in 13 prefectures of Yunnan Province (Fig. 1), including 3122 indigenous cases and 897 imported cases. Indigenous dengue outbreaks were reported in Xishuangbanna (2013 and 2015), Dehong (2013–2015), and Lincang (2015) Prefectures, which are located southwest of the province along the Laos and Myanmar borders. In Gengma County (Lincang Prefecture), indigenous dengue infections occurred in rural villages. However, in Jinghong City (Xishuangbanna Prefecture) and Ruili City (Dehong Prefecture), the endemic of indigenous dengue cases mainly occurred in urban areas. Sporadic imported dengue cases were also observed in Kunming, Qujing, Yuxi, Baoshan, Zhaotong, Lijiang, Puer, Chuxiong, Honghe, and Dali Prefectures (Table 1).

In 2013, the first (emergent) indigenous dengue outbreak occurred in Xishuangbanna; 1331 cases were reported, including 1269 in Jinghong City (1253 indigenous and 16 imported cases), 45 in Mengla County (34 indigenous and 11 imported cases), and 17 imported cases in Menghai County. In 2015, a re-emerging, large-scale indigenous DF outbreak was reported in Xishuangbanna, which was triggered by imported cases (patients) from Laos and Myanmar. A total of 1131 cases were reported, including 1089 indigenous cases and 42 imported cases. Importantly, 1046 of the indigenous cases and 8 of the imported cases were reported in Jinghong City.

Since 2013, epidemics of DF have been reported annually in Dehong Prefecture, with one large-scale outbreak occurring in Ruili City. From 2013 to 2015, a total of 1262 clinically/laboratory-confirmed dengue cases were reported in Ruili City, of which 593 were indigenous and 669 were imported. Almost all of the imported cases came from various neighboring Myanmar cities, particularly Mujie. The following is a breakdown of these cases by year: 238 (145 indigenous and 93 imported) in 2013; 297 (139 indigenous and 158 imported) in 2014; and 710 (309 indigenous and 418 imported) in 2015.

In 2015, emerging indigenous DF was reported in Gengma County in Lincang Prefecture. This outbreak included 96 indigenous and 104 imported cases. Imported patients originated from the neighboring Myanmar cities of Gungnong and Lashio.

Seasonal distribution of dengue cases

The monthly distribution of reported dengue cases is shown in Fig. 2a–f, which includes indigenous and imported cases. Distinct and regular seasonal features in the fluctuations of both types of cases were seen during epidemic years. Sporadic imported dengue cases were observed and reported during January–May, a slight increase was seen in June, cases generally peaked in September or October (depending on the year), and then cases gradually subsided in November (Fig. 2b–d).

In Ruili City, indigenous cases peaked in September, while imported cases peaked in October (Fig. 2a). June to December was an epidemic period for indigenous cases in Ruili City, Jinghong City, and Gengma County, with a peak occurring in July, August, September, or October according to the city and year. In Ruili City, the epidemic period for indigenous cases began earlier and extended longer with each passing year: August–November (2013), July–November (2014), and June–December (2015) (Fig. 2b–d). In Jinghong City, the epidemic periods for indigenous cases were August–November (2013) and

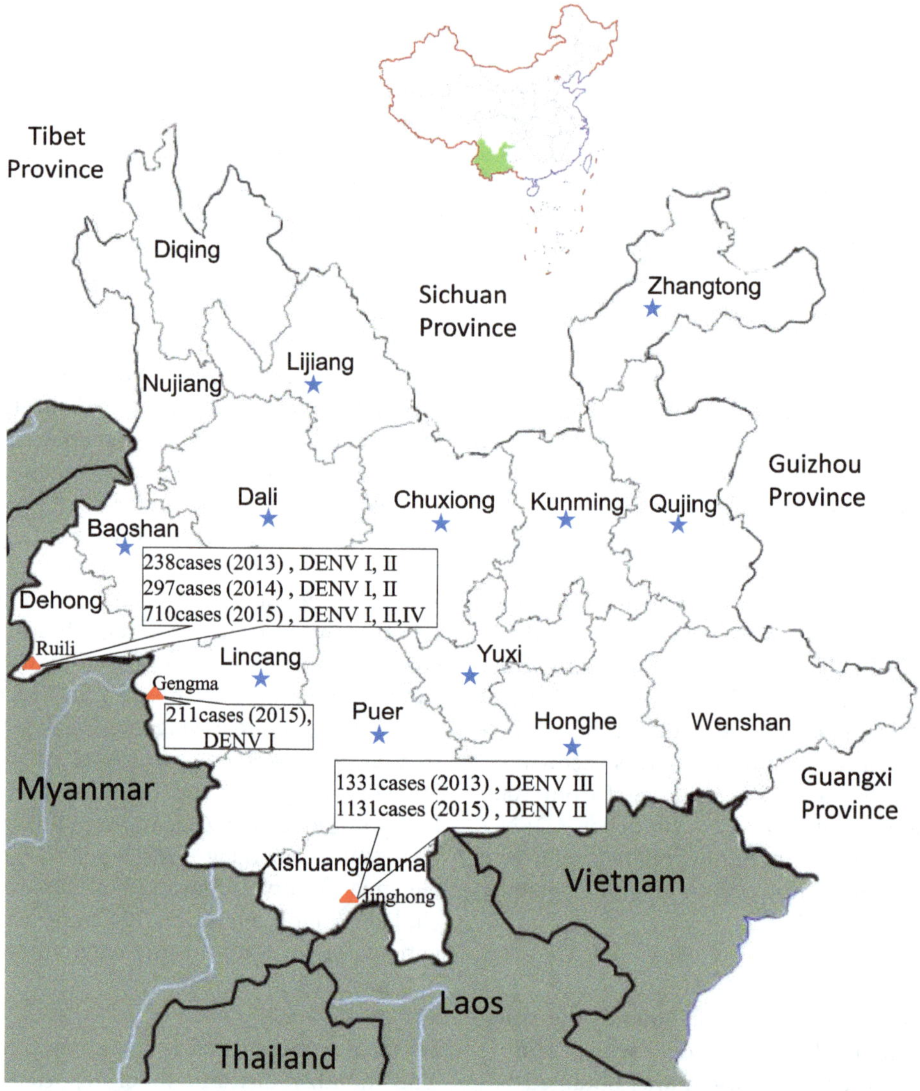

Fig. 1 Regional distribution of dengue fever cases in Yunnan Province, China, 2013–2015. The *green* region is Yunnan Province, which comprises 16 prefectures and is located in Southwest China. The cities with large-scale dengue outbreaks are highlighted using *red* triangles (including indigenous and imported cases), and sporadic imported cases of dengue fever evaluated in this paper are highlighted using blue pentagrams. The maps were generated and modified with Photoshop CS 8.0.1

July–December (2015) (Fig. 2e). The epidemic period for indigenous cases in Gengma County was July–November (2015) (Fig. 2f) (Additional file 1).

Demographic distribution

Of the 3634 DF cases from the cities of Ruili and Jinghong, 49.26% (1790) were male patients and 50.74% (1844) were female patients. Approximately 66.40% of the patients were adults (20–49 years of age) (Fig. 3b and d).

In Ruili City, 53.37% (661) of the DF cases were male patients and 46.43% (573) were female patients. The youngest patient was 6 months of age and the oldest was 86 years of age; 804 of these patients were 20–49 years of age, which accounted for 65.15% of all Ruili City DF cases. In 2013, a main peak appeared in the 30–39-year-old group; in 2014 and 2015, a main peak appeared in the 20–29-year-old group, while a secondary peak appeared in the 40–49-year-old group (Fig. 3a and b). The results of one-way ANOVA showed that there were significant differences ($P < 0.001$) according to age; the case constituent ratio (%) of the 20–49-year-old groups (20-, 30-, and 40-year-old groups) was significantly different among groups by Tukey's multiple comparison test ($P < 0.001$). There were no observed differences in age ($P > 0.05$) between 20- to 30- and 30- to 40-year-old groups, and no observed differences in the 0–19-year-old groups (0- vs 5- vs 10- vs 15-year-old groups, $P > 0.05$).

Table 1 Regional distribution of dengue fever cases in Yunnan Province, China, 2013 to 2015

Prefecture	2013		2014		2015		Total
	Indigenous	Imported	Indigenous	Imported	Indigenous	Imported	
Kunming	0	20	0	16	0	16	52
Qujing	0	0	0	1	0	5	6
Yuxi	0	1	0	0	0	2	3
Baoshan	0	2	0	3	0	6	11
Zhaotong	0	0	0	2	0	2	4
Lijiang	0	1	0	0	0	1	2
Puer	0	1	0	0	0	6	7
Lincang	0	0	0	1	96	104	201
Chuxiong	0	0	0	1	0	0	1
Honghe	0	0	0	0	0	3	3
Wenshan	0	0	0	0	0	0	0
Xishangbanna	1287	44	0	0	1089	42	2462
Dali	0	1	0	2	2	0	5
Dehong	145	93	139	158	309	418	1262
Nujiang	0	0	0	0	0	0	0
Diqing	0	0	0	0	0	0	0
Total							4019

In Jinghong City, 52.96% (1271) of the DF cases were female patients and 47.04% (1129) were male patients. The youngest patient was 5 months of age and the oldest patient was 89 years of age; approximately 67.04% of these patients were in the young adults group (20–49 years of age) (Fig. 3c and d). There were significant differences according to age (one-way ANOVA, $P < 0.001$); the case constituent ratio (%) of the 20–49-year-old groups (20-, 30-, and 40-year-old groups) was significantly different by Tukey's multiple comparison test ($P < 0.001$). There were no observed differences in age ($P > 0.05$) between 20-, 30-, and 40-year-old groups, and no observed differences in the 0–19-year-old groups (0- vs 5- vs 10- vs 15-year-old groups, $P > 0.05$).

Occupational distribution of DF patients

Of the 3634 DF cases from the cities of Ruili and Jinghong, the most common occupational group was business and service personnel (30.82%). The next most common group of patients was housekeepers, unemployed, and retired personnel (22.07%), followed by peasants and peasant workers (11.70%) and school-age children (9.41%).

Dengue diagnosis, virus identification, and amplification of CprM and E genes

A total of 165 samples were available to amplify and sequence the *CprM* gene from 232 DENV NS1 antigen-positive sera, which were randomly collected from DF patients in Yunnan Province, 2013–2015 (Table 2). Among 90 randomly-selected acute-phase sera (within 5 days of disease onset) that were positive for DENV NS1 antigen and used for *CprM* gene amplification, 88 DENV isolates were successfully obtained after inoculation and culture in C6/36 cells. These isolates were reverse transcribed by RT-PCR, followed by sequencing of *CprM* (Additional file 2) and *E* genes, and the sequences were submitted to the NCBI GenBank database (GenBank accession numbers: KX262914–KX262958 and KX056445–KX056474).

Phylogenetic analysis of isolated DENV and homologous strains reported in Yunnan and Guangdong Provinces and Southeast Asian countries

Phylogenetic analysis was performed based on the sequences obtained, including reference sequences from the NCBI GenBank database. This analysis indicated that DENV strains of all four serotypes were present in indigenous cases in Yunnan Province: DENV-1, DENV-2, and DENV-4 in Ruili City from 2013 to 2015; DENV-2 and DENV-3 in Xishuangbanna Prefecture in 2013 and 2015; and DENV-1 in Gengma County in 2015 (Table 2).

Homological analysis showed that DENV-1 found in Ruili City (2013–2015) and Gengma County (2015) was genotype I, which was the predominant genotype circulating in Southeast Asian countries. The phylogenetic tree revealed that DENV-1 genotype I showed 3 subclades and was named provisional genotype I/subclades 1–3 in DENV-1 (Fig. 4). The isolates of provisional genotype I/subclade 1 circulating in 2014 and 2015 were

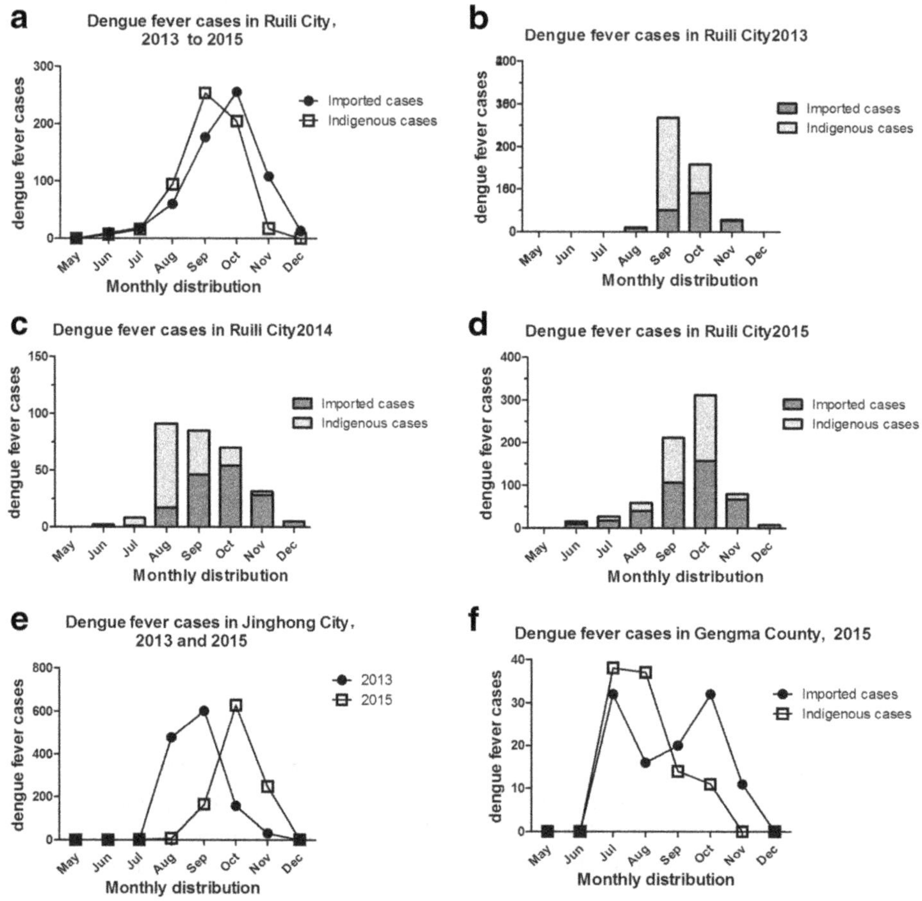

Fig. 2 Monthly distribution of dengue fever cases in Yunnan Province, China, 2013–2015. **a** Monthly distribution of all indigenous and imported dengue fever cases in Ruili City, 2013–2015. **b**–**d**. Monthly distribution of indigenous and imported dengue fever cases in Ruili City in 2013 **b**, 2014 **c**, and 2015 **d**. **e** Monthly distribution of indigenous dengue fever cases in Jinghong City, 2013 and 2015. *There were more indigenous cases than imported cases in Jinghong, thus analysis of monthly distribution only included indigenous dengue fever cases. **f** Monthly distribution of indigenous dengue fever cases in Gengma County, 2015

closely related to viruses from Thailand and Myanmar. The isolates of subclade 2 circulating in Ruili City and Gengma County (2015) clustered with viruses from Guangdong Province (2006). The isolates of subclade 3, which were circulating in Ruili City (2013–2015), were closely related to viruses from Guangdong Province and Myanmar and clustered with viruses from Sri Lanka (2009).

Phylogenetic analysis indicated DENV-2 from Yunnan Province had a different genotype. The isolates from Ruili City during 2013–2015 were categorized into 5 subclades, which were classified as DENV-2 Asian I genotype, and clustered with viruses from Thailand and Myanmar. The isolates from Jinghong City (2015) formed a tight cluster and were identified as DENV-2 Cosmopolitan genotype (or genotype IV), which is closely related to viruses from India and China (Fig. 5).

All isolates from Jinghong City and Mengla County in Xishuangbanna Prefecture in 2013 formed a tight cluster in the phylogenetic tree (Fig. 6) and were classified as DENV-3 genotype II. These isolates were closely related to viruses from Thailand, Myanmar, Bangladesh, Vietnam, and China. The seven isolates from Ruili City in 2015 were identified as DENV-4 genotype I (Fig. 6) and clustered with viruses from Thailand (1991).

Discussion

Since 2000, sporadic imported cases of DF have been reported almost annually in Yunnan Province [24]. In 2008, an epidemic of DF imported from Mujie City, Myanmar was reported in Ruili City, Yunnan Province [25]. In 2008, a smaller epidemic of 12 cases of indigenous DF occurred in Nansan (Zhengkang County) and Manghai (Mangshi County), which are located in southwestern Yunnan Province and border Myanmar, the suspected source of imported DF cases. In the current study, we confirmed that a large-scale indigenous DF outbreak emerged during 2013–2015 in Jinghong

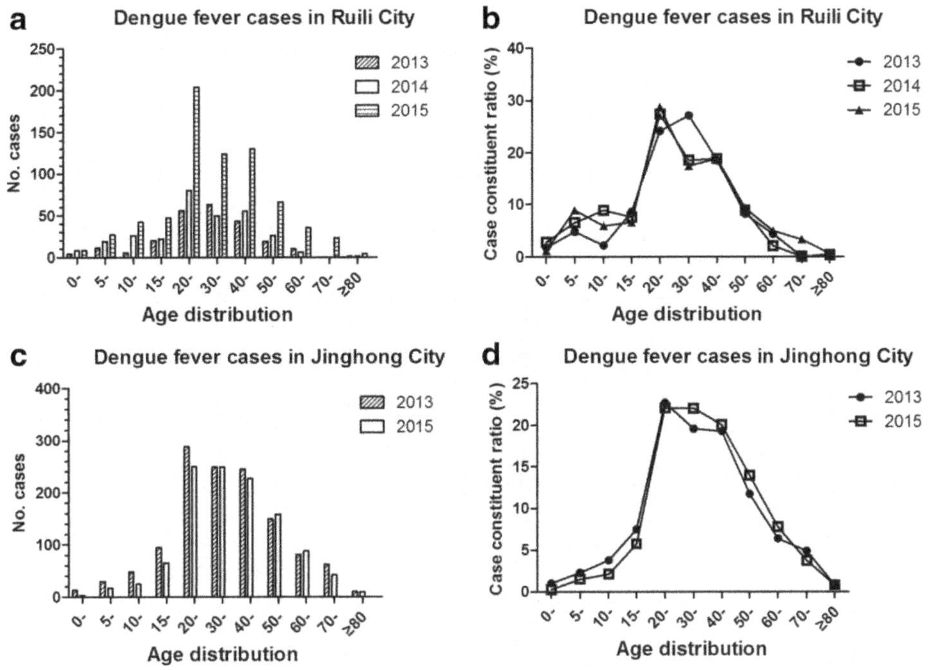

Fig. 3 Age distribution of dengue fever cases in Yunnan Province of China, 2013–2015. Age distribution **a** and case constituent ratio **b** of age composition of dengue fever cases in Ruili City, 2013–2015. Age distribution **c** and case constituent ratio **d** of age composition of dengue fever cases in Jinghong City, 2013–2015

City, Ruili City, and Gengma County, each of which share borders with Laos and Myanmar. In Jinghong City, Xishuangbanna Prefecture, indigenous DF outbreaks of DENV-3 (2013) and DENV-2 (2015) occurred. DENV-1 and DENV-2 emerged annually in Ruili City during 2013–2015, and DENV-4 emerged in 2015. An indigenous DF outbreak of DENV-1 also emerged in Gengma County in 2015.

All dengue infection cases reported in Yunnan Province during 2013–2015 were DF, and not dengue hemorrhagic fever (DHF). In Thailand, DHF was first recognized in 1949 [30]. Annually, DF/DHF cases are mostly observed in the 5–9-year-old group and the number of cases in the 5–14-year-old group accounts for 70–75% of all reported cases in Thailand [30, 31]. With respect to the age distribution of dengue cases in Yunnan Province, a

Table 2 Serotype Identification and Amplification of the *CprM* Gene of dengue fever cases in Yunnan Province, China, 2013 to 2015

Prefecture	2013		2014		2015		Total
	Indigenous	Imported	Indigenous	Imported	Indigenous	Imported	
Kunming		***2/4***[a]					***2/4***
		I (2)[b]					I (2)
Lincang					***5/8***	***8/10***	***13/18***
					I (5)	I (8)	I (13)
Dehong	***7/10***	***2/5***	***22/37***	***27/42***	***35/38***	***26/33***	***119/165***
	I (2)	I (1)	I (19)	I (26)	I (16)	I (10)	I (74)
	II (5)	II (1)	II (3)	II (1)	II (17)	II (11)	II (38)
					IV (2)	IV (5)	IV (7)
Xishangbanna	***11/12***	***1/3***			***17/25***	***2/5***	***31/45***
	III (11)	III (1)			II (17)	II (2)	II (19) III (12)

The denominator was the number of the positive acute serum of DENV NS1 antigen to Amplification of the *CprM*, and the numerator was the number of positive acute serum of Amplificating the DENV *CprM* in the test samples. [b]: I, II, III and IV is the 4 distinct serotypes: DENV-1, DENV-2, DENV-3 and DENV-4, respectively; the number in the bracket is the number of DENV serotype

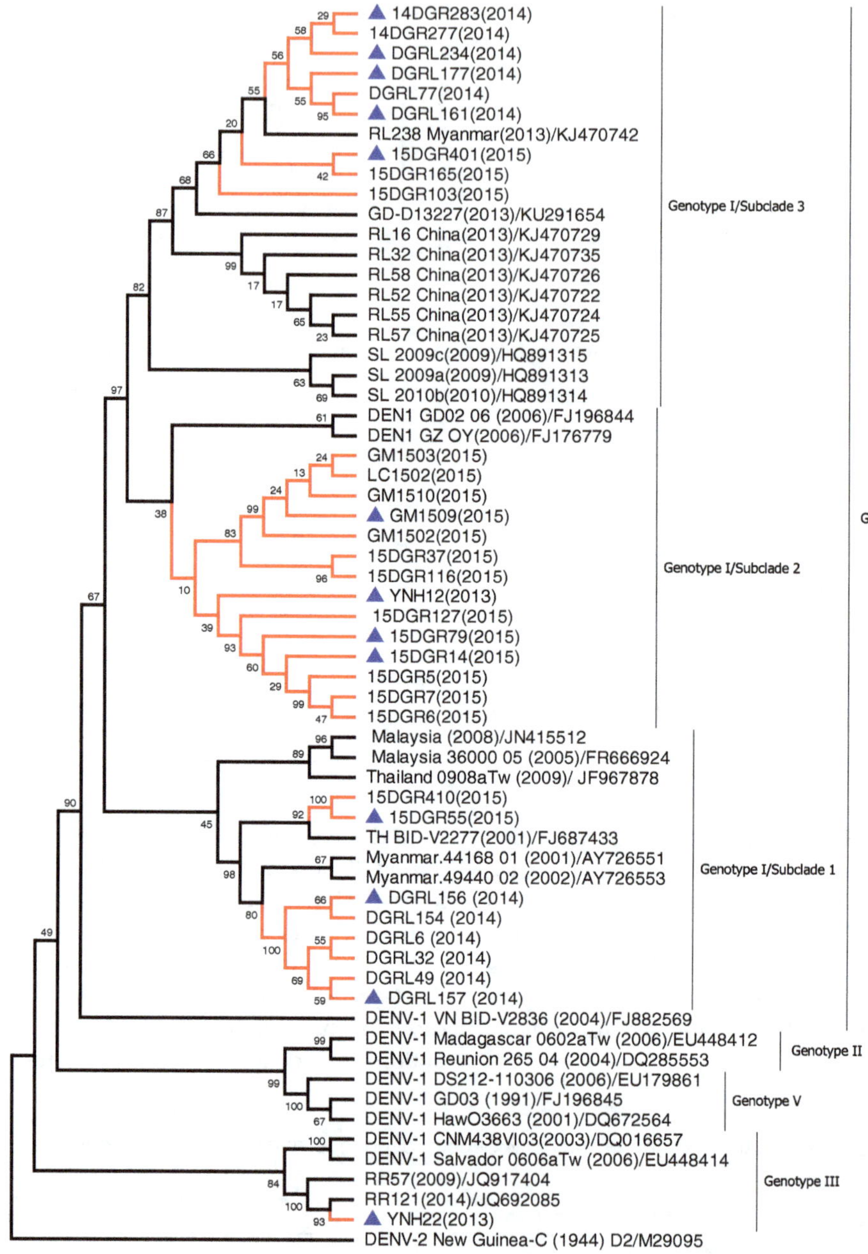

Fig. 4 Phylogenetic analysis of isolated DENV-1 *E* gene sequences with homologous strains reported in Yunnan Province. The phylogenetic tree was generated in MEGA version 6 (www.megasoftware.net) using the neighbor-joining method with 1000 bootstrap replicates. Viruses isolated from indigenous and imported cases evaluated in this paper are highlighted using red branches (isolates from imported cases are labeled with *blue* triangles). The isolates RL16–RL58, DGRL6–DGRL283, and 15DGR5–15DGR410 were isolated from Ruili City in 2013, 2014, and 2015, respectively. The isolates GM1502–GM1510 and LC1502 were isolated from Gengma County and Linxiang County of Lincang Prefecture in 2015. The isolates YNH22 andYNH12 were isolated from Kunming Prefecture in 2013

comparatively higher incidence (66.40% of all DF patients) of infection was observed in the 20–49-year-old group. In the 0–14-year-old group, the number of cases accounted for 3.89–7.08% of all reported cases in Jinghong City and 8.62–18.15% in Ruili City. This pattern differed from that observed in many dengue-endemic areas in Southeast Asian countries such as Thailand, in which children were most commonly infected [2, 32]. These results indicated that epidemic dengue in Yunnan Province has emerged in new geographic regions. In 2015, epidemic transmission of dengue in Gengma County occurred in rural villages. However, in Jinghong City and Ruili City, epidemic transmission occurred in large, tropical, urban centers and was part of the urban endemic/epidemic cycle, which is the

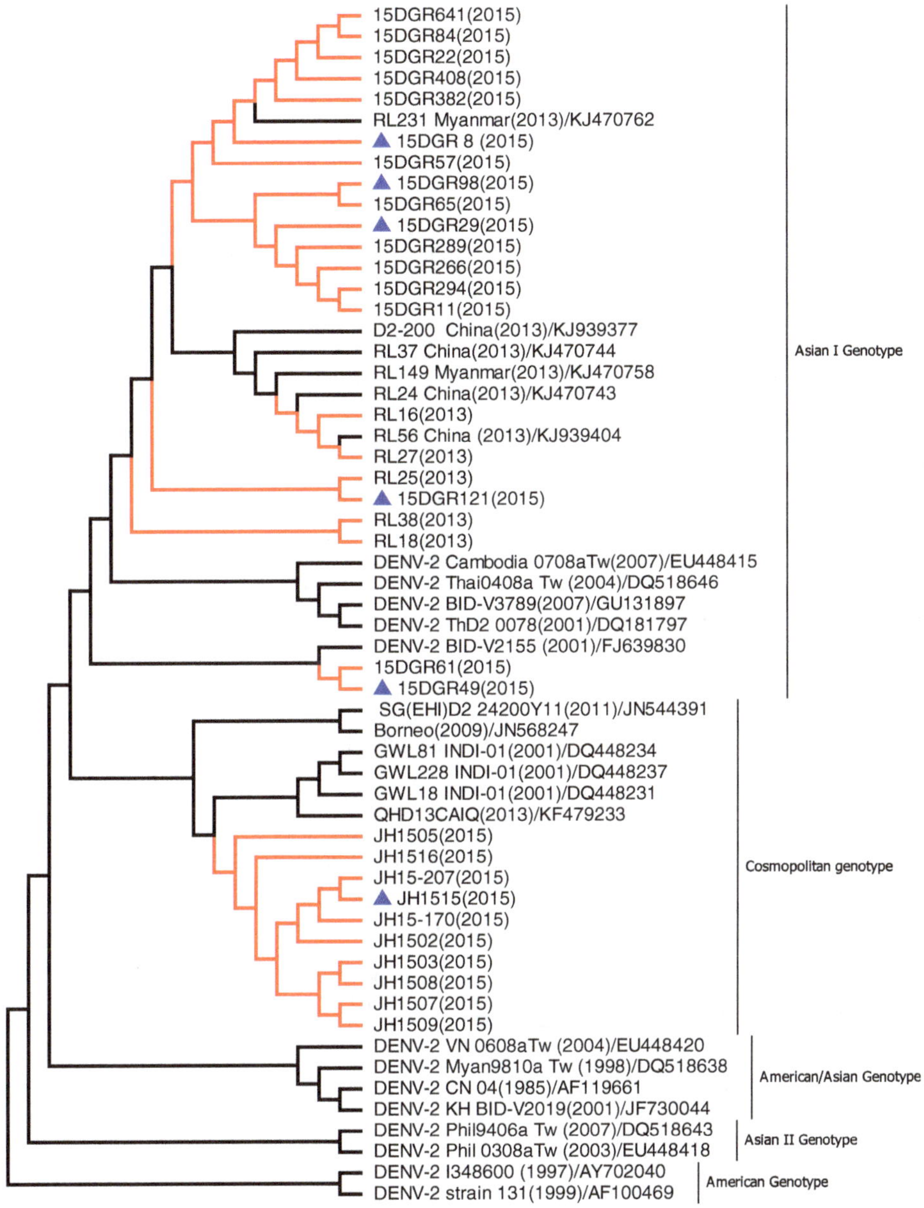

Fig. 5 Phylogenetic analysis of isolated DENV-2 *E* gene sequences with homologous strains reported in Yunnan Province. The phylogenetic tree was generated in MEGA version 6 using the neighbor-joining method with 1000 bootstrap replicates. Viruses isolated from indigenous and imported cases evaluated in this paper are highlighted using red branches (isolates from imported cases are labeled with *blue* triangles). The isolates RL16–RL54 and 15DGR8–15DGR641 were isolated from Ruili City of Dehong Prefecture in 2013 and 2015, respectively. The isolates JH1502–JH15-207 were isolated from Jinghong City of Xishuangbanna Prefecture in 2015

most important transmission cycle from a public health standpoint [32].

As four major drivers, failure to control *Ae. aegypti* mosquitoes in urban environments, lifestyle changes, urbanization, and globalization have increased the incidence and geographic spread of epidemic dengue [6]. Yunnan Province contains both tropical and subtropical regions with a 4060-km border with Southeast Asian countries. Previous investigations have confirmed that *Ae. albopictus* mosquitoes are widely distributed in the province [33, 34]; before 2004, however, *Ae. aegypti* mosquitoes were not found in this region. In 2004, *Ae. aegypti* mosquitoes were found only in the Jiegao Port area of Ruili City; by 2009, investigations of mosquito vectors again confirmed that *Ae. aegypti* mosquitoes were distributed locally around Jinghong Port (a port on the Lancang River, also known as the Mekong River) [35]. These results revealed that *Ae. aegypti* has expanded geographically from Southeast Asian countries to ports along the China-Myanmar and China-Laos borders through transport and cargo vessels.

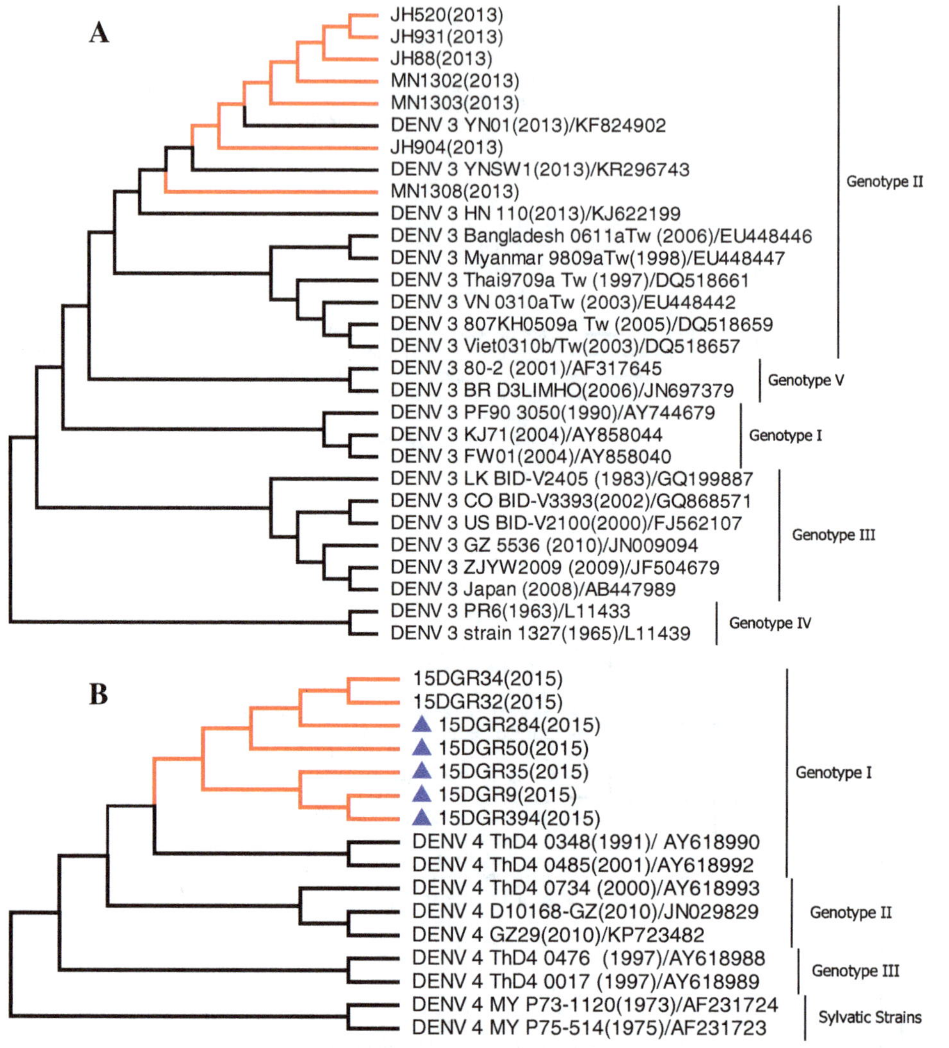

Fig. 6 Phylogenetic analysis of isolated DENV *E* gene sequences with homologous strains reported in Yunnan Province. The phylogenetic tree was generated in MEGA version 6 using the neighbor-joining method with 1000 bootstrap replicates. Viruses isolated from indigenous and imported cases evaluated in this paper are highlighted using red branches (isolates from imported cases are labeled with *blue* triangles). The isolates JH88–JH931 and MN1302–MN1308 were isolated from Jinghong City and Mengla County of Xishuangbanna Prefecture in 2013, respectively; the isolates 15DGR9–15DGR394 were isolated from Ruili City of Dehong Prefecture in 2015. **a** DENV-3, **b** DENV-4

In recent years, population densities and geographic distribution of *Ae. aegypti* have increased, especially in urban areas of Yunnan Province [35]. In 2013, investigations of mosquito vectors by the Xishuangbanna CDC and Ruili CDC revealed that the population densities of *Ae. aegypti* are greater than those of *Ae. albopictus*. The constituent ratios of *Ae. aegypti* and *Ae. albopictus* in Ruili City were 82.06% and 18.94%, respectively; in Jinghong City, they were 59.89% and 40.11%, respectively. Comprehensive analysis indicated that the indigenous dengue outbreak in Yunnan Province may be closely related to the expansion and invasion of *Ae. aegypti* in this region. Both *Ae. aegypti* and *Ae. albopictus* can transmit DENV to humans, and their presence in urban areas of Yunnan Province increases the risk of indigenous transmission. In Ruili City, the epidemic period for indigenous cases began earlier and extended longer with each passing year from 2013 to 2015. This may be affected or correlated with meteorological factors such as warming and precipitation enhancement in the rainy season, which has increased mosquito population densities and resulted in failure to control mosquitoes.

The two most common occupational groups identified among DF patients were business and service personnel (30.82%) and housekeepers, unemployed, and retired personnel (22.07%). It is important to note that residents work and live in environments that are densely populated with *Ae. aegypti* during the day, which increases exposure to infectious mosquito bites and DENV.

The emergence of DHF is associated with introduction of multiple strains of each serotype and the development of hyperendemicity in the region [6, 36]. Phylogenetic analysis indicated that DENV strains of all four serotypes have been identified in indigenous cases in Yunnan Province. During 2013–2015, DENV-1 genotype I, DENV-2 Asian I genotype, and DENV-4 genotype I were identified in Ruili City. The dengue epidemic pattern observed in Ruili City demonstrated hypoendemic characteristics: circulation of DENV-1 and DENV-2 over consecutive years. Multiple strains of each serotype were introduced, which may increase the risks of DHF emergence in Ruili City. All isolates from Xishuangbanna Prefecture in 2013 were classified as DENV-3 genotype II and isolates in 2015 were classified as DENV-2 Cosmopolitan genotype (or genotype IV). Fortunately, DENV-3 genotype II and DENV-2 Asian I genotype were not detected in dengue cases from Xishuangbanna Prefecture in 2015.

Conclusions

The present study suggested that multiple DENV serotypes are endemic in countries bordering Yunnan Province such as Laos, Thailand, and Myanmar. Imported DF patients from Laos and Myanmar were the primary cause of DF epidemics in Yunnan Province, and *Ae. aegypti* and *Ae. albopictus* remain widely distributed in urban regions of the tropics. These factors increase the risk of indigenous dengue transmission and indigenous DF epidemics or pandemics in Yunnan Province. Such evidence indicated that Ruili City is increasingly exhibiting features of an endemic area, as suggested by sustained DENV and the co-existence of multiple serotypes in this area. To prevent future dengue outbreaks and the spread of disease to other regions, joint dengue prevention and control measures should be strengthened in the China-Myanmar and China-Laos border regions of Yunnan Province. In particular, a sound laboratory-based disease surveillance system of imported patients and integrated vector control management are required in both of these regions.

Abbreviations

CDC: Center for Disease Control and Prevention; CPE: Cytopathic effects; CprM: Capsid/premembrane region; DENV: Dengue virus; DF: Dengue fever; DHF: Dengue hemorrhagic fever; E: Envelope

Funding

This work was financially sponsored by the National Key Basic Research Program of China (2016YFC1200100), the Key Programs (nos. BWS14J025 and AWS11L009), the Science and Technology Programs of Military (nos. 15QNP035 and CWS12J075), the General Financial Grant (nos. 2015 M582907 and 2016 T91009) from the China Postdoctoral Science Foundation, and the Youth Fund Program (no. 81101618) from the National Natural Science Foundation of China.

Authors' contributions

F-QZ and Q-SF are co-corresponding authors, who conceived and designed the research. T-SH and H-LZ wrote and revised the manuscript. T-SH, TT, LZ, GC, and JY performed the experiments. H-LZ, YF, J-HF, JZ, H-BL, Y-YL, Y-HL, X-XY, and H-CL performed sample collections and prepared figures. All authors read and approved the final manuscript.

Competing interests

The authors declare that they have no competing interests.

Consent to publication

Not applicable.

Author details

[1]Center for Disease Control and Prevention, Chengdu Military Region, 168 Daguan Road, Kunming 650032, People's Republic of China. [2]Yunnan Institute of Endemic Diseases Control and Prevention, Dali, Yunnan, People's Republic of China. [3]Xishuangbanna Center for Disease Control and Prevention, Jinghong, Yunnan, People's Republic of China. [4]Ruili Center for Disease Control and Prevention, Ruili, Yunnan, People's Republic of China. [5]Lincang Center for Disease Control and Prevention, Lincang, Yunnan, People's Republic of China. [6]The Postdoctoral Programme of Kunming General Hospital, Chengdu Military Region, Kunming, People's Republic of China.

References

1. Kraemer MU, Sinka ME, Duda KA, Mylne AQ, Shearer FM, Barker CM, Moore CG, Carvalho RG, Coelho GE, Van Bortel W, et al. The global distribution of the arbovirus vectors *Aedes aegypti* and Ae albopictus. elife. 2015;4:e08347.
2. WHO: Geneva. Dengue: Guidelines for Diagnosis, Treatment, Prevention and Control: New Edition. WHO and the Special Programme for Research and Training in Tropical Diseases 2009:3–16.
3. Wang E, Ni H, Xu R, Barrett AD, Watowich SJ, Gubler DJ, Weaver SC. Evolutionary relationships of endemic/epidemic and sylvatic dengue viruses. J Virol. 2000;74(7):3227–34.
4. Bhatt S, Gething PW, Brady OJ, Messina JP, Farlow AW, Moyes CL, Drake JM, Brownstein JS, Hoen AG, Sankoh O, et al. The global distribution and burden of dengue. Nature. 2013;496(7446):504–7.
5. Massad E, Coutinho FA. The cost of dengue control. Lancet. 2011; 377(9778):1630–1.
6. Gubler DJ. Dengue, Urbanization and Globalization: The Unholy Trinity of the 21(st) Century. Trop Med Health. 2011;39(4 Suppl):3–11.
7. Wilder-Smith A, Gubler DJ. Geographic expansion of dengue: the impact of international travel. Med Clin N Amer. 2008;92(6):1377–90. x
8. Wilder-Smith A, Schwartz E. Dengue in travelers. N Engl J Med. 2005; 353(9):924–32.
12. Malla S, Thakur GD, Shrestha SK, Banjeree MK, Thapa LB, Gongal G, Ghimire P, Upadhyay BP, Gautam P, Khanal S, et al. Identification of all dengue serotypes in Nepal. Emerg Infect Dis. 2008;14(10):1669–70.
13. Thant KZ, Tun MM, Parquet Mdel C, Inoue S, Lwin YY, Lin S, Aye KT, Khin PT, Myint T, Htwe K, et al. Molecular Epidemiology of Dengue Viruses Co-circulating in Upper Myanmar in 2006. Trop Med Health. 2015;43(1):21–7.
14. Trent DW, Grant JA, Monath TP, Manske CL, Corina M, Fox GE. Genetic variation and microevolution of dengue 2 virus in Southeast Asia. Virology. 1989;172(2):523–35.
15. Nguyen NH, Tran VB, Morris GE. Nucleotide sequences from the capsid and pre-protein regions of dengue viruses from Vietnam. Biochem Soc Trans. 1997;25(1):54S.
16. Russell PK, Van Quy D, Nisalak A, Simasathien P, Yuill TM, Gould DJ. Mosquito vectors of dengue viruses in South Vietnam. AmJTrop Med Hyg. 1969;18(3):455–9.
17. Dubot-Peres A, Vongphrachanh P, Denny J, Phetsouvanh R, Linthavong S, Sengkeopraseuth B, Khasing A, Xaythideth V, Moore CE, Vongsouvath M, et al. An epidemic of dengue-1 in a remote village in rural Laos. PLoS Negl Trop Dis. 2013;7(8):e2360.

18. Vu TT, Holmes EC, Duong V, Nguyen TQ, Tran TH, Quail M, Churcher C, Parkhill J, Cardosa J, Farrar J, et al. Emergence of the Asian 1 genotype of dengue virus serotype 2 in viet nam: in vivo fitness advantage and lineage replacement in South-East Asia. PLoS Negl Trop Dis. 2010;4(7):e757.
19. Jing QL, Yang ZC, Luo L, Xiao XC, Di B, He P, Fu CX, Wang M, Lu JH. Emergence of dengue virus 4 genotype II in Guangzhou, China, 2010: survey and molecular epidemiology of one community outbreak. BMC Infect Dis. 2012;12:87.
20. Luo L, Liang HY, Hu YS, Liu WJ, Wang YL, Jing QL, Zheng XL, Yang ZC. Epidemiological, virological, and entomological characteristics of dengue from 1978 to 2009 in Guangzhou, China. J Vector Ecol. 2012;37(1):230–40.
21. Shen SQ, Wei HX, Fu YH, Zhang H, Mo QY, Wang XJ, Deng SQ, Zhao W, Liu Y, Feng XS, et al. Multiple Sources of Infection and Potential Endemic Characteristics of the Large Outbreak of Dengue in Guangdong in 2014. Sci Rep. 2015;5:16913.
22. Wang B, Li Y, Feng Y, Zhou H, Liang Y, Dai J, Qin W, Hu Y, Wang Y, Zhang L, et al. Phylogenetic analysis of dengue virus reveals the high relatedness between imported and local strains during the 2013 dengue outbreak in Yunnan, China: a retrospective analysis. BMC Infect Dis. 2015;15:142.
23. Wang B, Yang H, Feng Y, Zhou H, Dai J, Hu Y, Zhang L, Wang Y, Baloch Z, Xia X. The distinct distribution and phylogenetic characteristics of dengue virus serotypes/genotypes during the 2013 outbreak in Yunnan, China: Phylogenetic characteristics of 2013 dengue outbreak in Yunnan, China. Infect Genet Evol. 2016;37:1–7.
24. Wu JY, Lun ZR, James AA, Chen XG. Dengue Fever in mainland China. AmJTrop Med Hyg. 2010;83(3):664–71.
25. Zhang HL, Fu SH, Deng Z, Yuan J, Jiang HY, Li MH, Gao XY, Wang JL, Liu YH, Yin ZL, et al. An outbreak of imported dengue fever from Myanmar to the border of China, with its viral molecular epidemiological features. Zhonghua liu xing bing xue za zhi. 2013;34(5):428–32.
26. Guo X, Yang H, Wu C, Jiang J, Fan J, Li H, Zhu J, Yang Z, Li Y, Zhou H, et al. Molecular Characterization and Viral Origin of the First Dengue Outbreak in Xishuangbanna, Yunnan Province, China, 2013. AmJTrop Med Hyg. 2015; 93(2):390–3.
27. Lanciotti RS, Calisher CH, Gubler DJ, Chang GJ, Vorndam AV. Rapid detection and typing of dengue viruses from clinical samples by using reverse transcriptase-polymerase chain reaction. J Clin Microbiol. 1992;30(3):545–51.
28. Tamura K, Stecher G, Peterson D, Filipski A, Kumar S. MEGA6: Molecular Evolutionary Genetics Analysis version 6.0. Mol Biol Evol. 2013;30(12):2725–9.
29. Chew MH, Rahman MM, Hussin S. Molecular epidemiology and phylogenetic analysis of Dengue virus type-1 and 2 isolated in Malaysia. Pak J Med Sci. 2015;31(3):615–20.
30. Yongyuth W. Dengue Control through Schoolchildren in Thailand. Dengue Bull. 1997;21:52–65.
31. WHO and the Special Programme for Research and Training in Tropical Diseases. Dengue guidelines for diagnosis, treatment, prevention and control: new edition[R]. Geneva: WHO; 2009. pp. 3-16.
32. Gubler DJ. Dengue and dengue hemorrhagic fever. Clin Microbiol Rev. 1998;11(3):480–96.
33. Wang Piyu WC, Canglin Z. Survey of transmission vectors of dengue fever in some areas in Yunnan Province, China. Trop Med. 2006;6(11):1933–4. (in Chinese)
34. Zhang Hailin ZD, Zhuqing M, et al. Characterized distribution of *Aedes albopictus* and their relation with arbovirus in Yunnan Province. Chin J Vector Biol Control. 2001;12(2):103–5. (in Chinese)
35. Yang Mingdong JJ, Yu-ting Z, Hongning Z. Distribution survey on *Aedes aegypti* in the border areas of Yunnan province, China. Chin J Vector Biol Control. 2015;26(4):406–8. (in Chinese)
36. Gubler DJ, Trent DW. Emergence of epidemic dengue/dengue hemorrhagic fever as a public health problem in the Americas. Infect Agents Dis. 1993;2(6):383–93.

13

A household-based survey of knowledge, attitudes and practices towards dengue fever among local urban communities in Taiz Governorate, Yemen

Thaker A. A. Alyousefi[1], Rashad Abdul-Ghani[2,3], Mohammed A. K. Mahdy[2,3*], Samira M. A. Al-Eryani[2], Abdulsalam M. Al-Mekhlafi[2], Yahia A. Raja[4], Shamusul Azhar Shah[5] and John C. Beier[6]

Abstract

Background: Yemen has witnessed several dengue fever outbreaks coincident with the social unrest and war in the country. The aim of the present study was to describe the knowledge, attitudes and practices (KAPs) of at-risk urban populations residing in Taiz, southwest of Yemen. In addition, factors possibly associated with poor preventive practices were investigated.

Methods: A household-based, cross-sectional survey was conducted in three urban districts encompassing 383 households. Data on the socio-demographic characteristics and KAPs of the participating household heads were collected using a pre-designed, structured questionnaire. The association of socio-demographic characteristics, knowledge and attitudes of the population with poor preventive practices against dengue fever was then analyzed using logistic regression.

Results: More than 90.0 % of respondent household heads had correct knowledge about fever, headache and joint pain as common signs and symptoms of dengue fever. Moreover, muscular pain and bleeding were perceived by more than 80.0 % of the respondents as being associated with dengue fever; however, only 65.0 % of the respondents reported skin rash as a sign of dengue fever. More than 95.0 % of respondents agreed about the seriousness and possible transmission of dengue fever; however, negative attitudes regarding the facts of being at risk of the disease and that the infection is preventable were expressed by 15.0 % of respondents. Despite the good level of knowledge and attitudes of the respondent population, poor preventive practices were common. Bivariate analysis identified poor knowledge of dengue signs and symptoms (OR = 2.1, 95 % CI = 1.24–3.68; $P = 0.005$) and its vector (OR = 2.1, 95 % CI = 1.14–3.84; $P = 0.016$) as factors significantly associated with poor preventive practices. However, multivariable analysis showed that poor knowledge of the vector is an independent predictor of poor preventive practices of the population (adjusted OR = 2.1, 95 % CI = 1.14–3.84; $P = 0.018$).

(Continued on next page)

* Correspondence: alsharaby9@yahoo.com
Department of Parasitology, Faculty of Medicine and Health Sciences, Sana'a University, Sana'a, Yemen
Tropical Disease Research Center, University of Science and Technology, Sana'a, Yemen
Full list of author information is available at the end of the article

(Continued from previous page)

Conclusion: The majority of people in urban communities of Taiz have a clear understanding of most signs/symptoms of dengue fever as well as positive attitudes towards the seriousness and possible transmissibility of dengue fever. However, negative attitudes regarding their perception of the risk and possible prevention of the infection are prevailing among a small proportion of the population and need to be targeted by educational campaigns. It appears that the good level of the population knowledge of the signs/symptoms of dengue fever and the factors contributing to the spread and control of its vectors did not translate into good practices.

Keywords: Dengue fever, Knowledge, Attitude, Practice, Taiz, Yemen

Background

Dengue fever is a systemic arboviral disease caused by the dengue virus and transmitted by infected female *Aedes* mosquitoes, mainly *Ae. aegypti* (primary vector) [1]. Infections can also be transmitted through blood transfusion, organ transplantation and possibly vertically from mother to child [2–6]. Although infection with dengue virus may be asymptomatic [7, 8], it may lead to a wide spectrum disease that ranges from non-severe fever to potentially fatal clinical manifestations [1]. Globally, 294 million inapparent and 96 million apparent dengue infections were estimated in 2010 [7]. Dengue virus has five serotypes [9], and infection with a certain serotype usually confers a lifelong serotype-specific immunity, but a temporary immunity to other serotypes [10, 11]. Moreover, more frequent and severe complications can occur in subsequent infection with a different serotype [10, 11]. Due to the absence of effective antiviral agents [1, 12], efforts focus on interrupting human-vector contact through targeting the adult vector and its immature stages by eliminating its breeding habitats in and near households [1]. Nevertheless, the incidence of dengue fever epidemics is escalating, and its endemic transmission expands to a wider geographical range [7]. It is noteworthy that the recombinant live-attenuated tetravalent dengue vaccine (CYD-TDV), commercially known as Dengvaxia®, was the first licensed vaccine against dengue, given as three doses at 0, 6 and 12 months [13]; however, its pooled efficacy over 25 months from the first dose was reported to be 65.6 % based on data derived from Phase 3 clinical trials from endemic countries in Asia and Latin America, with varying degrees of protection according to the virus serotype, age, disease severity and serostatus at vaccination [14]. Therefore, the Strategic Advisory Group of Experts on Immunization recommends the introduction of CYD-TDV only in high-endemicity settings, after careful assessment, where seroprevalence rates of the virus are 70 % or greater in the age group to be targeted by vaccination [15].

Dengue fever is a preventable infection, and success of dengue control depends largely on good knowledge, attitudes and practices (KAPs) of targeted communities towards the disease and its preventive measures. Community involvement after educational campaigns could be an effective approach to the prevention and control of dengue. In line with this view, it has been shown that community education could be more effective than insecticide spraying alone in reducing mosquito breeding habitats [16].

In 2003, AlHoot [17] reported IgG and IgM seronegativity for dengue fever among febrile and apparently healthy individuals from different localities in Yemen. Despite the increasing outbreaks of dengue fever in Yemen, very few studies have been published to document these outbreaks. Dengue fever outbreaks caused by dengue virus serotype 3 were reported in Al-Mukalla city, east of Yemen [18, 19]. Moreover, a case of imported dengue virus serotype 3 was also reported from an Italian man returning from a locality near Al-Mukalla in 2010 [20]. In Hodeidah, west of Yemen, 29.0 % (116/400) of hospitalized patients with fever and, at least, two signs or symptoms of dengue or dengue-like diseases were reported to be infected with dengue fever virus, predominantly of serotype 2 [21]. There is a lack of KAP studies on dengue fever among Yemeni people. Saied et al. [22] concluded that rural populations in Hodeidah governorate have an unclear understanding of dengue fever transmission, negative attitudes towards several features of the disease and poor practices against it.

The present social unrest and war in Yemen, particularly in Taiz, contribute to the incidence of dengue fever outbreaks (Ministry of Health and Population, unpublished data). Moreover, there is a need for documented proof on the KAPs of local populations in Taiz on the infection and its prevention. Therefore, the present study aimed at describing the KAPs of local urban communities in Taiz city towards dengue fever.

Methods

Study area and ethical clearance

This community-based, cross-sectional KAP study was conducted in the urban area of Taiz, a hinterland governorate in the southwest of Yemen, in the period from August to October 2015. Tiaz is located at the geographical coordinates of 13°34′44″N 44°01′19″E at an altitude of about 1400 m above the Red Sea level (Fig. 1). It is the most populous governorate in the country, with a

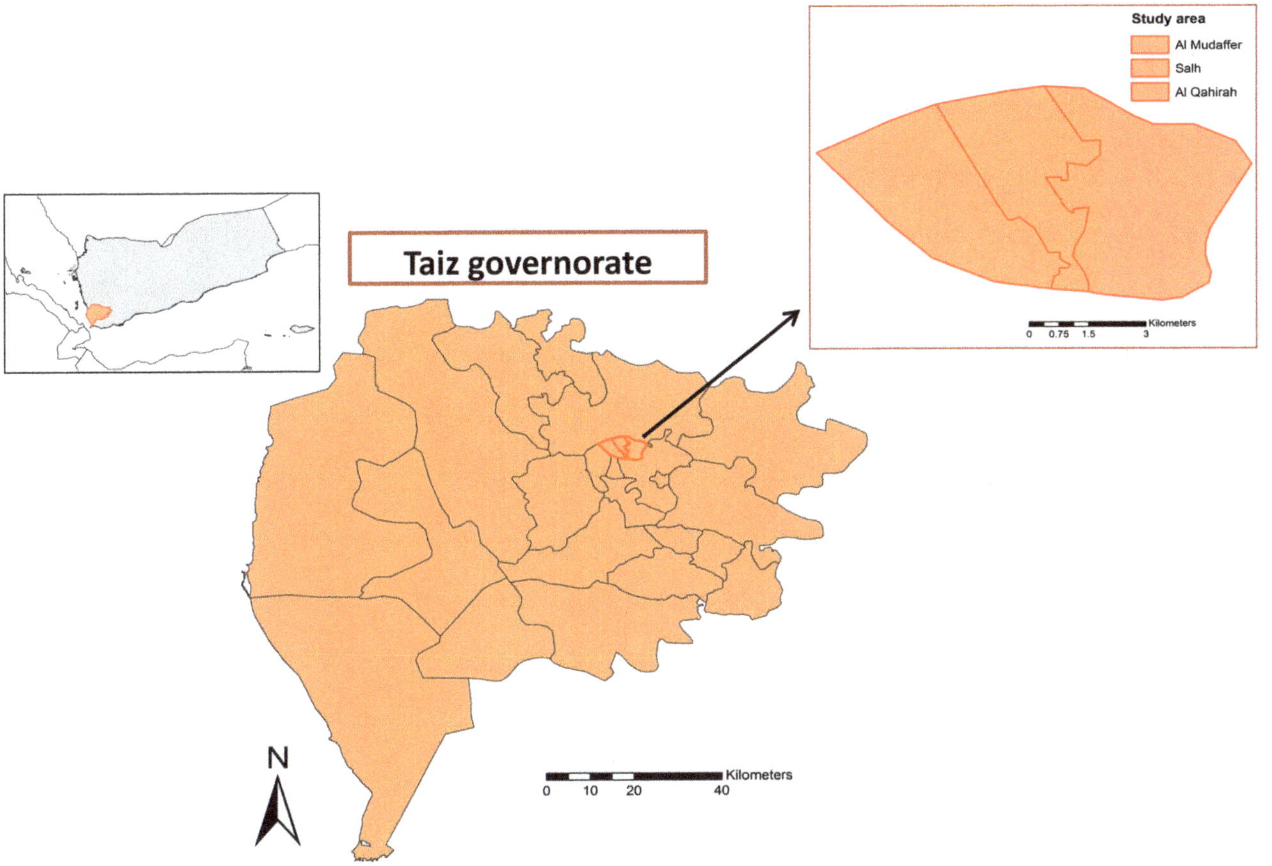

Fig. 1 Map of Yemen and Taiz governorate showing the study area

total population of more than 3 million people. Of them, about 684,000 people live in urban areas [23].

The study protocol was approved by the Ethics Committee of the Faculty of Medicine and Health Sciences, University of Science and Technology, Sana'a, Yemen. Participation was on a voluntary basis, and informed consent was obtained from participants after explanation of the study objectives.

Sample size and sampling strategy

According to the latest census, the total number of households in the urban areas of Taiz is 113,000 households [23]. The present study targeted 71,303 households in three urban dengue-endemic districts; namely, Al Qahirah, Al Mudhaffar and Salh. The sample size was calculated using Epi Info™ version 7.1.3 (Centers for Disease Control, Atlanta, US), using the following parameters: population size of 71,303 households, 5 % confidence limits and 95 % confidence level. The expected frequency of the outcome was considered 50 % because the study covered several potential variables. Accordingly, the minimum sample size calculated was 382 households. Households were randomly selected and household heads were invited to participate in the study after obtaining their informed consent. If the household head was not present or refused to participate, the head of the next household was included until reaching the sample size required.

Data were collected using a structured questionnaire through face-to-face interviews. Interviewers were trained before conducting the survey to ensure that the questionnaires were well understood by the surveyors, avoiding the difference in the definitions and interpretations of concepts used. The questionnaire included closed-ended questions about socio-demographic data, knowledge of the symptoms, transmission and vector of dengue fever, attitudes and practices of the respondents towards dengue fever.

Statistical analysis

Data were verified and analyzed using the IBM SPSS Statistics version 21.0 for Windows (IBM Corp., Armonk, NY, USA). Variables were presented as proportions, and the differences were tested using Pearson's chi-square test. To identify the predictors of poor practices, independent and dependent variables were converted into scores and categorized as poor and good. Scores of "one" and "zero" were given to the correct and incorrect knowledge or practices, respectively. For attitudes, the answers "disagree", "not sure", "agree" and "strongly agree" were given the scores of 1, 2, 3 and 4, respectively. Knowledge and practices were considered poor if the score was lower than or equal to the half of the total score (3, 2.5 and 4 for knowledge of symptoms, transmission and mosquito, respectively, and 4 for practices). Similarly, attitudes were considered negative if the score was lower than or equal to the half of the total score, which was 4.5. The associations between independent and dependent variables were tested using Pearson's chi-square test. The odds ratio (OR) and its 95 % confidence interval (CI) were also reported. Variables with P-values less than or equal to 0.2 were further analyzed by multivariable analysis using a forward conditional stepwise logistic regression model.

Results

Socio-demographic characteristics of the study respondents

Respondent distribution according to socio-demographic characteristics is shown in Table 1. Of the respondents, 48.6 % were females, 18.0 % were illiterate and 37.5 % had a paid job.

Table 1 Socio-demographic characteristics of the study respondents ($N = 383$)[a]

Variable	Respondent distribution n (%)
Age (years)	
< 30	142 (40.1)
40–30	127 (35.9)
41–50	50 (14.1)
51–60	26 (7.3)
> 60	9 (2.5)
Sex	
Male	197 (51.4)
Female	186 (48.6)
Educational level	
Illiterate	65 (18.0)
Primary school	56 (15.5)
Secondary school	96 (26.6)
University	144 (39.9)
Paid job	
Yes	75 (37.5)
No	125 (62.5)

[a]31, 22 and 183 of respondents did not indicate their age, education and job, respectively

Correct knowledge of respondent household heads on dengue fever

Table 2 summarizes the correct knowledge of household heads on dengue fever signs and symptoms, its transmission and the practices that can contribute to the spread of its vector mosquitoes. The majority of the 383 respondents correctly perceived that fever (98.7 %), headache (94.8 %) and joint pain (95.8 %) are main signs and symptoms of dengue fever. In addition, more than 80.0 % of respondents correctly identified pain behind the eyes, muscular pain and bleeding as signs and symptoms of dengue fever. However, skin rash was the least frequent symptom of the disease correctly identified by the respondents, being recognized by 65.0 % of them.

Regarding the recognized mode of dengue transmission, 84.6 % of respondents knew that the black mosquito is the vector transmitting dengue fever. Of whom, only 70.7 % knew that these mosquitoes are day-biters. In addition, about three-quarters of the respondents knew the possibility of dengue fever transmission via blood transfusion. On the other hand, comparable proportions of respondents, ranging between 68.1 and 85.1 %, had correct conceptions that flies, contact with infected people, eating contaminated food or drinking contaminated water have no role in the transmission of dengue fever (Table 2).

Stagnant water and keeping water in uncovered containers were recognized by more than 90.0 % of respondents as factors contributing to the spread of dengue-transmitting vector mosquitoes. In addition, more than 90.0 % of respondents knew that using mosquito nets, window screening, covering water containers, drying stagnant water and rubbish disposal are preventive measures that could contribute to reducing the spread of vector mosquitoes. However, cutting trees near houses, smoldering and using repellent creams as preventive measures that could reduce the spread of vector mosquitoes were recognized by 87.0, 77.2 and 70.1 % of respondents, respectively.

Attitudes of respondent household heads towards dengue fever

Table 3 shows the positive attitudes of respondent household heads towards dengue fever. The majority of respondents agreed about the seriousness of dengue fever and its transmissibility, 97.7 and 96.3 %, respectively. Lower positive attitude rates of 75.5 and 84.6 % were expressed regarding the facts of being at risk of contracting dengue fever and that the infection can be prevented, respectively.

Good practices of respondent household heads towards dengue fever

Table 4 summarizes good preventive practices against dengue-transmitting mosquitoes among respondent household heads. Covering water containers was the most common good practice among 94.8 % of respondent

Table 2 Correct knowledge of household heads about dengue fever in urban communities of Taiz governorate, Yemen ($N = 383$)

Knowledge items	Correct Knowledge	
	n	% (95 % CI)
Dengue fever signs and symptoms		
Fever	378	98.7 (97–99)
Headache	363	94.8 (92–97)
Joint pain	367	95.8 (93–97)
Muscle pain	314	82.0 (78–86)
Eye pain	337	88.0 (84–91)
Skin rash	249	65.0 (60–70)
Bleeding	309	80.7 (76–84)
Dengue fever transmission		
Flies do not transmit dengue	309	80.7 (76–84)
Contact with infected patients does not transmit dengue	326	85.1 (81–88)
Drinking contaminated water does not transmit dengue	264	68.9 (64–73)
Eating contaminated food does not transmit dengue	298	77.8 (73–82)
Dengue is transmitted by blood transfusion	292	76.2 (72–80)
Dengue is transmitted by black mosquitoes[a]	324	84.6 (81–88)
Mosquitoes bite at daytime	229	70.7 (66–75)
Factors mentioned to increase mosquito spread		
Stagnant water	312	96.3 (94–98)
Keeping water containers opened	296	91.4 (88–94)
Factors mentioned to reduce mosquito spread		
Using mosquito nets	300	92.6 (89–95)
Using window screens	311	96.0 (93–98)
Insecticide spraying	295	91.0 (87–94)
Covering water containers	299	92.3 (89–95)
Drying stagnant water	292	90.1 (86–93)
Using repellent creams	227	70.1 (65–75)
Smoldering	250	77.2 (72–81)
Rubbish disposal	309	95.4 (93–97)
Cutting trees near houses	282	87.0 (83–90)

[a]Sample size is 324 for the rest of questions

Table 3 Positive attitudes of household heads towards dengue fever in the urban communities of Taiz governorate, Yemen ($N = 383$)

Attitude items	Positive attitude	
	n	% (95 % CI)
Dengue fever is a serious disease	374	97.7 (96–99)
Dengue is a transmissible disease	369	96.3 (94–98)
I am at risk of dengue fever	289	75.5 (71–79)
Dengue fever can be prevented	324	84.6 (81–88)

CI confidence interval

household heads; followed by window screening (77.5 %), drying water collections around houses (72.1 %) and owning mosquito nets (65.0 %). However, about a half of the respondents did not follow good practices of insecticide spraying or sleeping under mosquito nets. Using creams and fans for repelling mosquitoes were the least frequent practices mentioned by the respondent household heads, being reported by 31.3 and 16.2 % of respondents, respectively.

Analysis of socio-demographic factors, knowledge and attitudes associated with poor practices

Factors possibly associated with poor preventive practices were analyzed by bivariate and multivariable analyses (Table 5). Using bivariate analysis, poor knowledge

Table 4 Good preventive practices of household heads against dengue fever in the urban communities of Taiz governorate, Yemen ($N = 383$)

Practice items	Good practice	
	n	% (95 % CI)
Insecticide spraying	186	48.6 (44–54)
Having mosquito nets	249	65.0 (60–70)
Sleeping under mosquito nets	183	47.8 (43–53)
Using fans for repelling mosquitoes	62	16.2 (13–20)
Window screening	297	77.5 (73–81)
Drying water collections around houses	276	72.1 (67–76)
Covering water containers	363	94.8 (92–97)
Using creams for repelling mosquitoes	120	31.3 (27–36)

CI confidence interval

of dengue signs and symptoms (OR = 2.1, 95 % CI = 1.24–3.68; $P = 0.005$) and its vector (OR = 2.1, 95 % CI = 1.14–3.84; $P = 0.016$) were significantly associated with poor preventive practices among respondents. However, multivariable analysis showed that poor knowledge of dengue vector (adjusted OR = 2.1, 95 % CI = 1.14–3.84; $P = 0.018$) was an independent factor associated with poor preventive practices among respondents (Table 5).

Table 5 Analysis of socio-demographic factors, knowledge and attitudes associated with poor practices

Variable	Poor practices			
	N	n (%)	OR (95 % CI)	*P* value
Age (years)				
> 50	35	15 (42.9)	Reference	
30-50	177	90 (50.8)	1.4 (0.66–2.87)	0.389
< 30	142	61 (43.0)	1.0 (0.48–2.12)	0.991
Sex				
Female	186	93 (50.0)	Reference	
Male	197	88 (44.7)	0.8 (0.54–1.21)	0.296
Education				
University	144	64 (44.4)	Reference	
Secondary school	96	44 (45.8)	1.0 (0.59–1.82)	0.908
Primary school	56	30 (53.6)	1.2 (0.58–2.32)	0.667
Uneducated	65	35 (53.8)	1.3 (0.67–2.54)	0.436
Paid job				
Yes	75	30 (40.0)	Reference	
No	125	47 (37.6)	0.9 (0.50–1.63)	0.736
Knowledge of signs and symptoms				
Good	316	139 (44.0)	Reference	
Poor	67	42 (62.7)	2.1 (1.24–3.68)	0.005
Knowledge of transmission				
Good	323	158 (48.9)	Reference	
Poor	60	23 (38.3)	0.7 (0.37–1.14)	0.132
Knowledge of vector*				
Good	272	118 (43.4)	Reference	
Poor	52	32 (61.5)	2.1 (1.14–3.84)	0.016
Attitudes				
Positive	339	157 (46.3)	Reference	
Negative	44	24 (54.5)	1.4 (0.74–2.61)	0.303

Scores ≤ the half of total scores were considered poor or negative; *identified as an independent predictor of poor practices using multivariable analysis (Adjusted OR = 2.1, 95 % CI = 1.14–3.84; $P = 0.018$)

Discussion

Globally, dengue fever is the most common vector-borne viral infection in the current century [24]. It tends to be of urban and peri-urban distribution, though it occurs in rural areas [25]. With the increasing incidence of dengue outbreaks in Yemen, the present study describes the KAPs of at-risk populations pertaining to dengue fever in three urban districts of Taiz. KAP surveys are of utmost importance in determining effective evidence-based prevention and control strategies through changing poor KAPs. Up to the best of our knowledge, this is the first study on the KAPs of Yemeni people in urban areas towards dengue.

In the present study, most urban community respondents were able to correctly identify fever, headache, joint pain, muscle pain, pain behind the eyes and bleeding as prominent signs and symptoms of dengue fever. However, skin rash was the least frequent symptom correctly recognized by the respondents. This is in agreement with a recent study on the KAPs of rural communities that reported the awareness of more than 90.0 % of respondents of the dengue fever symptoms [22]. Fever was the most frequently identified clinical presentation by the respondents, and this finding is consistent with previous studies from different countries [22, 26–29]. Because fever can be a sign of several febrile diseases endemic in Yemen such as malaria, people have to be educated about some other specific signs not sufficiently perceived by local populations such as rash and bleeding. Raising awareness about these signs and symptoms could help them distinguish dengue fever from other febrile infectious diseases, taking into consideration that only about two-thirds were able to correctly identify rash as a symptom of dengue.

In comparison to the recognition of dengue fever signs and symptoms, the perceived knowledge of the respondents about transmission of dengue fever by the black mosquito, a term used locally for describing the *Aedes* mosquitoes, was relatively lower (82.2 %). The lower level of knowledge among urban populations of Taiz that mosquitoes are vectors of dengue fever is comparable to that (83.4 %; 671/804) recently reported by Saied et al. [22] among Yemeni rural populations. In contrast, higher levels of knowledge were reported from northern Thailand (98.0 %), Nepal (92.0 %) and Pakistan (86.9 %) [28, 30, 31]. Of the respondents reporting that black mosquitoes transmit dengue fever, about two-thirds realized that these mosquitoes mainly transmit dengue fever during the daytime. This finding is higher than that recently reported among rural communities in Hodeidah, where about a third of the respondents perceived the daytime transmission of dengue fever [22]. In fact, malaria prevalence in the study areas could contribute to mistaken beliefs about the transmission of dengue fever by the same vector *Anopheles* mosquito. Therefore, differences in the characteristics, biting behaviors and habitat between malaria and dengue vector mosquitoes should be considered when tailoring educational campaigns to local communities about the prevention and control of dengue fever. Blood transfusion has been recently recognized as a possible mode of dengue fever transmission [4, 32, 33]; however, it was correctly identified by about three-quarters of the respondents as a source of dengue fever transmission.

Despite the low illiteracy rate (18.0 %) of the respondents in the present study, about 20 % of household heads have misconceptions about the modes of dengue fever transmission, including flies, contact with infected people, drinking contaminated water or eating contaminated food. In a recent study among rural populations in Hodeidah governorate, Saied et al. [22] reported that about 52.2 % (420/804) of the study population believe that dengue can be transmitted through contact with infected people. Such misconceptions may affect the practices of local populations for the prevention and control of the disease, which could be either poor or insufficient. Therefore, correction of mistakenly perceived modes of transmission should be considered to guide the health authorities for adapting forthcoming interventions for promoting best practices among populations of endemic areas. These misconceptions about the transmission modes have also been reported from other countries. In Jamaica, 33.5 and 28.2 % out of 188 parents of children attending child health clinics in an endemic area believe that dengue fever can be transmitted by flies and ticks, respectively [27]. Similarly, a recent KAP study in Nepal reported that 32.0, 42.0, 51.0 and 56.0 % of 589 participants in a cross-sectional survey in central Nepal believe that dengue fever can be transmitted by flies, by ticks, through food and water or by direct contact, respectively [31]. These mistaken beliefs about the modes of transmission may account for the negative attitude of 15.4 % of the respondents that dengue fever is not preventable.

The present study shows that the majority of the respondents (>90.0 %) recognized the role of stagnant water and keeping water in uncovered water containers as factors contributing to the spread of vector mosquitoes. This finding is comparable to that reported in a study in Nepal, where more than 90.0 % of lowland and highland populations identified stagnant water collections around houses as the breeding sites of mosquitoes [31]. Moreover, more than 90.0 % of the respondents were aware of the role of using mosquito nets, window screening, covering water containers, drying stagnant water and rubbish disposal as preventive measures that could contribute to reducing the spread of vector mosquitoes. However, fewer rates of perception were found regarding the role of cutting trees near houses, evaporation and smoldering and using repellent creams as preventive measures contributing to the reduction of dengue-transmitting mosquitoes. Apart from the good knowledge of people about the factors contributing to the spread of vector mosquitoes and the preventive measures to their reduction, the intriguing issue is the translation of such knowledge into practice, which was not evident among the respondents in the present study. Therefore, it is vital to seal the existing gap between knowledge and practices after gaining a better understanding of the reasons for not translating perceived knowledge into preventive practices.

The agreement that dengue fever is dangerous and can be transmitted among the population by the respondents of the present study is consistent with previous studies from other Asian countries [31, 34], where good attitudes towards the seriousness and/or transmissibility nature of dengue fever were found. In the present study, the negative attitudes among about 15.0 % of respondents from urban communities as regards not being exposed to the risk of dengue fever and that dengue fever is preventable are in line with the negative attitudes recently reported among the rural communities towards the prevention of dengue fever in Hodeidah governorate [22]. It is noteworthy that differences among various studies in relation to the attitudes of surveyed communities could be attributed to several factors, including the socio-economic status, educational levels and cultural aspects. Therefore, the success of future educational campaigns in fixing the gaps imposed by such negative attitudes of local populations pertaining to the risk and possible prevention of dengue could largely contribute to the control of the disease.

With the exception of the good practices of covering water containers, window screening and drying water collections around houses, other preventive practices are still not adopted by about a half of respondents. It is noteworthy that socio-demographic factors including age, educational level and paid job status were not predictors of poor practices in the present study. This finding could be attributed to the high literacy rate among urban residents and that the responses were obtained from the household heads. This is in contrast to the finding by Saied et al. [22], where a low educational level was a predictor of poor practices against dengue fever among rural populations in Yemen.

In the present study, a strong link exists between poor knowledge of respondents and their poor preventive practices as shown by bivariate analysis and confirmed by multivariable analysis. Poor knowledge of the vector mosquitoes was the independent factor significantly associated with poor practices of the respondents. This finding is consistent with that recently reported by Saied et al. [22] who found an association between knowledge and practices pertaining to the prevention of dengue fever among rural populations in Hodeidah. Similar associations between knowledge and practices have been recently reported from northern Thailand [28], Nepal [31] and Laos [35]. However, the association between knowledge and practices in the present study is in line with those from Jamaica [27], rural Malaysia [34] and Thailand [36], where good knowledge did not translate into good practices to reduce vector populations.

Despite being the first to uncover the KAPs of urban communities of Taiz towards dengue, the findings of the present survey have to be cautiously interpreted for several considerations. The small sample size may limit the precision of certain bivariate relationships between variables. Therefore, comparison across certain risk factors might not have enough sample or power. In addition, the present community survey adopted a 50.0 % cut-off score to divide good and poor knowledge because there was no similar knowledge questionnaires used previously. The questionnaires were mainly about general prevention knowledge but certainly could not cover the various and specific community correctness score. This might have a potential limitation when interpreting certain knowledge items. In other words, it is not necessary that one answer should be correct for all participants. For instance, bed nets may be valuable for infants but not working-age adults in reducing the risk of dengue infection. It is noteworthy that in spite of such limitations, the present findings unveil the existing gaps in the KAPs of urban communities in endemic areas of Taiz and highlight the need for further large-scale studies that consider the possible limitations for the sake of a better generalizability of results.

Conclusions

In conclusion, the majority of people in urban communities of Taiz have a clear understanding of fever, headache, joint pain and pain behind the eyes as common signs and symptoms of dengue fever. However, a considerable proportion exhibits vague perception of other signs and symptoms, including muscle pain, skin rash and bleeding as being associated with dengue fever. Although the majority of people in urban communities of Taiz show positive attitudes towards the seriousness and possible transmissibility of dengue fever, negative attitudes regarding their perception of the risk and possible prevention of the infection are prevailing among a small proportion of urban communities and need to be targeted by educational campaigns. It appears that the good level of the population knowledge of the signs/symptoms of dengue fever and the factors contributing to the spread and control of its vectors did not translate into good practices. Large-scale educational campaigns for changing poor KAPs of populations in endemic areas should be launched to augment the negligible efforts to control dengue fever. In addition, there is a need for conducting future intervention studies to address the existing gaps in the knowledge and practices related to the prevention of dengue fever.

Abbreviations

CI: confidence interval; CYD-TDV: recombinant live-attenuated tetravalent dengue vaccine; KAP: knowledge, attitudes and practices; OR: odds ratio; SPSS: Statistical Package for the Social Sciences

Acknowledgments

The authors acknowledge the help of the Charitable Society for Social Welfare, Sana'a during the survey. They also would like to thank community people for participating in this study.

Funding

Not applicable.

Authors' contributions

TAAA, MAKM, RA and YAR designed the study. TAAA conducted the field survey. MAKM analyzed the data. RA and MAKM drafted the manuscript. TAAA, SMAA, AMA, YAR, SAS and JCB revised the manuscript. All authors approved the final submitted version of the manuscript.

Competing interests

The authors declare that there is no competing interest.

Consent for publication

Not applicable.

Author details

[1]Department of Hematology, Faculty of Medical Sciences, Al-Razi University, Sana'a, Yemen. [2]Department of Parasitology, Faculty of Medicine and Health Sciences, Sana'a University, Sana'a, Yemen. [3]Tropical Disease Research Center, University of Science and Technology, Sana'a, Yemen. [4]Faculty of Public Health and Informatics, Umm Al-Qura University, Mecca, Saudi Arabia. [5]Department of Community Health, Universiti Kebangsaan Malaysia Medical Centre, Kuala Lumpur, Malaysia. [6]Department of Public Health Sciences, University of Miami Miller School of Medicine, Miami, FL, USA.

References

1. World Health Organization. Dengue: guidelines for diagnosis, treatment, prevention and control. Geneva: TDR/WHO; 2009.
2. Wilder-Smith A, Chen LH, Massad E, Wilson ME. Threat of dengue to blood safety in dengue-endemic countries. Emerg Infect Dis. 2009;15:8–11.
3. Stramer SL. The potential threat to blood transfusion safety of emerging infectious disease agents. Clin Adv Hematol Oncol. 2015;13:420–2.
4. Stramer SL, Hollinger FB, Katz LM, Kleinman S, Metzel PS, Gregory KR, et al. Emerging infectious disease agents and their potential threat to transfusion safety. Transfusion. 2009;49 Suppl 2:1S–29S.
5. Weerakkody RM, Palangasinghe DR, Dalpatadu KP, Rankothkumbura JP, Cassim MR, Karunanayake P. Dengue fever in a liver-transplanted patient: a case report. J Med Case Rep. 2014;8:378.
6. Wiwanitkit V. Unusual mode of transmission of dengue. J Infect Dev Ctries. 2010;4:51–4.
7. Bhatt S, Gething PW, Brady OJ, Messina JP, Farlow AW, Moyes CL, et al. The global distribution and burden of dengue. Nature. 2013;496:504–7.
8. Endy TP, Anderson KB, Nisalak A, Yoon IK, Green S, Rothman AL, et al. Determinants of inapparent and symptomatic dengue infection in a prospective study of primary school children in Kamphaeng Phet, Thailand. PLoS Negl Trop Dis. 2011;5:e975.
9. Normile D. Surprising new dengue virus throws a spanner in disease control efforts. Science. 2013;342:415.
10. OhAinle M, Balmaseda A, Macalalad AR, Tellez Y, Zody MC, Saborio S, et al. Dynamics of dengue disease severity determined by the interplay between viral genetics and serotype-specific immunity. Sci Transl Med. 2011;3: 114ra28.
11. Murphy BR, Whitehead SS. Immune response to dengue virus and prospects for a vaccine. Annu Rev Immunol. 2011;29:587–619.
12. Halstead SB. Dengue vaccine development: a 75 % solution? Lancet. 2012; 380:1535–6.
13. World Health Organization. Questions and answers on dengue vaccines. http://www.who.int/immunization/research/development/dengue_q_and_a/en/. Accessed 26 May 2016.
14. Hadinegoro SR, Arredondo-García JL, Capeding MR, Deseda C, Chotpitayasunondh T, Dietze R, et al. Efficacy and long-term safety of a dengue vaccine in regions of endemic disease. N Engl J Med. 2015;373: 1195–206.
15. The Strategic Advisory Group of Experts (SAGE) on immunization. SAGE meeting of April 2016. http://www.who.int/immunization/sage/meetings/2016/april/en/. Accessed 26 May 2016.
16. Espinoza-Gomez F, Hernandez-Suarez CM, Coll-Cardenas R. Educational campaign versus malathion spraying for the control of *Aedes aegypti* in Colima, Mexico. J Epidemiol Community Health. 2002;56:148–52.
17. AlHoot MA. Epidemiological study on dengue fever in Yemen. Sana'a: Sana'a University [Master thesis]; 2003.
18. Madani TA, el Abuelzein TM, Al-Bar HM, Azhar EI, Kao M, Alshoeb HO, et al. Outbreak of viral hemorrhagic fever caused by dengue virus type 3 in Al-Mukalla, Yemen. BMC Infect Dis. 2013;13:136.
19. Bin Ghouth AS, Amarasinghe A, Letson GW. Dengue outbreak in Hadramout, Yemen, 2010: an epidemiological perspective. Am J Trop Med Hyg. 2012;86:1072–6.
20. Ravanini P, Huhtamo E, Hasu E, Rosa F, Costantino S, Crobu MG, et al. Imported dengue virus serotype 3, Yemen to Italy, 2010. Emerg Infect Dis. 2011;17:929–31.
21. Rezza G, El-Sawaf G, Faggioni G, Vescio F, Al Ameri R, De Santis R, et al. Co-circulation of dengue and chikungunya viruses, Al Hudaydah, Yemen, 2012. Emerg Infect Dis. 2014;20:1351–4.
22. Saied KG, Al-Taiar A, Altaire A, Alqadsi A, Alariqi EF, Hassaan M. Knowledge, attitude and preventive practices regarding dengue fever in rural areas of Yemen. Int Health. 2015;7:420–5.
23. Central Statistical Organization. The general population, housing and establishment census. Sana'a: CSO; 2004.
24. Gubler DJ. Epidemic dengue/dengue hemorrhagic fever as a public health, social and economic problem in the 21st century. Trends Microbiol. 2002;10:100–3.
25. Van Kleef E, Bambrick H, Hales S. The geographic distribution of dengue fever and the potential influence of global climate change. TropIKA.net 2010. http://journal.tropika.net/scielo.php?script=sci_arttext&pid=S2078-86062010005000001. Accessed 6 Jan 2016.
26. Gupta P, Kumar P, Aggarwal OP. Knowledge, attitude and practices related to dengue in rural and slum areas of Delhi after the dengue epidemic of 1996. J Commun Dis. 1998;30:107–12.
27. Shuaib F, Todd D, Campbell-Stennett D, Ehiri J, Jolly PE. Knowledge, attitudes and practices regarding dengue infection in Westmoreland, Jamaica. West Indian Med J. 2010;59:139–46.
28. Van Benthem BH, Khantikul N, Panart K, Kessels PJ, Somboon P, Oskam L. Knowledge and use of prevention measures related to dengue in northern Thailand. Trop Med Int Health. 2002;7:993–1000.
29. Acharya A, Goswami K, Srinath S, Goswami A. Awareness about dengue syndrome and related preventive practices amongst residents of an urban resettlement colony of south Delhi. J Vector Borne Dis. 2005;42:122–7.
30. Itrat A, Khan A, Javaid S, Kamal M, Khan H, Javed S, et al. Knowledge, awareness and practices regarding dengue fever among the adult population of dengue hit cosmopolitan. PLoS One. 2008;3:e2620.
31. Dhimal M, Aryal KK, Dhimal ML, Gautam I, Singh SP, Bhusal CL, et al. Knowledge, attitude and practice regarding dengue fever among the healthy population of highland and lowland communities in central Nepal. PLoS One. 2014;9:e102028.
32. Stramer SL, Linnen JM, Carrick JM, Foster GA, Krysztof DE, Zou S, et al. Dengue viremia in blood donors identified by RNA and detection of dengue transfusion transmission during the 2007 dengue outbreak in Puerto Rico. Transfusion. 2012;52(8):1657–66.
33. Pozzetto B, Memmi M, Garraud O. Is transfusion-transmitted dengue fever a potential public health threat? World J Virol. 2015;4:113–23.
34. Hairi F, Ong CH, Suhaimi A, Tsung TW, bin Anis Ahmad MA, Sundaraj C, et al. A knowledge, attitude and practices (KAP) study on dengue among selected rural communities in the Kuala Kangsar district. Asia Pac J Public Health. 2003;15:37–43.
35. Mayxay M, Cui W, Thammavong S, Khensakhou K, Vongxay V, Inthasoum L, et al. Dengue in peri-urban Pak-Ngum district, Vientiane capital of Laos: a community survey on knowledge, attitudes and practices. BMC Public Health. 2013;13:434.
36. Koenraadt CJ, Tuiten W, Sithiprasasna R, Kijchalao U, Jones JW, Scott TW. Dengue knowledge and practices and their impact on *Aedes aegypti* populations in Kamphaeng Phet, Thailand. Am J Trop Med Hyg. 2006;74:692–700.

14

Epidemiological risk factors for adult dengue in Singapore: an 8-year nested test negative case control study

Chee Fu Yung[1,4*], Siew Pang Chan[2,3], Tun Linn Thein[4], Siaw Ching Chai[4] and Yee Sin Leo[2,4,5,6]

Abstract

Background: Understanding changes in the ecology and epidemiology of dengue is important to ensure resource intensive control programmes are targeted effectively as well as to inform future dengue vaccination strategies.

Methods: We analyzed data from a multicentre longitudinal prospective study of fever in adults using a nested test negative case control approach to identify epidemiological risk factors for dengue disease in Singapore. From April 2005 to February 2013, adult patients presenting with fever within 72 h at selected public primary healthcare clinics and a tertiary hospital in Singapore were recruited. Acute and convalescent blood samples were collected and used to diagnose dengue using both PCR and serology methods. A dengue case was defined as having a positive RT-PCR result for DENV OR evidence of serological conversion between acute and convalescent blood samples. Similarly, controls were chosen from patients in the cohort who tested negative for dengue using the same laboratory methods.

Results: The host epidemiological factors which increased the likelihood of dengue disease amongst adults in Singapore were those aged between 21 and 40 years old (2 fold increase) while in contrast, Malay ethnicity was protective (OR 0.57, 95%CI 0.35 to 0.91) against dengue disease. Spatial factors which increased the odds of acquiring dengue was residing at a foreign workers dormitory or hostel (OR 3.25, 95 % CI 1.84 to 5.73) while individuals living in the North-West region of the country were less likely to get dengue (OR 0.50, 95%CI 0.29 to 0. 86). Other factors such as gender, whether one primarily works indoors or outdoors, general dwelling type or floor, the type of transportation one uses to work, travel history, as well as self-reported history of mosquito bite or household dengue/fever were not useful in helping to inform a diagnosis of dengue.

Conclusions: We have demonstrated a test negative study design to better understand the epidemiological risk factors of adult dengue over multiple seasons. We were able to discount other previously speculated factors such as gender, whether one primarily works indoors or outdoors, dwelling floor in a building and the use of public transportation as having no effect on one's risk of getting dengue.

Keywords: Dengue, Epidemiology, Test-negative, Risk factors, Public health, Adult, Singapore

* Correspondence: cheefu.yung@gmail.com
[1]Infectious Disease Service, Department of Paediatrics, KK Women's and Children's Hospital, Singapore, Singapore
[4]Communicable Disease Centre, Institute of Infectious Diseases and Epidemiology, Tan Tock Seng Hospital, Singapore, Singapore
Full list of author information is available at the end of the article

Background

Globally, dengue is the most widespread arbovirus that currently infects approximately 390 million people per year [1]. There are four antigenically distinct dengue virus serotypes (DENV-1, DENV-2, DENV-3 and DENV-4). Although the majority of cases resolve uneventfully, in a number of cases, progression to severe dengue or dengue haemorrhagic shock can occur resulting in death. There is no effective treatment for dengue. Currently, the mainstay of dengue prevention strategy relies on surveillance systems to allow early case detection, larval and breeding site source reduction of the main vector *Aedes aegypti* mosquito.

The epidemiology of dengue in Singapore evolved from a childhood disease with significant morbidity and mortality in the 1960s into a period of low dengue incidence between 1974 and 1985 following the introduction of vector source reduction, public health education and law enforcement in the 1970s. Despite continued implementation of these control measures resulting in a national *Aedes spp* House index (HI), which is a measure of the percentage of houses positive for *Aedes spp* breeding, below 1 %, Singapore has experienced a resurgence of dengue since 1986 [2, 3]. The success of vector control activities likely resulted in the reduction of herd immunity in older age groups as well as a fall in force of infection [4]. Dengue became a disease affecting primarily adults with children being spared although serologic surveys have shown that they remain highly susceptible [5]. Previous analysis of case notification data have also found that the prevalence of dengue in women were lower than men as indicated by a male to female disease ratio of 1.6:1 [3, 6, 7] It has been postulated that the reason for such a pattern of dengue epidemiology could be due to a shift in dengue transmission from the home to outside the home [2].

Understanding changes in the ecology and epidemiology of dengue is important for development of more effective control programs [8]. Mosquito control programmes are resource intensive. In Singapore, it was estimated that vector control cost approximately US$50 million per year [9]. Evidence to guide the use and prioritisation of such funds will be invaluable. Dengue being a mosquito-borne disease exhibits demographic as well as spatial and temporal variations in their distribution [10]. However, there is a paucity of long term studies identifying epidemiological risk factors for dengue transmission over multiple years. Understandably most published work describing such risk factors are based on dengue case notification data (clinical and/or laboratory confirmed) from surveillance systems and incidence rate derived from population census [7, 11–13]. Such data and epidemiological analysis have significant limitations. Firstly, it is impossible to exclude selection bias resulting from differences between cases that present to healthcare and those that do not. Secondly, no surveillance system can capture all dengue cases so misclassification of population denominators as non-cases is a constant limitation. Thirdly, the time element is often poorly unaccounted for although dengue epidemiology is season dependent and the force of infection of dengue is known to have temporal variations [14].

The test negative study design has primarily been used and validated to assess vaccine effectiveness [15, 16]. Controls are selected from individuals who also presented to clinicians with similar symptoms to cases and hence were tested for the same disease of interest but found to be negative. In classic case control studies, controls are routinely selected from patients presenting to the same healthcare facility as cases but with a distinct condition from the disease of the cases being studied. For case control results to be valid, controls should belong to the same source population from which cases are identified [17]. They should be individuals who theoretically would have been cases had they acquired the targeted disease or condition of interest. Therefore, test negative controls have significant advantages over classic controls. They provide assurance as being from the same source population as cases would have presented to healthcare and would have been cases if their aetiology had been the disease being studied.

In this paper, we analyzed data from a multicentre longitudinal prospective study of fever in adults using a nested test negative approach to identify epidemiological risk factors for dengue disease over 8 years (2005 to 2013) in Singapore.

Methods

Patients

From April 2005 to February 2013, adult patients aged > = 18 years presenting with acute onset fever (> = 37.5 C) or a history of fever (> = 37.5C) within 72 h at selected public primary healthcare clinics and a tertiary hospital in Singapore were recruited. Details of the cohort were published previously [18]. The epidemiological data collected included home address region (as well as dwelling type and floor level if living in multi-storey flat), healthcare recruitment site, travel history in the past 2 weeks, nature of work and primary means of transportation to work (Table 1). There were three scheduled visits: Visit 1 at 1–3 days post fever onset, Visit 2 at 4–7 days post fever onset and visit 3 during convalescence at 3–4 weeks post fever onset. Venous blood was collected at each visit.

Laboratory diagnosis

Blood samples were used to diagnose dengue using both PCR and serology methods. RT-PCR was used to detect DENV RNA as previously described [19]. Results were analyzed with the LightCycler software version 3.5.

Table 1 Characteristics of cases and controls

Variable	Category	Case		Control	
		n	%	n	%
Total		395		1308	
Age group	<21	13	3.3	140	10.7
	21 to 30	130	32.9	396	30.3
	31 to 40	97	24.6	238	18.2
	41 to 50	76	19.2	235	18.0
	51 to 60	55	13.9	197	15.1
	61 and above	24	6.1	102	7.8
Gender (Female/Male)	Female	142	35.9	503	38.5
Ethnicity	Chinese	265	67.1	781	59.7
	Malay	33	8.4	240	18.3
	Indian	57	14.4	193	14.8
	Other	40	10.1	94	7.2
Home address region	SW	52	13.4	204	15.8
	C	204	52.4	646	50.0
	NW	62	15.9	264	20.4
	NE	61	15.7	158	12.2
	SE	10	2.6	20	1.5
Country of origin (Singapore/Others)	Singapore	248	62.8	909	69.5
Healthcare recruitment site	A	217	54.9	807	61.7
	B	12	3.0	24	1.8
	C	34	8.6	180	13.8
	D	28	7.1	63	4.8
	E	33	8.4	193	14.8
	F	71	18.0	41	3.1
Medical history (Diabetes/Hypertension/IHD/Malignancy/Steroid treatment) [No/Yes]	No	338	85.6	1099	84.1
Self-reported history of past dengue infection (No/Yes)	No	378	96.7	1235	95.0
Dwelling type	Multistorey public flats	291	73.7	1082	82.8
	Multistorey private flats	18	4.6	64	4.9
	Landed houses	35	8.9	83	6.4
	Foreign (construction) workers dormitory/hostel	51	12.9	77	5.9
Dwelling floor level	mean floor	6	4[a]	7	4[a]
Travel history (No/Yes)	No	342	86.6	1101	84.3
Type of employment (Indoor/Outdoor/Both) and Primary mode of transportation to work (Public-train or bus/Private-taxi or car/Walking)	Unemployed	90	22.8	269	20.7
	Indoor & Public	90	22.8	410	31.6
	Indoor & Private	24	6.1	84	6.5
	Indoor & Walking	10	2.5	41	3.2
	Outdoor & Public	37	9.4	108	8.3
	Outdoor & Private	24	6.1	51	3.9
	Outdoor & Walking	19	4.8	29	2.2
	Both & Public	52	13.2	208	16.0
	Both & Private	35	8.9	80	6.2
	Both & Walking	14	3.5	19	1.5
Self-reported history of mosquito bite (No/Yes)	No	291	73.7	994	76.5
Self-reported history of household dengue (No/Yes)	No	372	94.4	1294	99.2
Self-reported history of household fever (No/Yes)	No	295	74.7	1076	82.6

[a]Standard Deviation

Reactions with high crossover point (Cp) or ambiguous melting curve results were further analyzed by 2 % agarose gel electrophoresis, to confirm the presence of the correctly sized amplicon. Serology testing for IgM and IgG antibodies against DENV was performed using commercially available ELISAs (Panbio, Brisbane, Australia) according to manufacturer's instructions.

Definitions

To ensure high sensitivity and specificity thus minimizing bias from misclassification, cases and controls were classified using strict laboratory criteria. A dengue case was defined as having a positive RT-PCR result for DENV OR evidence of serological conversion between acute and convalescent blood samples. Similarly, controls were chosen from patients in the cohort whom we could be confident that they did not have dengue. This was defined as having a negative RT-PCR result for DENV OR no evidence of serological conversion between acute and convalescent blood samples.

Statistical analysis

Variables percentage proportions between cases and controls were calculated. Data with continuous variables were compared using two tailed *t*-test. Multilevel regression analysis incorporating time by month and year was used for multivariable analysis. First we developed a full model of dengue which included all independent variables: predetermined age categories, gender, ethnicity, home address region, country of birth, healthcare recruitment site, past medical history, self-reported history of past dengue infection, dwelling type, dwelling floor level, travel history, nature of work, transportation to work, self-reported history of mosquito bite, self-reported history of household dengue and self-reported history of household fever. Backward stepwise regression was performed to identify independent predictor variables of dengue disease. We fixed age and gender but other variables were only retained in the model if $P < 0.05$. All statistical analysis was performed using STATA, version 13. We estimated that a sample size of 395 cases and 10 % exposed controls would allow us to detect highest odds ratio (OR) < 1 of 0.4 and smallest OR > 1 of 2, with α at 0.05 and β of 0.1.

Results

A total of 3246 patients were recruited for the prospective cohort study. 1508 were excluded because they were RT-PCR negative and also did not return for the convalescent visit 3. Another 35 patients were also excluded as they were RT-PCR negative and did not demonstrate IgG seroconversion despite being IgM positive at Visit 1. The remaining 1703 patients fulfilled our case definitions for cases and controls and were used for subsequent analysis (Fig. 1). Summary demographics and epidemiological characteristics between the study cases and controls are shown in Table 1. Overall, cases and controls were fairly similar. The temporal distribution of study dengue cases also resembled the national notification of dengue cases as shown in Fig. 2.

In the full model where all variables were included, statistically significant odds ratios for dengue disease were found for housing type and healthcare recruitment site variables only (Table 2). However, after backward stepwise analysis where age and gender were fixed, only ethnicity, home address region and housing type remained as relevant variables in the model. Individuals aged between 21 and 30 years (OR 2.12, 95 % CI 1.11 to 4.05) and 21 to 40 years (OR 2.28, 95 % CI 1.16 to 4.47) were found to have significantly higher odds of dengue disease compared to those < 21 years. The point estimate OR in individuals aged > 41 years showed a downward trend signifying lower risk of dengue disease although the 95 % CI were not statistically significant. There was no difference in odds of dengue by gender. Geographically, apart from residents in the North West region of Singapore who had a lower risk of dengue (OR 0.50, 95 % CI 0.29 to 0.86), the rest of the island had similar risk. Interestingly, Malay ethnicity was found to be protective against dengue

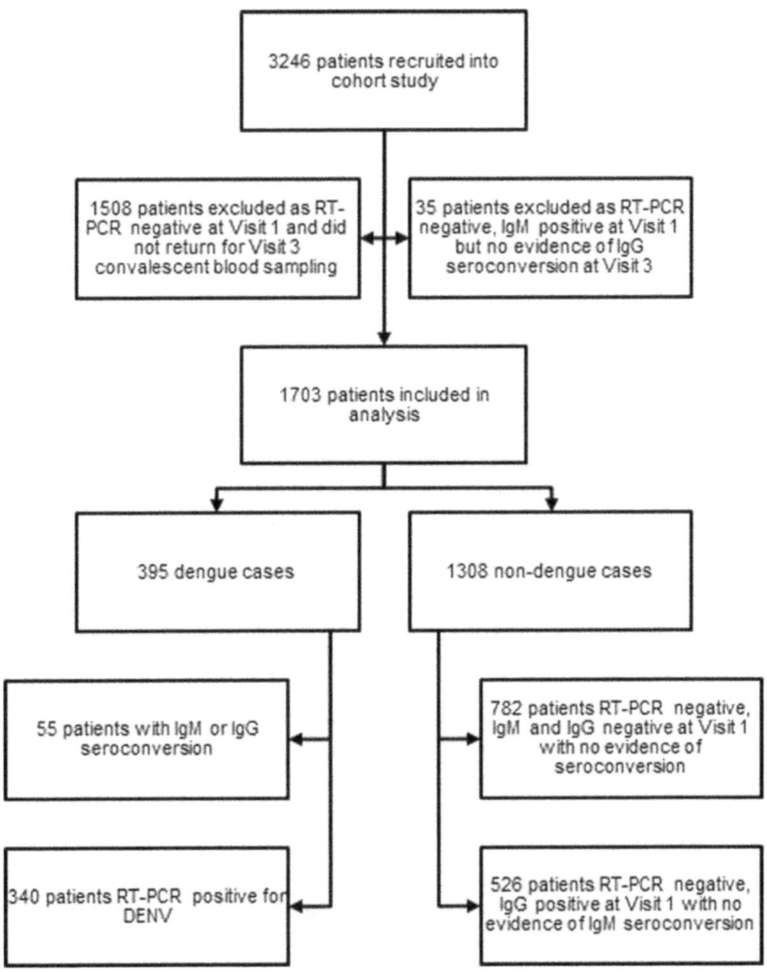

Fig. 1 Consort diagram of cases and controls used in the study

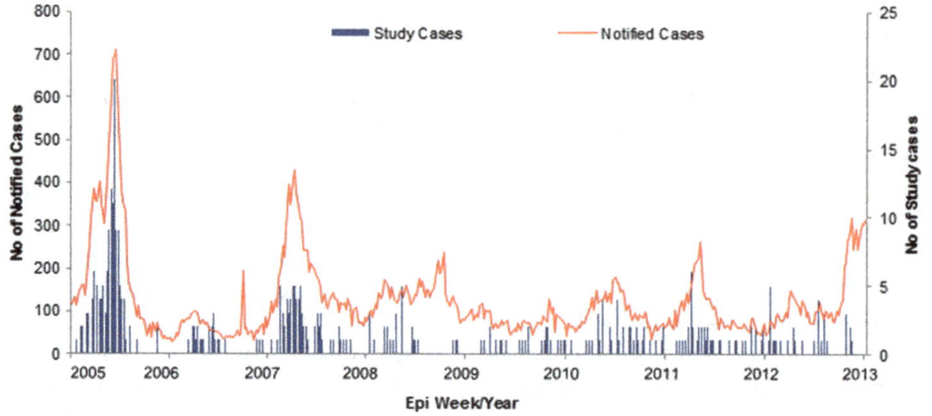

Fig. 2 Distribution of dengue study cases and national notification cases, 2005 to 2013

disease with an OR 0.57, 95 % CI 0.35 to 0.91 when compared to Chinese ethnicity. We also found that individuals residing at foreign worker dormitory/hostels were more likely to be diagnosed with having dengue compared to those residing in multi-storey public flats (OR 3.25, 95 % CI 1.84 to 5.73).

Discussion

The host epidemiological factors which increase the likelihood of dengue disease amongst adults in Singapore were found to be age, particularly if one was aged between 21 and 40 years old while in contrast, Malay ethnicity was found to lower the odds of dengue disease. Spatial epidemiological factors which increased the risk of dengue was residing at a foreign workers dormitory or hostel while individuals living in the North West region of the country had a lower risk of dengue. We also confirmed that there were no differences in odds of dengue disease by gender. Other factors such as whether one primarily works indoors or outdoors, unemployed status, dwelling type or floor, the type of transportation one uses to work, travel history, as well as self-reported history of mosquito bite or household dengue/fever were not useful in helping to inform a diagnosis of dengue. We have demonstrated a test negative control study design incorporating temporal adjustment using multi-level analysis to better understand the epidemiological risk factors of dengue over multiple seasons.

Our results defined a clear and specific age group with increased risk of dengue over the past 8 years in Singapore. Individuals aged 21 to 40 years old have the highest risk of acquiring the disease amongst adults. This is likely to be the age group with the highest risk for the whole population as serologic studies have confirmed very low rates of infection in children compared to adults [5, 20]. Furthermore, the point odds ratios of dengue in age categories above 40 years clearly showed a downward trend. This has important implications for future roll out of a dengue vaccine. The leading dengue vaccine candidate is a recombinant live, attenuated, tetravalent dengue vaccine (Sanofi Pasteur) which demonstrated overall efficacy of 56 · 5 % [21]. However, these results were based on trial cohorts composed of children in settings with high paediatric dengue incidences. Strategically, one would normally aim to deploy a vaccine at an age before the highest risk of infection or disease. Our epidemiological study show that if a dengue vaccine were deployed during the first year of life, in a setting with older age of first infection such as Singapore, the benefits of the vaccine would not be detectable until 20 years later. Currently, we do not know if protection will persist that long. A rise in median age of infection reported in developing countries like Thailand, Vietnam and anecdotally across Asia suggests that Singapore's epidemiology may not be unique in the near future [12, 22–25]. Furthermore, older age of dengue disease was also commonly reported in non-endemic subtropical regions in Taiwan and China who have large seasonal outbreaks following importation of the virus [13, 26]. Therefore, a pre-school leaving or even an adult dengue vaccination strategy may need to be considered as a more rational and cost effective approach for these settings. The challenge is there is unlikely to be efficacy data for adults in the near future to help inform policy decisions. Hence any roll out would require close monitoring to assess efficacy as well as safety. In addition, adult vaccination strategies are renowned to be logistically very difficult to implement and achieve high coverage. This has been demonstrated in countries where adult influenza and pneumococcal vaccination programmes have been rolled out. For a vector borne disease like dengue, high coverage to reduce the reproductive number to < 1 should be an important target to ensure herd protection in the population with the ultimate objective of disease elimination.

Surveillance data routinely reports higher number of dengue cases and clusters in the eastern and central

Table 2 Multilevel logistic regression analysis of dengue epidemiological risk factors

Variable	Category	Full model		Stepwise model	
		OR	95 % CI	AOR	95%CI
Gender	Female	1.00		1.00	
	Male	1.05	0.72 to 1.53	0.95	0.70 to 1.31
Age Group	< 21	1.00		1.00	
	21 to 30	**2.56**	**1.24 to 5.29**	**2.12**	**1.11 to 4.05**
	31 to 40	**3.01**	**1.39 to 6.53**	**2.28**	**1.16 to 4.47**
	41 to 50	2.53	1.17 to 5.47	1.83	0.92 to 3.62
	51 to 60	2.35	1.04 to 5.34	1.62	0.79 to 3.31
	61 and above	1.68	0.63 to 4.51	1.18	0.51 to 2.72
Ethnicity	Chinese	1.00		1.00	
	Malay	**0.47**	**0.28 to 0.79**	**0.57**	**0.35 to 0.91**
	Indian	0.69	0.43 to 1.12	0.73	0.47 to 1.14
	Other	0.63	0.33 to 1.22	0.82	0.47 to 1.44
Home address region	South-west	1.00		1.00	
	Central	0.63	0.28 to 1.39	0.65	0.42 to 1.02
	North-west	**0.38**	**0.15 to 0.98**	**0.50**	**0.29 to 0.86**
	North-east	0.74	0.32 to 1.77	1.20	0.71 to 2.03
	South-east	1.21	0.36 to 4.12	1.25	0.44 to 3.54
Housing type	Multistorey public flats	1.00		1.00	
	Multistorey private flats	0.80	0.37 to 1.73	0.73	0.35 to 1.52
	Landed houses	0.99	0.28 to 3.55	1.44	0.82 to 2.55
	Foreign workers dormitory/hostel	**3.03**	**1.51 to 6.06**	**3.25**	**1.84 to 5.73**
Country of origin	Singapore	1.00			
	Others	0.92	0.61 to 1.38		
Healthcare recruitment site	A	1.00			
	B	**4.27**	**1.15 to 15.95**		
	C	0.65	0.24 to 1.74		
	D	**3.60**	**1.52 to 8.54**		
	E	1.61	0.69 to 3.76		
	F	**2.38**	**1.08 to 5.26**		
Self-reported history of past dengue infection	No	1.00			
	Yes	0.63	0.28 to 1.41		
Medical history (Diabetes/Hypertension/HD/Malignancy/ Steroid treatment)	No	1.00			
	Yes	0.58	0.34 to 0.99		
Dwelling floor level	Level 1	1.00			
	Every 1 level up	0.95	0.91 to 0.99		
Travel history	No	1.00			
	yes	0.87	0.55 to 1.37		
Type of employment (Indoor/Outdoor/Both) and Primary mode of transportation to work (Public-train or bus/Private-taxi or car/Walking)	Unemployed	1.00			
	Indoor & Public	0.51	0.31 to 0.82		
	Indoor & Private	0.87	0.42 to 1.80		
	Indoor & Walking	0.70	0.28 to 1.78		

Table 2 Multilevel logistic regression analysis of dengue epidemiological risk factors *(Continued)*

	Outdoor & Public	0.70	0.35 to 1.41
	Outdoor & Private	1.41	0.63 to 3.11
	Outdoor & Walking	0.68	0.24 to 1.91
	Both & Public	0.68	0.38 to 1.21
	Both & Private	0.43	0.19 to 0.98
	Both & Walking	0.81	0.23 to 2.88
Self-reported history of mosquito bite	No	1.00	
	Yes	0.91	0.62 to 1.35
Self-reported history of household dengue	No	1.00	
	Yes	1.02	0.23 to 4.52
Self-reported history of household fever	No	1.00	
	Yes	1.22	0.83 to 1.80

Figures in **bold** are statistically significant, $P < 0.05$
OR Odds Ratio, *AOR* Adjusted Odds Ratio, *CI* Confidence Interval

regions of Singapore [27]. Our analysis suggests that this is probably an artefact of higher population densities in these regions than actual higher dengue transmission. We postulate that our finding of lower risk of dengue in the North West region compared to the rest of the island could also be attributed to the difference in level of urbanization with subsequent variations in mosquito vector species. The North West region of Singapore is significantly less developed than the rest of the island with large areas of forests still present. This would count against the main vector of dengue, the *Aedes Aegypti* species which is known to thrive in urban settings rather than forested areas [28–31]. Unfortunately, we do not have vector surveillance data to verify this and cannot rule out other factors influencing spatial dengue risk. We did find the odds of dengue disease to be more than 3 times higher in individuals living at foreign workers dormitories or hostels compared to multi-storey public flats where the majority of the local population resides. Such settings could be high-risk areas for dengue epidemics. Dengue transmission has been shown to vary at the neighbourhood level within an urban setting in Thailand [32]. Therefore, the densely occupied nature of such dormitories or hostels in combination with low herd immunity since a significant proportion of foreign workers come from countries where dengue is not endemic may be the reason for this. However, the workers mostly work at construction sites and these have been known to be high risk areas by authorities with mosquito breeding found in about 10 % of sites inspected in 2013 [33]. Singapore has introduced tough legislation for guilty contractors including stop-work orders, prosecution in court and requirements to employ environmental control officer at large construction sites. It is difficult to disentangle the actual site of dengue infection for this cohort although individuals with dengue during the highly infectious fever phase are more likely to be resting at home. Strategies including both educational and source reduction activities targeted at occupants as well as owners of foreign worker residential sites may need to be considered as part of public health efforts to control dengue.

We were not able to identify any difference in odds of dengue disease by factors such as gender, working outdoors, being unemployed and type or level of dwelling. Previous studies have suggested that dengue transmission in Singapore have shifted to outside the home environment based on a jump in seroprevalence from 1 % in < 6 years old to about 7 % in 6 to 15 years which is the age for formal schooling in Singapore [5]. Similarly, it was also hypothesized that lower reported females incidence could be explained by the same dynamics when factoring differences in male and female proportions in the workforce [6]. However, the pediatric seroprevalence data did not have participants older than 15 years and participants were recruited from a single hospital setting. Large seroprevalence studies carried out in adults > 18 years old have shown that > 5 % increases in seroprevalence for 5 to 10 year age categories should be expected [20, 34]. Gender differences in health seeking behaviour and employment rates where producing a medical certificate is a requirement if one is unwell in Singapore could have accounted for dengue gender variations found in routine notification data. Since our controls were individuals who also presented to healthcare but tested negative for dengue, our results were not vulnerable to these biases. Furthermore, an adult serologic survey using samples from a representative National Health Survey also did not find that those who spent more time at home e.g. homemaker or retired as being more likely to be positive for recent dengue infection [34]. Outbreak reports using notification data from the two large outbreaks (2005 and

2007) covered by the study period had conflicting reports of increased risk of dengue by dwelling types [7]. The scarcity of landed properties in Singapore makes landed properties an important socioeconomic profile which may affect health service seeking behaviour and access. Our study design using robust controls confirmed that the type and floor level one resides in does not influence one's risk of dengue disease. This lends support to the homogenous success of national vector control activities and the known significant vertical flight range of the *Aedes* mosquito [35].

Clinically, we were able to confirm that self-reported history of mosquito bite or household dengue/fever and travel history elicited during consultations were not useful in predicting a diagnosis of dengue amongst febrile patients, confirming the known challenges in clinical dengue diagnosis. Interestingly, we did identify Malay ethnicity as being almost 40 % less likely to have dengue compared to Chinese ethnicity amongst adults presenting with fever. Serologic surveys support this finding, with Malay ethnicity identified as the ethnic group with the lowest seropositivity [20, 34]. A genetic predisposition to dengue fever or severe dengue is suspected and studies in Vietnam and Cuba have found a possible role for HLA class 1 allele [36, 37]. A recent study in neighbouring Malaysia which has a similar ethnic mix to Singapore identified HLA-B*13 and HLA-B*18 as being associated with dengue susceptibility and protection respectively amongst patients with Malay ethnicity.

In this study we were not able to account for the role of dengue infection. We used febrile adults presenting to healthcare with a confirmed diagnosis of dengue as a proxy for dengue transmission. However, surveillance notification data are also subject to the same limitation. Although serologic surveys can identify dengue infection especially seroprevalence, available tests are limited by their ability to identify actual date of infection. We also assumed that our study cohort was representative of dengue epidemiology in Singapore. Comparing our incidence to national notification data covering the same period showed similar distribution which would support our assumption (Fig. 2). We were not able to investigate serotype specific differences which may be present in view of known variations in viral competence. DENV-1 and DENV-2 were the predominant circulating serotypes during the study period.

Conclusions

Our results provided invaluable insights into deciphering the epidemiology of adult dengue in urban settings. We demonstrated the use of test negative controls which minimized biases associated with notification data routinely used for studying dengue epidemiological risk factors. In Singapore, the age group most likely to acquire dengue disease was found to be between 21 to 40 years but Malay ethnicity was found to be protective against dengue. We also identified living in a foreign worker dormitory/hostel as a significant epidemiological risk factor for dengue disease. Spatially, the risk of dengue was significantly lower in the North West region of Singapore compared to the rest of the island possibly due to its lower level of urbanization resulting in reduced *Aedes Aegypti* prevalence. We confirmed that gender, employment, use of public transportation, dwelling type as well as floor did not affect one's odds of getting dengue. Our findings have important implications in informing clinical diagnosis of adult dengue, prioritising vector control activities as well as future roll out of a licensed dengue vaccine.

Acknowledgement
We would like to thank colleagues at Environmental Health Institute (EHI), National Environment Agency, Singapore for their laboratory support.
We are also grateful to the patients who volunteered as well as the EDEN study teams for their contributions.

Funding
None.

Authors' contributions
Conceived and designed the study: CFY. Acquire data: CFY SPC TLT SCC YSL. Analysis and interpretation of data: CFY SPC. Drafting and revision of the paper: CFY SPC TLT SCC YSL. All authors read, agreed and approved the final manuscript.

Competing interests
The authors declare that they have no competing interest.

Consent for publication
Not applicable.

Author details
[1]Infectious Disease Service, Department of Paediatrics, KK Women's and Children's Hospital, Singapore, Singapore. [2]Department of Medicine, Yong Loo Lin School of Medicine, National University of Singapore, Singapore, Singapore. [3]Faculty of Science, Technology and Engineering, La Trobe University, Melbourne, Australia. [4]Communicable Disease Centre, Institute of Infectious Diseases and Epidemiology, Tan Tock Seng Hospital, Singapore, Singapore. [5]Lee Kong Chian School of Medicine, Nanyang Technological University Singapore, Singapore, Singapore. [6]Saw Swee Hock School of Public Health, National University Singapore, Singapore, Singapore.

References

1. Bhatt S, Gething PW, Brady OJ, Messina JP, Farlow AW, et al. The global distribution and burden of dengue. Nature. 2013;496:504–7.
2. Ooi EE, Goh KT, Gubler DJ. Dengue prevention and 35 years of vector control in Singapore. Emerg Infect Dis. 2006;12:887–93.
3. Goh KT. Dengue-a remerging infectious disease in Singapore. Dengue in Singapore Singapore: Institute of Environmental Epidemiology, Ministry of the Environment. 1998. p. 33–49

4. Egger JR, Ooi EE, Kelly DW, Woolhouse ME, Davies CR, et al. Reconstructing historical changes in the force of infection of dengue fever in Singapore: implications for surveillance and control. Bull World Health Organ. 2008;86:187–96.
5. Ooi EE, Hart TJ, Tan HC, Chan SH. Dengue seroepidemiology in Singapore. Lancet. 2001;357:685–6.
6. Ooi EE. Changing pattern of dengue transmission in Singapore. Dengue Bulletin. 2001;25:40–4.
7. Ler TS, Ang LW, Yap GS, Ng LC, Tai JC, et al. Epidemiological characteristics of the 2005 and 2007 dengue epidemics in Singapore - similarities and distinctions. Western Pac Surveill Response J. 2011;2:24–9.
8. Morrison AC, Zielinski-Gutierrez E, Scott TW, Rosenberg R. Defining challenges and proposing solutions for control of the virus vector Aedes aegypti. PLoS Med. 2008;5:e68.
9. Carrasco LR, Lee LK, Lee VJ, Ooi EE, Shepard DS, et al. Economic impact of dengue illness and the cost-effectiveness of future vaccination programs in Singapore. PLoS Negl Trop Dis. 2011;5:e1426.
10. Naish S, Dale P, Mackenzie JS, McBride J, Mengersen K, et al. Spatial and temporal patterns of locally-acquired dengue transmission in northern Queensland, Australia, 1993–2012. PLoS One. 2014;9:e92524.
11. Burke DS, Nisalak A, Johnson DE, Scott RM. A prospective study of dengue infections in Bangkok. Am J Trop Med Hyg. 1988;38:172–80.
12. Thai KT, Binh TQ, Giao PT, Phuong HL, le Hung Q, et al. Seroprevalence of dengue antibodies, annual incidence and risk factors among children in southern Vietnam. Trop Med Int Health. 2005;10:379–86.
13. Lin CH, Schioler KL, Jepsen MR, Ho CK, Li SH, et al. Dengue outbreaks in high-income area, Kaohsiung City, Taiwan, 2003–2009. Emerg Infect Dis. 2012;18:1603–11.
14. Reiner Jr RC, Stoddard ST, Forshey BM, King AA, Ellis AM, et al. Time-varying, serotype-specific force of infection of dengue virus. Proc Natl Acad Sci U S A. 2014;111:E2694–2702.
15. Orenstein EW, De Serres G, Haber MJ, Shay DK, Bridges CB, et al. Methodologic issues regarding the use of three observational study designs to assess influenza vaccine effectiveness. Int J Epidemiol. 2007;36:623–31.
16. De Serres G, Skowronski DM, Wu XW, Ambrose CS. The test-negative design: validity, accuracy and precision of vaccine efficacy estimates compared to the gold standard of randomised placebo-controlled clinical trials. Euro Surveill. 2013;18(37). http://dx.doi.org/10.2807/1560-7917.ES2013.18.37.20585.
17. Rothman KJ GS, Lash TL. Case–control studies. Modern Epidemiology. 3rd ed. Philadelphia: Lippincott Williams & Wilkins; 2008. p. 111–28.
18. Low JGOE, Tolfvenstam T, Leo YS, Hibberd ML, Ng LC, Lai YL, Yap GS, Li CS, Vasudevan SG, Ong A. Early Dengue infection and outcome study (EDEN) - study design and preliminary findings. Ann Acad Med Singapore Nov. 2006;35(11):783–9.
19. Lai YL, Chung YK, Tan HC, Yap HF, Yap G, et al. Cost-effective real-time reverse transcriptase PCR (RT-PCR) to screen for Dengue virus followed by rapid single-tube multiplex RT-PCR for serotyping of the virus. J Clin Microbiol. 2007;45:935–41.
20. Ang LW, Cutter J, James L, Goh KT. Seroepidemiology of dengue virus infection in the adult population in tropical Singapore. Epidemiol Infect. 2015;143:1585–93. doi:10.1017/S0950268814002507.
21. Capeding MR, Tran NH, Hadinegoro SR, Ismail HI, Chotpitayasunondh T, Chua MN, et al. Clinical efficacy and safety of a novel tetravalent dengue vaccine in healthy children in Asia: a phase 3, randomised, observer-masked, placebo-controlled trial. Lancet. 2014;384(9951):1358–65.
22. Malavige GN, Velathanthiri VG, Wijewickrama ES, Fernando S, Jayaratne SD, et al. Patterns of disease among adults hospitalized with dengue infections. QJM. 2006;99:299–305.
23. Simmons CP, Farrar J. Changing patterns of dengue epidemiology and implications for clinical management and vaccines. PLoS Med. 2009;6:e1000129.
24. Thai KT, Nishiura H, Hoang PL, Tran NT, Phan GT, et al. Age-specificity of clinical dengue during primary and secondary infections. PLoS Negl Trop Dis. 2011;5:e1180.
25. Wichmann O, Hongsiriwon S, Bowonwatanuwong C, Chotivanich K, Sukthana Y, et al. Risk factors and clinical features associated with severe dengue infection in adults and children during the 2001 epidemic in Chonburi, Thailand. Trop Med Int Health. 2004;9:1022–9.
26. Liang WJ, He JF, Luo HM, Zhou HQ, Yang F, Zheng K. Epidemiological analysis of dengue fever in Guangdong province, 2001–2006. South Chin J Prev Med. 2007;33:4–7.
27. (Last accessed: 7th October 2014) National Environment Agency, Singapore. Dengue Website: http://www.dengue.gov.sg/
28. Thongsripong P, Green A, Kittayapong P, Kapan D, Wilcox B, et al. Mosquito vector diversity across habitats in central Thailand endemic for dengue and other arthropod-borne diseases. PLoS Negl Trop Dis. 2013;7:e2507.
29. Tsuda Y, Suwonkerd W, Chawprom S, Prajakwong S, Takagi M. Different spatial distribution of Aedes aegypti and Aedes albopictus along an urban–rural gradient and the relating environmental factors examined in three villages in northern Thailand. J Am Mosq Control Assoc. 2006;22:222–8.
30. Braks MA, Honorio NA, Lourencqo-De-Oliveira R, Juliano SA, Lounibos LP. Convergent habitat segregation of Aedes aegypti and Aedes albopictus (Diptera: Culicidae) in southeastern Brazil and Florida. J Med Entomol. 2003;40:785–94.
31. Mogi M, Khamboonruang C, Choochote W, Suwanpanit P. Ovitrap surveys of dengue vector mosquitoes in Chiang Mai, northern Thailand: seasonal shifts in relative abundance of Aedes albopictus and Ae. aegypti. Med Vet Entomol. 1988;2:319–24.
32. Salje H, Lessler J, Endy TP, Curriero FC, Gibbons RV, et al. Revealing the microscale spatial signature of dengue transmission and immunity in an urban population. Proc Natl Acad Sci U S A. 2012;109:9535–8.
33. Ng LC, Ho D. Challenges of dengue control. Ann Acad Med Singapore. 2013;42:696–7.
34. Yew YW, Ye T, Ang LW, Ng LC, Yap G, et al. Seroepidemiology of dengue virus infection among adults in Singapore. Ann Acad Med Singapore. 2009;38:667–75.
35. Liew C, Curtis CF. Horizontal and vertical dispersal of dengue vector mosquitoes, Aedes aegypti and Aedes albopictus, in Singapore. Med Vet Entomol. 2004;18:351–60.
36. Loke H, Bethell DB, Phuong CX, Dung M, Schneider J, et al. Strong HLA class I–restricted T cell responses in dengue hemorrhagic fever: a double-edged sword? J Infect Dis. 2001;184:1369–73.
37. Sierra B, Alegre R, Perez AB, Garcia G, Sturn-Ramirez K, et al. HLA-A, –B, –C, and -DRB1 allele frequencies in Cuban individuals with antecedents of dengue 2 disease: advantages of the Cuban population for HLA studies of dengue virus infection. Hum Immunol. 2007;68:531–40.

15

Evaluation of the importance of fever with respect to dengue prognosis according to the 2009 WHO classification

Caroline Tukasan[1], Nathália Barbosa Furlan[1], Cássia Fernanda Estofolete[2], Maurício Lacerda Nogueira[2*] and Natal Santos da Silva[1,2,3*]

Abstract

Background: The 2009 revised World Health Organization (WHO) guidelines for dengue describe fever as the core symptom. Accordingly, the diagnosis of non-febrile patients is complicated. The aim of this study was to evaluate the importance of fever in patients with dengue according to the 2009 revised WHO classification.

Methods: In this study, we assessed 30,670 dengue cases using enzyme-linked immunosorbent assay, detection of the non-structural protein 1, or polymerase chain reaction for diagnostic confirmation. Fisher's exact test was used to evaluate associations between fever and related clinical manifestations. The Mann–Whitney *U* test was used to assess the association of dengue classification with fever and time to treatment. The effects of fever and time to treatment on the risk of progression were analyzed using an ordinal logistic regression to stereotype the model.

Results: Disease classification was found to associate significantly with both fever and time to treatment (both $P < 0.001$). Non-febrile patients were nearly four-fold more likely to exhibit "dengue without warning signs" than "severe dengue" (odds ratio [OR] = 3.74; 95% confidence interval [CI]: 3.20–4.36). Patients who received treatment within 7 days were twice as likely to have "dengue without warning signs" as opposed to "severe dengue" when compared to those who waited >7 days (OR = 2.23; 95% CI: 1.78–2.80). However, this difference was negligible in the multivariate analysis (OR = 1.02; 95% CI: 0.98–1.07).

Conclusions: Fever is a risk factor for disease progression in patients with dengue. However, non-febrile patients should not be neglected because this may delay treatment and could lead to more severe disease.

Keywords: Dengue fever, Severe dengue, Dengue epidemiology, WHO 2009 classification

Background

Dengue is an infectious disease that exhibits acute evolution [1]. The incidence of dengue has increased across all age groups [2] to become a clear public health problem [3]. The causative dengue virus (DENV) belongs to the *Flaviviridae* family within the *Flavivirus* genus [4], and harbors RNA genetic material that encodes three structural (capsid [C], membrane protein [M] and glycoprotein for the viral envelope [E]) and seven non-structural (NS1, NS2a, NS2b, NS3, NS4a, NS4b and NS5) proteins [5] essential for viral replication in host cells [4, 6]. DENV is transmitted by a bite from a female *Aedes aegypti* mosquito [7] that caries one of the four virus serotypes [4]. The viremic period of the disease is defined as the period during which dengue virus can be detected in the blood of an infected human [6]. Following inoculation of the virus into the host, the incubation period may vary from 4 to 10 days [8, 9], after which various clinical signs and symptoms will emerge [9]. Infection with a specific virus serotype initiates permanent,

* Correspondence: mnogueira@famerp.br; natalss@gmail.com
[2]Laboratório de Pesquisas em Virologia, Faculdade de Medicina de São José do Rio Preto, São José do Rio Preto, São Paulo, Brazil
[1]Faculdade de Medicina, União das Faculdades dos Grandes Lagos, São José do Rio Preto, São Paulo, Brazil
Full list of author information is available at the end of the article

or homotypic, immunity against that serotype [5, 6, 9]. Reinfection with a different strain may induce a cross-reaction in which existing antibodies from the first infection bind but do not abolish the virus; this process generally leads to more severe disease [5, 10].

The 1997 World Health Organization (WHO) guidelines on dengue presented three disease categories: dengue fever, dengue hemorrhagic fever, and dengue shock syndrome [3]. Investigations intended to classify the disease and facilitate the initiation of treatment are necessary when a patient is suspected to have dengue. Patients with dengue fever usually presents with an abrupt-onset high fever [11] and two or more other symptoms, such as headache, retro-orbital pain, myalgia, and arthralgia. Laboratory tests may indicate leukopenia and thrombocytopenia without plasma leakage. In addition to the classic symptoms of dengue fever, patients with dengue hemorrhagic fever present with a positive result on the tourniquet test and signs of spontaneous bleeding. This disease is divided into four grades, of which grades three and four are defined as dengue shock syndrome, indicated by the presence of signs of circulatory deficiency such as a weak pulse and hypotension, or even an absent pulse and blood pressure, as a result of plasma leakage [8].

Owing to difficulties with the application of this classification to patients with more severe symptoms, the WHO revised its guidelines in 2009 to include three categories: dengue without warning signs, dengue with warning signs, and severe dengue [2, 3, 12]. Symptoms of dengue with warning signs may include abdominal pain, vomiting, fluid retention, bleeding from mucous membranes, lethargy, and hepatomegaly. Laboratory tests may indicate an increase in erythrocytes with thrombocytopenia. Patients with severe dengue experience plasma leakage, bleeding, and organ failure [2, 3, 8]. Notably, fever is the core symptom of both classifications. Patients who do not present with fever or who develop fever later are difficult to classify according to these guidelines. Furthermore, dengue may present with symptoms similar to other acute febrile illnesses, especially those caused by other arboviruses such as the Zika and Chikungunya viruses, which were both recently detected in Brazil (in 2015 and 2014, respectively), thus contributing to the complicated diagnosis of dengue [13].

The main objective of the present study was to evaluate the importance of fever in patients with dengue, to analyze clinical data related to fever, and to assess associations between fever and the severity indices listed in the 2009 revised WHO guidelines.

Methods

This study evaluated 30,670 confirmed cases of dengue identified in São José do Rio Preto, São Paulo, Brazil between April 1998 and June 2012 (before the emergence of the Zika and Chikungunya viruses in Brazil). Patient information was collected from medical forms of the dengue surveillance system (SINAN, Information System for Notifiable Diseases) associated with the Brazilian Ministry of Health (Additional file 1). This service requires notification of all suspected cases of this disease nationwide. Diagnostic confirmation was conducted in government laboratories via the enzyme-linked immunosorbent assay (ELISA)-based detection of specific IgM antibodies, detection of the non-structural protein 1 (NS1), or polymerase chain reaction (PCR).

The classification system proposed in the WHO 2009 guidelines was used as an ordinal dependent variable. The outcome was one of three different classification levels: dengue without warning signs, dengue with warning signs, and severe dengue. The presence of fever reported by the patient or measured at the time of medical examination was evaluated separately as an independent variable. The time to treatment from the onset of any dengue symptom was categorized as ≤7 days or >7 days and also analyzed as an independent variable. General clinical manifestations, such as headache, vomiting, arthralgia, myalgia, prostration, and diarrhea, were grouped as a single variable (general symptoms). Hemorrhagic manifestations were also included as an independent variable and included the clinical presentation of epistaxis, petechiae, rash, gingival bleeding, hematuria, gastrointestinal bleeding, menorrhagia, and positive tourniquet test. Ascites, pleural effusion, pericardial effusion, hematocrit elevation above the reference levels for sex and age, and the presence of hypoproteinemia were grouped as a plasma leakage variable. Organ failure, including myocarditis, neurological manifestations (as impaired consciousness), and liver failure (AST or ALT > =1000 IU/mL), as defined by WHO, were considered another variable [8]. All suspected cases of dengue which are notified to the Brazilian Ministry of Health are previously evaluated by a doctor or nurse. In our study we do not consider whether the patient was or was not referred to a hospital for both febrile cases as non-febrile.

Fisher's exact test was used to assess the associations of fever with sex, general symptoms, hemorrhagic manifestations, plasma leakage, organ failure, and time to treatment. The Mann–Whitney *U* test was used to verify associations of the WHO 2009 classification for dengue with fever and the time to treatment. An ordinal logistic regression to stereotype model was used to analyze the risk of progression to different levels in the WHO 2009 classification among patients with or without fever. Severe dengue was used as the reference category in the pairwise comparison for each classification. The time interval from symptom onset to presentation for medical care was also analyzed. Odds ratios (ORs) were defined as the ratio of the likelihood of dengue without warning signs or severe dengue in the first comparison and of the likelihood of dengue with warning signs or severe dengue in the second comparison. The quality-of-fit of the models was assessed using the deviance test. All statistical tests were performed using SPSS (version 19; SPSS, Inc., Chicago, IL, USA) and the free statistical program R (version 3.2.0, VGAM package rrvglm function; The R Project for Statistical Computing, Vienna, Austria), and a 5% significance level was implemented.

This study was authorized by the Ethical Committee of the União das Faculdades dos Grandes Lagos, São José do Rio Preto, São Paulo, Brazil. The requirement for informed patient consent was waived.

Results

Of the 30,670 patients with dengue recorded during the study period, fever information was not recorded in the medical forms to 15,914 patients; however, in 14,756 forms this information was present properly. Of these, 14.248 (96.6%) had fever and 508 (3.4%) had not. Only patients with adequate record about the occurrence of were evaluated statistically. 11,726 (79.5%) were aged between 15 and 60 years; 1702 (11.5%) were older than 60 years, and 1328 (9.0%) were aged 0–14 years. The study included 8711 (59.0%) female and 5996 (40.6%) male patients (information on sex was not available for 49 (0.3%) individuals).

Information about general symptoms was available for all 14,756 individuals. Of these, 14,717 (99.7%) exhibited general symptoms, whereas 39 (0.3%) patients reported no general complaints. Of the 14,744 patients with available information about hemorrhagic manifestations, 9320 (63.2%) presented with at least one hemorrhagic manifestation, whereas 5424 (36.8%) had no bleeding complaints patients (information on hemorrhagic manifestation was not available for 12 (0.1%) individuals). At least one form of plasma extravasation was reported in 427 (2.9%) patients, whereas 12,417 (84.1%) had no related complaints (information on plasma extravasation was not available for 1912 (13.0%) individuals). There were 5041 (34.2%) reports of organ dysfunction, whereas 8920 (60.4%) had no dysfunction complaints reported. Regarding the revised WHO classification, 1499 (10.2%), 12,889 (87.3%), and 368 (2.5%) patients were diagnosed with dengue without warning signs, dengue with warning signs, and severe dengue, respectively. The average time to treatment was 5.84 days (standard deviation, 5.25 days).

There was a significantly higher incidence of fever among women (n = 8348, 58.8%) vs. men (n = 5854, 41.2%; $P < 0.001$). Fever was also associated with an increased incidence of general symptoms ($P < 0.001$). In contrast, fever was not statistically significantly associated with hemorrhagic manifestations ($P = 0.261$) or plasma leakage ($P = 0.689$). Despite a significant association of fever with organ failure ($P = 0.011$) 150 patients who did not present with fever were diagnosed with failure of at least one of the studied organs. Fever was not statistically significantly associated with the time to treatment ($P = 0.133$; Table 1).

The Mann–Whitney test indicated a statistically significant association between fever and the WHO classification ($U = 3{,}160{,}348.5$; $P < 0.001$). A significant association was also observed between the time to treatment and WHO classification ($U = 43{,}705{,}568.5$; $P < 0.001$). The ordinal logistic regression was adjusted using the stereotype model, and weights were estimated as model parameters. The univariate analysis indicated that the significant association detected by the Mann–Whitney test represented an increased likelihood that non-febrile individuals would present with "dengue without warning signs" rather than "severe dengue"; this likelihood was nearly four-fold higher than that of febrile individuals (OR = 3.73; 95% confidence interval [CI]: 3 19–4.36). In contrast, the likelihood that patients with or without fever would present with "dengue with warning signs" or "severe dengue" was similar (OR = 1.04; 95% CI: 0.89–1.21).

Patients who presented for treatment within 7 days of symptom onset were twice as likely to be classified as having "dengue without warning signs" rather than "severe dengue", compared to those who presented for treatment more than 7 days after symptom onset. When these two variables were evaluated in the same

Table 1 Comparison between clinical variables and the presence of fever in patients with dengue

	Gender*		General symptomatology*		Hemorrhagic manifestations**		Plasma leakage†		Organ failure††		Time to treatment‡	
	Male n (%)	Female n (%)	Yes n (%)	No n (%)	Yes n (%)	No n (%)	Yes n (%)	No n (%)	Yes n (%)	No n (%)	≤7 days n (%)	>7 days n (%)
Fever												
Yes	5,854 (41.2)	8,348 (58.8)	13,960 (100.0)	0 (0)	8987 (63.1)	5250 (36.9)	411 (3.3)	11,985 (96.7)	4,891 (36.3)	8,581 (63.7)	11,132 (78.7)	3,008 (21.3)
No	142 (28.1)	363 (71.9)	469 (92.3)	39 (7.7)	333 (65.7)	174 (34.3)	16 (3.6)	432 (96.4)	150 (30.7)	339 (69.3)	380 (75.8)	121 (3.9)

Fisher's exact test: *$P < 0.001$, **$P = 0.261$, †$P = 0.689$, ††$P = 0.011$, ‡$P = 0.133$

multivariate analysis model, the magnitude of the association between patients without fever who presented with "dengue without warning signs" vs. "severe dengue" was retained (OR = 3.74; 95% CI: 3.20–4.36). However, the difference between patients who received treatment within 7 days or >7 days of symptom onset was negligible (OR = 1.02; 95% CI: 0.98–1.07) when "dengue without warning signs" and "severe dengue" were considered. All models exhibited good fit in the deviance test ($P > 0.05$; Table 2).

Table 2 Ordinal logistic regression (stereotype model)[a]

	Dengue without warning signs vs. severe dengue			Dengue with warning signs vs. severe dengue		
	β_1	Odds ratio	95% confidence interval	β_2	Odds ratio	95% confidence interval
Univariate						
Fever						
Yes[b]		1.00			1.00	
No	1.31	3.73	3.19–4.36	0.04	1.04	0.89–1.21
Time to treatment						
> 7 days[b]		1.00			1.00	
≤ 7 days	0.80	2.23	1.78–2.80	−0.09	0.92	0.73–1.15
Multivariate						
Fever						
Yes[b]		1.00			1.00	
No	1.32	3.74	3.20–4.36	0.04	1.04	0.89–1.22
Time to treatment						
> 7 days[b]		1.00			1.00	
≤ 7 days	0.02	1.02	0.98–1.07	0.0006	1.00	0.96–1.04

Deviance test: $P > 0.05$ for all models
[a]Dependent variable: 2009 World Health Organization guideline dengue classification
[b]Reference

Discussion

Previous literature reports have not utilized such a large number of patients with both clinically and laboratory confirmed dengue nor a stereotype model to evaluate the importance of fever as a trigger for the investigation of suspected dengue cases. Furthermore, the present study is the first to use the 2009 revised WHO classification system as an outcome measure. Although the results demonstrated a statistically significant association between fever and organ failure ($P = 0.011$), 150 patients without fever also experienced organ failure. Both univariate and multivariate logistic regression analyses indicated that patients without fever were less likely to have severe disease (OR = 3.73; 95% CI: 3.19–4.36 and OR = 3.74; 95% CI: 3.20–4.36, respectively). Furthermore, in the univariate analysis, patients who received treatment within 7 days were less likely to have severe disease when compared to those who received a delayed diagnosis and treatment (OR = 2.23; 95% CI: 1.78–2.80); however, this difference was negligible in the multivariate analysis (OR = 1.02; 95% CI: 0.98–1.07).

The presence of fever, as well as the tourniquet test [11], in suspected dengue carriers is often highly valued as a method of defining the continuity of the conducting case. Even the 2009 WHO guidelines emphasize the presence of fever as a starting point for dengue evaluation [8, 14]. However, the absence of fever, observed in 508 of our study participants, might reduce the demand for medical care. We note that our results highlight the fact that patients without fever were more likely to remain in the lower strata of the 2009 revised classification, and therefore those with fever presented with more severe cases of dengue [8, 11, 14].

Generally, fever has been present in most [15–17], if not all, patients participating in studies of dengue [18]; however, a lack of fever in patients with dengue might be an obstacle to the initiation of investigations and the classification of arbovirosis as dengue without warning signs, dengue with warning signs, or severe dengue. Fever might not be important in the detection of dengue, as shown by Ho et al. in a 2013 study of 581 patients from a hospital in Taiwan in which fever was found to have a moderate sensitivity (67.3%) and positive predictive value (71.7%) and a low specificity (12.3%) and negative predictive value (10.2%) [19]. Reliance on the presentation of fever for a dengue diagnosis might lead to delayed treatment and an increase in disease severity. Furthermore, in a study conducted in the State of Minas Gerais, Brazil, 5.1% of patients with dengue who were admitted to an intensive care unit had not presented with fever at any time prior to admission [20]. Additionally, asymptomatic or presymptomatic individuals might present a high risk of DENV transmission to mosquitos (OR = 5.10; CI: 1.76–57.51 and OR = 4.84; CI: 2:02–11:58, respectively) [21].

Detection of the Chikungunya and Zika viruses in Brazil in 2014 [22] and 2015 [13], respectively, has complicated the diagnosis of dengue based on the presence of fever because infections with these arboviruses yield similar clinical presentations [13]. In addition, cases of Zika might also present clinically as afebrile, as described in a study by Yap [23], leading to the misdiagnosis of dengue as Zika and possibly delaying the initiation of appropriate treatment, leading to further clinical complications. In our cohort of patients with dengue, delays in presentation for treatment were associated with a worse prognosis. Similar results were also found in another study that used a threshold of 4 days with regard to presentation for treatment [19, 24].

We note that we have implemented all precautions to eliminate potential errors that are common in very large retrospective databases, particularly with regard to the annotation of patient records. Additionally, we believe that correct and exhaustive debugging of our data, which involved the removal of conflicting information, increased the reliability of our obtained results and minimized the limitations associated with this type of study.

Conclusions

We conclude that the presence of fever in patients with dengue can be a risk factor for progression to more severe disease. However, patients who do not present with fever should not be neglected, as this might delay treatment, another factor associated with the development of severe disease.

Abbreviations

CI: Confidence interval; DENV: Dengue virus; ELISA: Enzyme-Linked Immunoassay; NS1: Nonstructural protein 1; NS2a: Nonstructural protein 2a; NS2b: Nonstructural protein 2b; NS3: Nonstructural protein 3; NS4a: Nonstructural protein 4a; NS4b: Nonstructural protein 4b; NS5: Nonstructural protein 5; OR: Odds ratio; PCR: Polymerase chain reaction; SINAN: Notifiable diseases information system; WHO: World Health Organization

Acknowledgments

We thank the Municipal Secretariat for Health of São José do Rio Preto for granting access to the database concerning dengue.

Funding

This work was supported by Fundação de Amparo à Pesquisa do Estado de São Paulo (FAPESP) [2013/21719-3] to MLN.

Authors' contributions

CT and NSS conceived the study; NSS and CFE designed the study protocol; NBF, NSS, and CT drafted the manuscript; and MLN and NSS critically revised the manuscript for intellectual content. All authors read and approved the final manuscript. NSS is the guarantor of the paper.

Competing interests

The authors declare that they have no competing interests.

Consent for publication

Not applicable.

Author details

[1]Faculdade de Medicina, União das Faculdades dos Grandes Lagos, São José do Rio Preto, São Paulo, Brazil. [2]Laboratório de Pesquisas em Virologia, Faculdade de Medicina de São José do Rio Preto, São José do Rio Preto, São Paulo, Brazil. [3]Laboratório de Modelagens Matemática e Estatística em Medicina, Faculdade de Medicina, União das Faculdades dos Grandes Lagos, São José do Rio Preto, São Paulo, Brazil.

References

1. Tuan NM, Nhan HT, Chau NV, Hung NT, Tuan HM, Tram TV, et al. Sensitivity and specificity of a novel classifier for the early diagnosis of dengue. PLoS Negl Trop Dis. 2015;9:e0003638.
2. Barniol J, Gaczkowski R, Barbato EV, da Cunha RV, Salgado D, Martínez E, et al. Usefulness and applicability of the revised dengue case classification by disease: multi-centre study in 18 countries. BMC Infect Dis. 2011;11:106.
3. Narvaez F, Gutierrez G, Perez MA, Elizondo D, Nuñez A, Balmaseda A, et al. Evaluation of the traditional and revised WHO classifications of Dengue disease severity. PLoS Negl Trop Dis. 2011;5:e1397.
4. Heilman JM, De Wolff J, Beards GM, Basden BJ. Dengue fever: a Wikipedia clinical review. Open Med. 2014;8:e105–15.
5. Singhi S, Kissoon N, Bansal A. Dengue and dengue hemorrhagic fever: management issues in an intensive care unit. J Pediatr (Rio J). 2007;83(2 Suppl):S22–35.
6. Schmid MA, Diamond MS, Harris E. Dendritic cells in dengue virus infection: targets of virus replication and mediators of immunity. Front Immunol. 2014;5:647.
7. Louis VR, Phalkey R, Horstick O, Ratanawong P, Wilder-Smith A, Tozan Y, et al. Modeling tools for dengue risk mapping - a systematic review. Int J Health Geogr. 2014;13:50.
8. World Health Organization (WHO). Dengue: guidelines for diagnosis, treatment, prevention and control. New edition. Geneva: WHO Press; 2009.
9. Milligan GN, Sarathy VV, Infante E, Li L, Campbell GA, Beatty PR, et al. A dengue virus type 4 model of disseminated lethal infection in AG129 mice. PloS one. 2015;10(5):e0125476.
10. Syenina A, Jagaraj CJ, Aman SA, Sridharan A, St John AL. Dengue vascular leakage is augmented by mast cell degranulation mediated by immunoglobulin Fcgamma receptors. Elife. 2015;4:e05291.
11. Mayxay M, Phetsouvanh R, Moore CE, Chansamouth V, Vongsouvath M, Sisouphone S, et al. Predictive diagnostic value of the tourniquet test for the diagnosis of dengue infection in adults. Trop Med Int Health. 2011;16:127–33.
12. Cavalcanti LP, Mota LA, Lustosa GP, Fortes MC, Mota DA, Lima AA, et al. Evaluation of the WHO classification of dengue disease severity during an epidemic in 2011 in the state of Ceara, Brazil. Memorias do Instituto Oswaldo Cruz. 2014;109:93–8.
13. Musso D, Cao-Lormeau VM, Gubler DJ. Zika virus: following the path of dengue and chikungunya? Lancet. 2015;386(9990):243–4.
14. Srikiatkhachorn A, Rothman AL, Gibbons RV, Sittisombut N, Malasit P, Ennis FA, et al. Dengue-how best to classify it. Clin Infect Dis. 2011;53:563–7.
15. Unnikrishnan R, Faizal BP, Vijayakumar P, Paul G, Sharma RN. Clinical and laboratory profile of dengue in the elderly. J Family Med Prim Care. 2015;4: 369–72.
16. Huang SY, Lee IK, Liu JW, Kung CT, Wang L. Clinical features of and risk factors for rhabdomyolysis among adult patients with dengue virus infection. Am J Trop Med Hyg. 2015;92:75–81.
17. Suleman M, Faryal R, Aamir UB, Alam MM, Nisar N, Sharif S, et al. Dengue outbreak in Swat and Mansehra, Pakistan 2013: An epidemiological and diagnostic perspective. Asian Pac J Trop Dis. 2016;9:380–4.
18. Hoffmeister B, Suttorp N, Zoller T. The revised dengue fever classification in German travelers: clinical manifestations and indicators for severe disease. Infection. 2015;43:21–8.
19. Ho TS, Wang SM, Lin YS, Liu CC. Clinical and laboratory predictive markers for acute dengue infection. J Biomed Sci. 2013;20:75.
20. Amancio FF, Heringer TP, de Oliveira CC, Fassy LB, de Carvalho FB, Oliveira DP, et al. Clinical profiles and factors associated with death in adults with dengue admitted to intensive care units, Minas Gerais. Brazil PloS One. 2015;10:e0129046.
21. Duong V, Lambrechts L, Paul RE, Ly S, Lay RS, Long KC, et al. Asymptomatic humans transmit dengue virus to mosquitoes. Proc Natl Acad Sci U S A. 2015;112:14688–93.
22. Gautret P, Simon F. Dengue, chikungunya and Zika and mass gatherings: What happened in Brazil, 2014. Travel Med Infect Dis. 2016;14:7–8.
23. Duffy MR, Chen TH, Hancock WT, Powers AM, Kool JL, Lanciotti RS, et al. Zika virus outbreak on Yap Island, Federated States of Micronesia. N Engl J Med. 2009;360:2536–43.
24. Thanachartwet V, Oer-Areemitr N, Chamnanchanunt S, Sahassananda D, Jittmittraphap A, Suwannakudt P, et al. Identification of clinical factors associated with severe dengue among Thai adults: a prospective study. BMC Infect Dis. 2015;15:420.

16

Serum neutrophil gelatinase-associated lipocalin and resistin are associated with dengue infection in adults

Kuan-Ting Liu[1,2,3], Yao-Hua Liu[2], Chun-Yu Lin[3,4], Ming-Ju Tsai[5], Ya-Ling Hsu[6], Meng-Chi Yen[2*†] and Po-Lin Kuo[1,7*†]

Abstract

Background: Dengue is a major health problem in tropical areas, including Taiwan. Dengue virus infection affects various types of cells and results in elevation of serum inflammatory molecules. Because these molecules may be associated with dengue virus infection, the aim of this study was to identify novel molecules in febrile patients with dengue infection. In addition, we determined whether these molecules were correlated with the count of leukocytes and platelets.

Methods: Febrile adults (Age >18 years old) who presented to the emergency department and were confirmed dengue virus infection were enrolled in this study. Serum from dengue patients and healthy controls was collected and serum level of sepsis-associated inflammatory molecules was measured by Luminex assay.

Results: Elevated level of macrophage migration inhibitory factor, soluble vascular cell adhesion molecule-1, sFasL, resistin and interferon-γ were detected in patients' serum. Higher levels of neutrophil gelatinase-associated lipocalin (NGAL) and resistin were detected in dengue patients with normal leukocyte count and all dengue patients, respectively. Furthermore, the serum level of NGAL, but not resistin, was correlated with cell count in dengue patients.

Conclusion: Our results revealed that resistin and NGAL are novel dengue-associated molecules. These results may help elucidate the regulatory mechanisms of anti-dengue immune responses.

Keywords: Dengue, Neutrophil gelatinase-associated lipocalin (NGAL), Resistin, Serum

Background

Dengue is a mosquito-borne viral disease caused by four serotypes of dengue virus and is endemic in tropical and subtropical areas including Southeast Asia [1]. A report from World Health Organization indicated the incidence of dengue fever has risen 30-fold in the past 50 years [2]. A recent study revealed that 390 million people were estimated to be infected with dengue per year [3]. According to the Taiwan National Infectious Disease Statistics System, more than 20,000 cases of dengue fever were diagnosed in southern Taiwan, including Kaohsiung city and Tainan city, since 2014 [4]. It is therefore a serious threat to public health in Taiwan and tropical countries.

Infection with any dengue serotype causes a wide spectrum of symptoms, ranging from a mild flu-like syndrome (dengue fever) to a severe syndrome (dengue hemorrhagic fever and dengue shock syndrome) [2]. Onset of fever is observed in dengue patients during the acute febrile phase of dengue. The acute phase of illness lasts for 3–7 days, and then the convalescent phase lasts for several days to several weeks [5, 6]. Because dengue virus infects various cell types, including peripheral leukocytes and endothelial cells [7], the levels of multiple cytokines and chemokines such as macrophage migration inhibitory factor (MIF), tumor necrosis factor alpha (TNF-α), interleukin (IL)-1β, and interferon-γ (IFN-γ),

* Correspondence: 1030605@ms.kmuh.org.tw; kuopolin@seed.net.tw
†Equal contributors
[2]Department of Emergency Medicine, Kaohsiung Medical University Hospital, Kaohsiung Medical University, No.100, Tzyou 1st Road, Kaohsiung 807, Taiwan
[1]Graduate Institute of Clinical Medicine, College of Medicine, Kaohsiung Medical University, No.100, Shih-Chuan 1st Road, Kaohsiung 807, Taiwan
Full list of author information is available at the end of the article

increase at different time points during the disease course [8–10]. The serum level of neutrophils-secreted elastase in patients with dengue shock syndrome is higher than in dengue patients without shock [11, 12]. In addition, dengue virus-infected patients have elevated levels of soluble intercellular cell adhesion molecule 1 (sICAM-1) and soluble vascular adhesion molecule-1 (sVCAM-1), which may regulate the activation and damage of endothelial cells [13]. Fas/Fas ligand (FasL) pathways participate in dengue virus-induced apoptosis of endothelial cells [14]. On the other hand, low platelet count and low leukocyte count are often observed in dengue patients [15, 16]. Platelets-secreted molecules may play a role in both dengue pathogenesis and inflammation regulation because dengue virus also alters platelets-leukocytes and platelets-endothelial cells interactions [17]. Activated platelets affect the production of IL-10 and TNF-α from mononuclear cells [18]. Because some of the aforementioned molecules were common markers in both sepsis and dengue [19], we were interested in whether other sepsis-associated molecules were also associated with dengue infection.

This study aimed to determine novel dengue-associated molecules in febrile patients. The Luminex assays were used for analyzing the sepsis-associated molecules in serum of dengue patients and healthy controls. In order to determine the potential association between these molecules and cell types (such as leukocytes and endothelial cells), the expression pattern of serum molecules in online available dataset was analyzed, either. Because low white blood cell count and low platelet count are clinical features of dengue, we also investigated whether the concentration of these molecules were correlated with white blood cell count and platelet count.

Methods

Sample collection

Adult patients (age >18 years old) who presented to the emergency department of Kaohsiung Medical University Hospital with fever (tympanic temperature >38.3 °C) from Sep 2014 to Dec 2014 were eligible for the study. After obtaining informed consent, 10 ml of blood was drawn and then the serum separated and stored in aliquots in −80 °C. Because dengue is a notifiable disease in Taiwan, serum should be collected from all patients with suspected dengue infection and sent to the Taiwan Centers for Disease Control (CDC), where final confirmation of the diagnosis was made (The commercial DENV Ag NS1 Strip [Bio-Rad] was used). Patients with dengue confirmed by CDC were selected and their sera were used for the following Luminex assay. The sera from healthy controls were also collected after obtaining informed consent.

Quantification of sepsis-associated molecules

The concentration of serum molecules was determined by using Luminex technology. MILLIPLEX MAP Human Sepsis Magnetic Bead Panel 1 (macrophage migration inhibitory factor [MIF], soluble intercellular adhesion molecule 1 [sICAM-1], soluble Fas [sFas], soluble Fas ligand [sFasL], soluble vascular cell adhesion molecule 1 [sVCAM-1], and total plasminogen activator inhibitor-I [tPAI-I]) (Millipore, Billerica, MA, USA), MILLIPLEX MAP Human Sepsis Magnetic Bead Panel 3 (lactoferrin, elastase 2, neutrophil gelatinase–associated lipocalin [NGAL], resistin, and thrombospondin-1) (Millipore, Billerica, MA, USA) and Magnetic Luminex Performance Assay (Human High Sensitivity Cytokine Base Kit A, interferon-γ [IFN-γ]) (R&D Systems, Minneapolis, MN, USA) were used for determining the serum levels of these molecules according to the manufacturer's instructions. Data was acquired on Luminex xMAP technology (Millipore, St Charles, MO, US). For concentration calculation, the calibration curve for each serum molecule was analyzed with a five parameter logistic curve fit curve through the Milliplex Analyst Software (Viagene Tech, Carlisle, MA, USA).

Collection of independent microarrays dataset regarding dengue virus infection

The publicly available microarray dataset was obtained from NCBI Gene Expression Omnibus datasets (GEO dataset, http://www.ncbi.nlm.nih.gov/gds/) [20]. Briefly, we searched "dengue" at GEO datasets and then the results were filtered by the criteria "human" and "expression profiling by array." After excluding the datasets from cell lines and peripheral blood mononuclear cells (PBMC) and datasets without healthy control, the dataset with GEO Series accession number of GSE51808 (http://www.ncbi.nlm.nih.gov/geo/query/acc.cgi?acc=gse51808) was chosen. The dataset contains healthy controls (9 healthy controls) and dengue patients (18 dengue fever patients and 10 dengue hemorrhagic fever patients) [21]. Expression values were adapted from GEO2R.

Statistical analysis

Differences between two independent groups were analyzed with student's T test (Two tailed). Comparisons between three groups were done with one-way ANOVA test, followed by Bonferroni's multiple comparison test. The results were expressed as the median and the inter quartile range. Correlation was estimated with Spearman's correlation. Graphs and statistical analysis were carried out using GraphPad Prism version 5.03 (GraphPad Software, San Diego, CA). P-value < 0.05 was considered significant.

Results

Identification of dengue-associated molecules in serum of dengue patients and healthy controls

Two hundred and seventy-four patients with non-severe dengue (145 males, median age is 42.5), and 33 healthy controls (20 males, median age is 37) were collected. Serum levels of MIF, sVCAM-1, sFasL, resistin and IFN-γ in dengue patients were significantly higher than those in healthy controls (Table 1). To the best of our knowledge, this is the first report describing the association between resistin and dengue infection. In order to compare the expression pattern of these molecules in patients' serum with the expression pattern of these molecules in whole blood cells, we obtained microarray data from Gene Expression Omnibus (GEO, accession number: GSE51808, gene expression profile in whole blood cells) [21]. As shown in Table 2, elevated mRNA levels of MIF and decreased mRNA level of thrombospondin-1 were observed in dengue patients (including dengue fever and dengue hemorrhagic fever). Different expression pattern was observed in serum of dengue patients and RNA expression of whole blood cells. In whole blood cells, there was no difference was found in resistin level in dengue patients compared with that in healthy control (Table 2).

Sepsis-associated molecules in patients with leukopenia and thrombocytopenia

We further investigated whether the concentration of these molecules were associated with blood cell counts in dengue patients since leukopenia (<4000/mm^3) and thrombocytopenia (<100,000/mm^3) are common clinical features of dengue. The levels of sVCAM-1 and IFN-γ were significantly higher in both leukopenic and thrombocytopenic dengue patients than in other dengue patients, whereas the levels of elastase 2, lactoferrin, NGAL, and thrombospondin-1 were significantly lower in both leukopenic and thrombocytopenic dengue patients than those in other dengue patients (Tables 3 and 4). The result implies that NGAL is a novel molecule which might associate with anti-dengue immune responses. Similar expression pattern of these molecules was observed in the leukopenic group and thrombocytopenic group. The results might suggest the level of elastase 2, lactoferrin, NGAL, and thrombospondin-1 associate with the number of leukocytes and platelets.

Correlation between those molecules with leukocyte and platelet count in dengue patients

Increased serum level of resistin was observed in dengue patients. Serum NGAL level was significantly higher in dengue patients without leukopenia or thrombocytopenia than those with leukopenia or thrombocytopenia (Fig. 1). In contrast, serum resistin level was similar in the groups of dengue patients classified by the presence of leukopenia or thrombocytopenia (Fig. 1). The results further suggest the NGAL level correlates with the number of blood cells. Further analyses showed that serum level of NGAL, but not resistin, was correlated with leukocyte and platelet count in dengue patients (Table 5). Elastase 2 and lactoferrin were correlated with leukocyte and platelet count, either.

Discussion

In 2014, there was a dengue fever outbreak in Taiwan and 96 % of patients were from Kaohsiung city [22]. A recent report indicates dengue virus 1 is dominant serotype [23]. Because patients were enrolled from Sep 2014 to Dec 2014 in Kaohsiung city, we supposed serotype I was predominant serotype in our study. Furthermore, a report indicated around 70 % of non-dengue virus 2 infection (dengue virus 1 and dengue virus 3) is primary infection

Table 1 Serum concentrations of sepsis-associated molecules in healthy donors and dengue patients

	Healthy controls ($n = 33$)	Dengue patients ($n = 274$)	P value
MIF	190.1 ± 27.83	753.6 ± 27.83	0.0046
sICAM-1	151,276 ± 12,035	381,200 ± 44,284	0.0776
sVCAM-1	487,114 ± 27,041	1,681,017 ± 30,861	<0.0001
sFasL	32.04 ± 1.657	76.04 ± 2.224	<0.0001
sFas	5428 ± 2622	5205 ± 325	0.8639
tPAI-1	117,506 ± 6263	122,256 ± 2207	0.4803
Elastase 2	76,746 ± 9427	73,292 ± 3601	0.7511
Lactoferrin	199,422 ± 22,270	244,062 ± 12,547	0.2263
NGAL	183,962 ± 16,769	272,870 ± 18,830	0.1047
Resistin	8778 ± 1099	17,451 ± 707.6	<0.0001
Thrombospondin-1	9,873,050 ± 214,185	9,749,456 ± 695,838	0.8513
IFN-γ	0.182 ± 0.003	5.377 ± 1.147	<0.0001

Note: Serum concentrations (pg/mL) of molecules were expressed in Mean ± SEM

Table 2 Gene expression between health donors and dengue patients (adapted from GEO dataset: GSE51808)

Gene symbol	Probe	Healthy (*n* = 9)	Dengue (*n* = 28)	*P* value
MIF	217871_PM_s_at	10.28 ± 0.05	11.29 ± 0.12	<0.0001
ICAM-1	202637_PM_s_at	7.34 ± 0.12	7.84 ± 0.16	0.0987
VCAM-1	203868_PM_s_at	3.39 ± 0.07	3.29 ± 0.08	0.4704
FasL	210865_PM_at	6.34 ± 0.30	6.07 ± 0.16	0.4339
Fas	216252_PM_x_at	8.51 ± 0.14	7.85 ± 0.19	0.0669
PAI-1	1568765_PM_at	4.92 ± 0.17	4.88 ± 0.09	0.6271
Elastase 2	206871_PM_at	4.65 ± 0.27	4.80 ± 0.30	0.7888
Lactoferrin	202018_PM_s_at	8.50 ± 0.42	9.43 ± 0.35	0.1748
NGAL	212531_PM_at	8.15 ± 0.18	8.76 ± 0.19	0.0975
Resistin	220570_PM_at	6.63 ± 0.38	7.01 ± 0.25	0.4565
Thrombospondin-1	215775_PM_at	3.90 ± 0.07	3.74 ± 0.05	0.0272
IFN-γ	210354_PM_at	5.80 ± 0.23	6.29 ± 0.16	0.1333

Note
The number in parentheses is the number of patients
The Dengue group includes patients with dengue fever (*n* = 18) and dengue hemorrhagic fever (*n* = 10)
Expression values of molecules were expressed in Mean ± SEM

in Taiwan [24]. It might imply that enrolled patients with primary infection were dominant. Our results showed the serum concentrations of MIF, sVCAM-1, sFasL, resistin, and IFN-γ were significantly higher in dengue patients than that in healthy controls. Previous studies have indicated that elevated serum levels of MIF, sVCAM-1, sFas, sFasL, and IFN-γ are associated with dengue [9, 10, 13, 14]. Similar expression pattern was observed in the present study. To the best of our knowledge, this is the first report describing elevated serum levels of resistin in dengue patients.

Previous studies have shown that elastase 2, lactoferrin, and NGAL are mainly secreted from neutrophils [25]. Elastase 2 and lactoferrin locate in azurophilic granules and specific granules, respectively [26]. Increasing serum levels of elastase 2 and lactoferrin are correlated with neutrophil degranulation and IL-8 is one of the important regulators for neutrophil degranulation in dengue-infected children [11, 27]. NGAL is a kind of protein inhibiting bacterial growth [28]. The role of NGAL is unclear in dengue infection. The plasma and urine NGAL level in rotavirus-induced dehydration is higher than that in healthy controls [29]. However, the function of NGAL is not well-known in dengue infection. In addition, NGAL is a biomarker for human acute kidney injury [30]. Although dengue hemorrhagic fever is reported to be a risk factor of acute kidney factor in children [31], the NGAL level does not reveal significant difference between dengue patients and healthy controls in adults. In this study, the dengue patients were enrolled after fever onset. We assumed that most of enrolled patients might be in the acute febrile phase and critical phase of dengue. Relatively low level of

Table 3 Serum concentrations of sepsis-associated molecules in dengue patients with different leukocyte counts

	Leukocyte count <4000/mm^3 (*n* = 158)	Leukocyte count >4000/mm^3 (*n* = 116)	*P* value
MIF	741.5 ± 86.56	770.1 ± 106.9	0.8338
sICAM-1	390,856 ± 63,423	368,049 ± 59,280	0.7996
sVCAM-1	1,861,371 ± 46,636	1,435,361 ± 34,827	<0.0001
sFasL	75.38 ± 2.79	76.94 ± 3.63	0.7295
sFas	5744 ± 502.9	4471 ± 337.5	0.0526
tPAI-1	120,103 ± 2986	125,189 ± 3258	0.2557
Elastase 2	60,422 ± 3308	90,821 ± 6909	<0.0001
Lactoferrin	200,423 ± 20,354	303,259 ± 21,099	<0.0001
NGAL	221,109 ± 8826	343,372 ± 42,051	0.0012
Resistin	17,016 ± 835	17,920 ± 1227	0.5706
Thrombospondin-1	8,699,875 ± 256,414	11,230,123 ± 321,044	<0.0001
IFN-γ	7.696 ± 1.91	2.219 ± 0.64	0.0180

Note: Serum concentrations (pg/mL) of molecules were expressed in Mean ± SEM

Table 4 Serum concentrations of sepsis-associated molecules in dengue patients with different platelet counts

	Platelet count <100,000/mm^3 (*n* = 83)	Platelet count >100,000/mm^3 (*n* = 191)	*P* value
MIF	816.7 ± 133.5	726.1 ± 77.27	0.5370
sICAM-1	463,596 ± 114,059	345,395 ± 39,751	0.2206
sVCAM-1	1,920,550 ± 45,670	1,576,926 ± 37,198	<0.0001
sFasL	73.75 ± 3.96	77.04 ± 2.76	0.4976
sFas	6274 ± 879	4741 ± 262	0.0299
tPAI-1	118,768 ± 4450	123,770 ± 2508	0.2984
Elastase 2	54,986 ± 4241	81,246 ± 4718	0.0007
Lactoferrin	173,218 ± 18,650	274,264 ± 15,551	0.0002
NGAL	206,081 ± 10,558	301,894 ± 26,368	0.0191
Resistin	18,640 ± 1213	16,934 ± 866	0.2687
Thrombospondin-1	7,557,301 ± 357,474	10,722,449 ± 232,877	<0.0001
IFN-γ	10.23 ± 3.45	3.26 ± 0.63	0.0051

Note: Serum concentrations (pg/mL) of molecules were expressed in Mean ± SEM

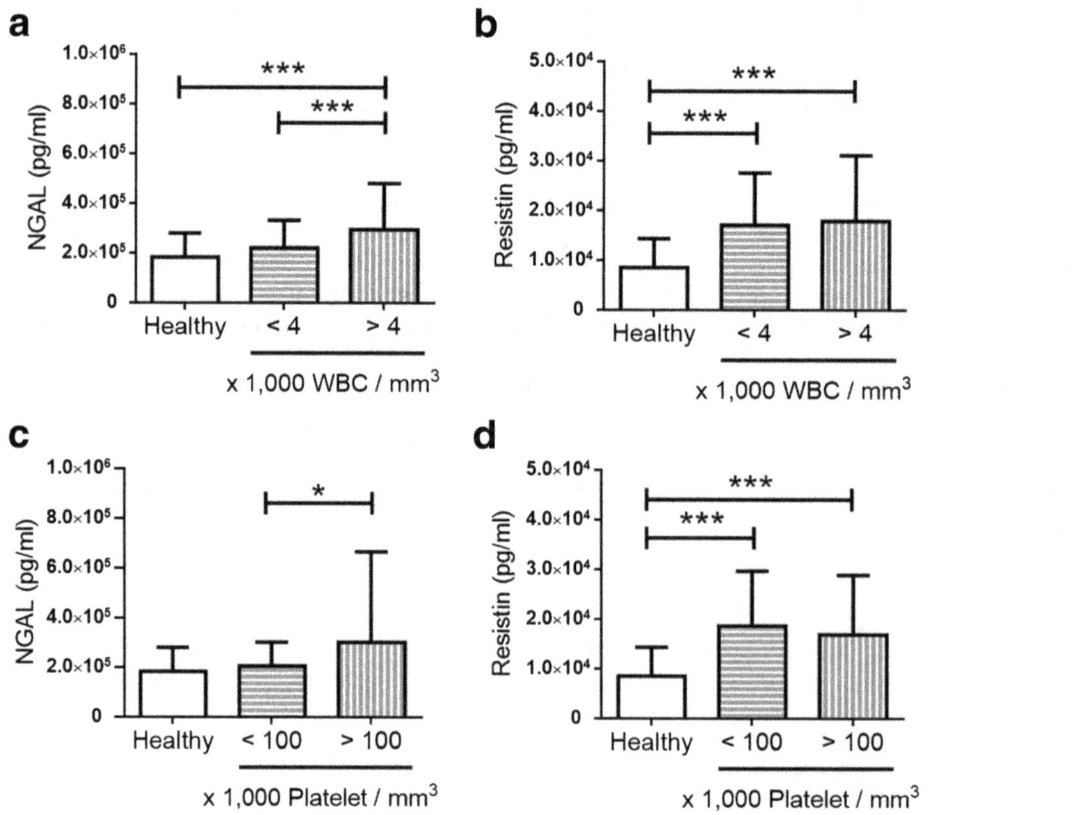

Fig. 1 The levels of NGAL and resistin in healthy controls and dengue patients with different cell count. *Bar graphs* showing the serum concentration of (**a**) NGAL and (**b**) resistin in healthy controls and dengue patients with different leukocyte count; (**c**) NGAL and (**d**) resistin in healthy controls and dengue patients with different platelet count. All quantitative data are expressed as means ± SD. * $p < 0.05$; *** $p < 0.0001$

Table 5 Correlation between serum molecules and the blood cell counts in dengue patients

Cell count	Molecules	Spearman's *R* value	*P* value
Leukocyte count	Elastase 2	0.2758	<0.0001
Leukocyte count	Lactoferrin	0.3508	<0.0001
Leukocyte count	NGAL	0.2764	<0.0001
Leukocyte count	Resistin	−0.0398	0.5120
Platelet count	Elastase 2	0.2774	<0.0001
Platelet count	Lactoferrin	0.3527	<0.0001
Platelet count	NGAL	0.2764	<0.0001
Platelet count	Resistin	−0.0420	0.4889

all three molecules was observed in dengue patients with leukopenia and thrombocytopenia (Tables 3 and 4). All molecules were significantly correlated with leukocyte and platelet count (Table 5). The highest virus titer is in the febrile phase of dengue (1–3 days post fever onset) and the number of leukocyte and platelet decreases is in critical phase (4–6 days post fever onset) [32]. It might suggest elastase 2, lactoferrin and NGAL play a role in anti-dengue immune responses in febrile phase.

Potts and colleagues report that dengue patients had lower platelet, white blood cell and neutrophil counts [33]. Although we did not count neutrophils in this study, we supposed serum levels of elastase 2, lactoferrin, and NGAL correlated with neutrophil counts in adult dengue patients. A recent study indicated that the concentration of the endothelial cell-related molecule VCAM-1 was negatively correlated with neutrophil count [34]. In Tables 3 and 4, the level of sVCAM-1, IFN-γ and three neutrophils-related molecules showed opposite expression pattern in the leukopenic group and thrombocytopenic group. Thrombospondin-1 which is an inflammatory molecule in activated platelet shows similar expression pattern with elastase 2, lactoferrin, and NGAL in this study [35]. It needs to further investigate whether these molecules involve in the regulation of the interaction between T cells, neutrophils, platelet, and endothelial cells during dengue infection in the future.

Resistin is a kind of adipokine and is involved in various inflammatory processes [36, 37]. Peripheral blood mononuclear cells (PBMCs), macrophages, and bone marrow cells are major sources of resistin in human [38]. Circulating levels of IL-6, IL-10 and IFN-γ associated with the level of resistin in an obese mouse model [39]. Pro-inflammatory cytokines, such as IL-6 and TNF-α induce mRNA expression of resistin in human PBMCs. Resistin is significantly correlated with IL-6 and ICAM-1 in patients with obstructive sleep apnea syndrome [40]. The present study showed that serum resistin level significantly increased in dengue patients. Our results indicated that resistin did not correlate with leukocyte and platelet count although human PBMC and macrophage are reported to secret resistin [38]. Persistent human papillomavirus infection increases the resistin level in plasma of older women [41]. However, the function of resistin in dengue virus and human papillomavirus infection is still unknown. In addition, we observed high expression level of resistin, MIF and sFasL in dengue patients and no significant correlation between these molecules and leukocyte and platelet count. It suggests that serum resistin and sFasL might be potential biomarkers for dengue infection since MIF is correlated with disease severity and clinical outcome in dengue [10].

Conclusion

We demonstrated that five inflammatory molecules were elevated in the serum from dengue patients. NGAL and resistin were novel dengue-associated molecules while NGAL might associate with anti-dengue immune responses and resistin might be a novel biomarker for dengue infection. Further investigation to determine their roles in dengue infection may contribute to the understanding the regulatory mechanism of anti-dengue immune responses.

Acknowledgements
None.

Funding
This study was supported by grants from the Ministry of Science and Technology (MOST 104-2320-B-037-014-MY3; MOST 104-2314-B-037-053-MY4; MOST 103-2320-B-037-006-MY3), the Kaohsiung Medical University "Aim for the Top 500 Universities Grant, Grant No. KMU-DT105010", and the Kaohsiung Medical University "Aim for the Top Universities Grant, Grant No. KMU-TP103A13".

Authors' contributions
KTL was involved in sample preparation and acquisition of data; YHL and CYL contributed to sample preparation; MJT and YLH helped the statistical analysis and correction; MCY and PLK designed the project and drafted the manuscript; MCY performed the laboratory analyses; PLK gave final approval of the version to be published. All authors read and approved the final manuscript.

Competing interests
The authors declare that they have no competing interests.

Consent for publication
Not Applicable.

Author details
[1]Graduate Institute of Clinical Medicine, College of Medicine, Kaohsiung Medical University, No.100, Shih-Chuan 1st Road, Kaohsiung 807, Taiwan. [2]Department of Emergency Medicine, Kaohsiung Medical University Hospital, Kaohsiung Medical University, No.100, Tzyou 1st Road, Kaohsiung 807, Taiwan. [3]School of Medicine, College of Medicine, Kaohsiung Medical University,

Kaohsiung 807, Taiwan. [4]Division of Infectious Diseases, Department of Internal Medicine, Kaohsiung Medical University Hospital, Kaohsiung Medical University, Kaohsiung 807, Taiwan. [5]Division of Pulmonary and Critical Care Medicine, Kaohsiung Medical University Hospital, Kaohsiung Medical University, Kaohsiung 807, Taiwan. [6]Graduate Institute of Medicine, College of Medicine, Kaohsiung Medical University, Kaohsiung 807, Taiwan. [7]Institute of Medical Science and Technology, National Sun Yat-Sen University, Kaohsiung 804, Taiwan.

References

1. Guzman MG, Harris E. Dengue. Lancet. 2015;385(9966):453–65.
2. WHO. Global strategy for dengue prevention and control. Geneva: World Health Organization; 2012.
3. Bhatt S, Gething PW, Brady OJ, Messina JP, Farlow AW, Moyes CL, Drake JM, Brownstein JS, Hoen AG, Sankoh O, et al. The global distribution and burden of dengue. Nature. 2013;496(7446):504–7.
4. Taiwan National Infectious Disease Statistics System. Taipei (Taiwan): Taiwan Centers for Disease Control 2015, c2015 (updated 2015 Sep 6; cited 2015 Sep 7), Available from http://nidss.cdc.gov.tw/en/.
5. Gubler DJ. Dengue and dengue hemorrhagic fever. Clin Microbiol Rev. 1998;11(3):480–96.
6. Bandyopadhyay S, Lum LCS, Kroeger A. Classifying dengue: a review of the difficulties in using the WHO case classification for dengue haemorrhagic fever. Trop Med Int Health. 2006;11(8):1238–55.
7. Oishi K, Saito M, Mapua CA, Natividad FF. Dengue illness: clinical features and pathogenesis. J Infect Chemother. 2007;13(3):125–33.
8. Suharti C, van Gorp ECM, Setiati TE, Dolmans WMV, Djokomoeljanto RJ, Hack CE, ten Cate H, van der Meer JWM. The role of cytokines in activation of coagulation and fibrinolysis in Dengue Shock Syndrome. Thromb Haemostasis. 2002;87(1):42–6.
9. Bozza FA, Cruz OG, Zagne SM, Azeredo EL, Nogueira RM, Assis EF, Bozza PT, Kubelka CF. Multiplex cytokine profile from dengue patients: MIP-1beta and IFN-gamma as predictive factors for severity. BMC Infect Dis. 2008;8:86.
10. Chen LC, Lei HY, Liu CC, Shiesh SC, Chen SH, Liu HS, Lin YS, Wang ST, Shyu HW, Yeh TM. Correlation of serum levels of macrophage migration inhibitory factor with disease severity and clinical outcome in dengue patients. Am J Trop Med Hyg. 2006;74(1):142–7.
11. Juffrie M, van der Meer GM, Hack CE, Haasnoot K, Sutaryo, Veerman AJP, Thijs LG. Inflammatory mediators in dengue virus infection in children: Interleukin-8 and its relationship to neutrophil degranulation. Infect Immun. 2000;68(2):702–7.
12. Long TH, Lynn DJ, Henn M, Birren BW, Lennon NJ, Phuong TL, Kien THD, Tham THN, Lanh NM, Farrar JJ, et al. The early whole-blood transcriptional signature of dengue virus and features associated with progression to dengue shock syndrome in vietnamese children and young adults. J Virol. 2010;84(24):12982–94.
13. Cardier JE, Rivas B, Romano E, Rothman AL, Perez-Perez C, Ochoa M, Caceres AM, Cardier M, Guevara N, Giovannetti R. Evidence of vascular damage in dengue disease: demonstration of high levels of soluble cell adhesion molecules and circulating endothelial cells. Endothelium. 2006; 13(5):335–40.
14. Liao H, Xu J, Huang J. FasL/Fas pathway is involved in dengue virus induced apoptosis of the vascular endothelial cells. J Med Virol. 2010; 82(8):1392–9.
15. Jayashree K, Manasa GC, Pallavi P, Manjunath GV. Evaluation of platelets as predictive parameters in dengue fever. Indian J Hematol Blo. 2011; 27(3):127–30.
16. Watt G, Jongsakul K, Chouriyagune C, Paris R. Differentiating dengue virus infection from scrub typhus in Thai adults with fever. Am J Trop Med Hyg. 2003;68(5):536–8.
17. Butthep P, Bunyaratvej A, Bhamarapravati N. Dengue virus and endothelial cell: a related phenomenon to thrombocytopenia and granulocytopenia in dengue hemorrhagic fever. Southeast Asian J Trop Med Public Health. 1993; 24 Suppl 1:246–9.
18. Gudbrandsdottir S, Hasselbalch HC, Nielsen CH. Activated platelets enhance IL-10 secretion and reduce TNF-alpha secretion by monocytes. J Immunol. 2013;191(8):4059–67.
19. Pierrakos C, Vincent JL. Sepsis biomarkers: a review. Crit Care. 2010;14(1):R15.
20. Barrett T, Wilhite SE, Ledoux P, Evangelista C, Kim IF, Tomashevsky M, Marshall KA, Phillippy KH, Sherman PM, Holko M, et al. NCBI GEO: archive for functional genomics data sets-update. Nucleic Acids Res. 2013;41(D1):D991–5.
21. Kwissa M, Nakaya HI, Onlamoon N, Wrammert J, Villinger F, Perng GC, Yoksan S, Pattanapanyasat K, Chokephaibulkit K, Ahmed R, et al. Dengue virus infection induces expansion of a CD14(+)CD16(+) monocyte population that stimulates plasmablast differentiation. Cell Host Microbe. 2014;16(1):115–27.
22. Wang SF, Wang WH, Chang K, Chen YH, Tseng SP, Yen CH, Wu DC, Chen YM. Severe dengue fever outbreak in Taiwan. Am J Trop Med Hyg. 2016;94(1):193–7.
23. Wang SF, Chang K, Lu RW, Wang WH, Chen YH, Chen M, Wu DC, Chen YM. Large Dengue virus type 1 outbreak in Taiwan. Emerg Microbes Infect. 2015;4(8):e46.
24. Lin CC, Huang YH, Shu PY, Wu HS, Lin YS, Yeh TM, Liu HS, Liu CC, Lei HY. Characteristic of dengue disease in Taiwan: 2002–2007. Am J Trop Med Hyg. 2010;82(4):731–9.
25. Miller LS, Cho JS. Immunity against Staphylococcus aureus cutaneous infections. Nat Rev Immunol. 2011;11(8):505–18.
26. Kolaczkowska E, Kubes P. Neutrophil recruitment and function in health and inflammation. Nat Rev Immunol. 2013;13(3):159–75.
27. Nuijens JH, Abbink JJ, Wachtfogel YT, Colman RW, Eerenberg AJM, Dors D, Kamp AJM, Vanschijndel RJMS, Thijs LG, Hack CE. Plasma elastase alpha-1-antitrypsin and lactoferrin in sepsis - evidence for neutrophils as mediators in fatal sepsis. J Lab Clin Med. 1992;119(2):159–68.
28. Corbin BD, Seeley EH, Raab A, Feldmann J, Miller MR, Torres VJ, Anderson KL, Dattilo BM, Dunman PM, Gerads R, et al. Metal chelation and inhibition of bacterial growth in tissue abscesses. Science. 2008;319(5865):962–5.
29. Celik T, Altekin E, Isguder R, Kenesari Y, Duman M, Arslan N. Evaluation of neutrophil gelatinase-associated lipocalin in pediatric patients with acute rotavirus gastroenteritis and dehydration. Ital J Pediatr. 2013;39:52.
30. Devarajan P. Neutrophil gelatinase-associated lipocalin: a promising biomarker for human acute kidney injury. Biomark Med. 2010;4(2):265–80.
31. Laoprasopwattana K, Pruekprasert P, Dissaneewate P, Geater A, Vachvanichsanong P. Outcome of dengue hemorrhagic fever-caused acute kidney injury in Thai children. The Pediatr. 2010;157(2):303–9.
32. WHO. Dengue guidelines for diagnosis, treatment, prevention and control. Geneva: World Health Organization; 2009.
33. Potts JA, Rothman AL. Clinical and laboratory features that distinguish dengue from other febrile illnesses in endemic populations. Trop Med Int Health. 2008;13(11):1328–40.
34. Liao B, Tang Y, Hu F, Zhou W, Yao X, Hong W, Wang J, Zhang X, Tang X, Zhang F. Serum levels of soluble vascular cell adhesion molecules may correlate with the severity of dengue virus-1 infection in adults. Emerg Microbes Infect. 2015;4(4):e24.
35. Lopez-Dee Z, Pidcock K, Gutierrez LS. Thrombospondin-1: multiple paths to inflammation. Mediators Inflamm. 2011;2011:296069.
36. Rajala MW, Lin Y, Ranalletta M, Yang XM, Qian H, Gingerich R, Barzilai N, Scherer PE. Cell type-specific expression and coregulation of murine resistin and resistin-like molecule-alpha in adipose tissue. Mol Endocrinol. 2002; 16(8):1920–30.
37. Patel L, Buckels AC, Kinghorn IJ, Murdock PR, Holbrook JD, Plumpton C, Macphee CH, Smith SA. Resistin is expressed in human macrophages and directly regulated by PPAR gamma activators. Biochem Biophys Res Commun. 2003;300(2):472–6.
38. Lazar MA. Resistin- and Obesity-associated metabolic diseases. Horm Metab Res. 2007;39(10):710–6.
39. Kepczynska MA, Wargent ET, Cawthorne MA, Arch JR, O'Dowd JF, Stocker CJ. Circulating levels of the cytokines IL10, IFNgamma and resistin in an obese mouse model of developmental programming. J Dev Orig Health Dis. 2013;4(6):491–8.
40. Harsch IA, Koebnick C, Wallaschofski H, Schahin SP, Hahn EG, Ficker JH, Lohmann T, Konturek PC. Resistin levels in patients with obstructive sleep apnoea syndrome - the link to subclinical inflammation? Med Sci Monitor. 2004;10(9):Cr510–5.
41. Baker R, Dauner JG, Rodriguez AC, Williams MC, Kemp TJ, Hildesheim A, Pinto LA. Increased plasma levels of adipokines and inflammatory markers in older women with persistent HPV infection. Cytokine. 2011;53(3):282–5.

17

Dengue type 4 in Rio de Janeiro, Brazil: case characterization following its introduction in an endemic region

Manoela Heringer[1], Thiara Manuele A Souza[1], Monique da Rocha Q Lima[1], Priscila Conrado G Nunes[1], Nieli Rodrigues da C Faria[1], Fernanda de Bruycker-Nogueira[1], Thaís Chouin-Carneiro[1], Rita Maria R Nogueira[2] and Flavia Barreto dos Santos[1*]

Abstract

Background: Due to the populations' susceptibility, DENV-4 introduction in 2010 led to the occurrence of explosive epidemics in the following years in Brazil. In 2011, DENV-4 was identified in Rio de Janeiro (RJ) and it was prevalent in 2012 and 2013. Here, we aimed to characterize clinical, epidemiological and laboratorial aspects of DENV-4 cases after this serotype introduction in an endemic scenario.

Methods: Dengue suspected cases (n = 3727) were received and analyzed from January 2011 to December 2013, during outbreaks occurred in RJ, Brazil. Samples were submitted to virological, serological and molecular methods for case confirmation. DENV-4 cases (n = 705) were characterized according to the type of infection, disease severity and, viremia levels and NS1 antigenemia were accessed. Representative strains were partial sequenced for genotyping.

Results: DENV-4 was identified in 44.2% (705/1593) of dengue positive cases, virus isolated in 48.7% of the cases. Anti-DENV IgM was detected in 39.4% of the cases, however an increased detection was observed in cases with ≥4 days of symptoms (57.0%). NS1 antigen was identified in 41.5% of DENV-4 cases however, after immune complexes dissociation, the detection significantly increased (87.6%). Females were more affected than males, so did children aged 11–15 years old. Primary cases were more frequently observed than secondary ones and most of them were classified as dengue. No differences on NS1 antigenemia and viraemia within the groups were observed. Despite the higher frequency of severe disease on individuals >65 years old, no differences were observed among the groups and type of infection. However, DENV-4 fatal cases were more frequent on secondary infections (57.1%). DENV-4 Genotype II was identified with a probable origin from Venezuela and Colombia.

Conclusions: It has been shown that laboratorial diagnosis is still a reliable tool for the disease surveillance, detecting and confirming emerging epidemics. Despite the occurrence of secondary infections, most DENV-4 cases presented a mild disease. As RJ is endemic for dengue, high rates of secondary infections would be expected. Despite the existence of two genotypes, only Genotype II was identified in our study.

Keywords: Dengue virus type 4, Laboratorial diagnosis, Phylogeny, Endemic, Rio de Janeiro, Brazil

* Correspondence: flaviab@ioc.fiocruz.br
[1]Viral Immunology Laboratory, Oswaldo Cruz Institute/FIOCRUZ, Av Brasil 4365, Manguinhos, Rio de Janeiro, RJ 21045-360, Brazil
Full list of author information is available at the end of the article

Background

Dengue is one of the most important arboviruses in the world and the World Health Organization (WHO) estimates that between 70 and 500 million people are annually infected worldwide [1]. Dengue viruses (DENV 1–4) belong to the family *Flaviviridae*, genus *Flavivirus* [2] and based on the analysis of the envelope gene sequences [3, 4] or complete sequencing of the viral genome [5], four genotypes are characterized for DENV-4: Genotype I represented by strains from Thailand, Philippines, Sri Lanka and Japan (from Southeast Asia); Genotype II represented by strains from Indonesia, Malaysia, Tahiti, the Caribbean and the Americas; Genotype III represented by recent strains in Thailand that were different from the others; and Genotype IV represented by wild strains of Malaysia [3–5].

After 63 years without reported cases in Brazil, reinfestation by vector *Aedes aegypti* in the 70's led to epidemics in Boa Vista, Roraima in 1981–1982 [6]. However, dengue became a public health problem in the country when the DENV-1 was identified in the serum of patients in an epidemic in the state of Rio de Janeiro (RJ) in 1986 [7]. The introduction of DENV-2 in 1990, also in the state of RJ [8], led to an increase in the disease severity and the first dengue hemorrhagic fever (DHF) cases were reported in the country [9]. DENV-3 introduction in RJ and in the country in 2000 caused one of the most severe epidemics reported in the country in 2002 [10, 11]. In 2007–2008, the country experienced the most severe epidemic in terms of morbidity and mortality, in addition to severe cases in children due to the DENV-2 re-emergence. RJ alone was responsible for 255,818 cases [12–14]. In 2009, DENV-1 re-emerged in the southeast region of the country and it was the serotype detected in 50.4% of the viral isolations, displacing DENV-2 and DENV-3 [15]. In July of 2010, DENV-4 was isolated in Roraima [16], 28 years after its first detection in that same State and soon this serotype spread other States, including RJ [17]. Despite the epidemic caused by DENV-1, DENV-4 could be isolated during the disease surveillance supported by the performed laboratorial diagnosis. Due to the populations' susceptibility to this newly introduced serotype, explosive epidemics in the country were a real threat. Furthermore, despite being known as a mild serotype, the impact of the emergence of DENV-4 in an endemic region where the other three serotypes were circulating was unknown. This study aimed to analyze the epidemiology of DENV-4 cases occurring in Rio de Janeiro after this serotype introduction, the role of the different laboratory methodologies for case confirmation, the association of viremia and NS1 antigenemia with disease severity and the surveillance of the circulating genotype.

Methods

Dengue suspected cases

Dengue suspected cases were received during a surveillance program performed by the Flavivirus Laboratory, Oswaldo Cruz Institute, FIOCRUZ, Regional Reference Laboratory for the Brazilian Ministry of Health, located in RJ, from January 2011 to December 2013. Acute serum samples (up to the 7th day after the onset of the symptoms) stored at –70 °C were submitted for virus isolation, RT-PCR and NS1 antigen capture ELISA. Convalescent samples (> the 7th day after the onset of the symptoms) stored at –20 °C were tested for MAC-ELISA and IgG-ELISA tests.

Dengue cases classification

Dengue confirmed cases were classified according to the 2009 WHO classification [18] and grouped as follows: dengue without warning signs: patients living in and/or traveling to dengue endemic area, presenting fever and two of the following symptoms: nausea, vomiting, rash, aches, pain, positive tourniquet test and leukopenia; dengue with warning signs (DWAS): dengue patients with any of the following warning signs: abdominal pain or tenderness, persistent vomiting, clinical fluid accumulation, mucosal bleeding, lethargy or restlessness, liver enlargement >2 cm, and an increase in hematocrit concurrent with rapid decrease in platelet count and severe dengue (SD): "dengue patients presenting at least one of the following:" severe plasma leakage (leading to shock and fluid accumulation with respiratory distress), severe bleeding evaluated by clinicians, severe involvement of liver by aspartate aminotransferase (AST) or alanine transferase (ALT) >1000 U, central nervous system with impaired consciousness, and severe involvement of the heart and other organs.

Virus isolation

Virus isolation was performed by inoculation into C6/36 *Aedes albopictus* cell line [19] and isolates were identified by indirect fluorescent antibody test (IFAT) using serotype-specific monoclonal antibodies [20].

Immunoglobulin M (IgM) antibody capture ELISA (MAC-ELISA)

The Panbio dengue IgM Capture ELISA (E-DEN01M, Brisbane, Australia) was used for the qualitative detection of anti-DENV IgM antibodies in serum for case confirmation according to the manufacturer's instructions.

Immunoglobulin G (IgG) antibody detection ELISA (IgG-ELISA)

The IgG-ELISA previously described [21] was performed for the characterization of dengue immune response as primary or secondary infections, in dengue cases previously confirmed by virus isolation, RT-PCR and/or MAC-ELISA.

Viral RNA extraction

Viral RNA was extracted from serum using QIAamp Viral RNA Mini kit (Qiagen, Hilden, Germany) following the manufacturer's instructions and stored at –70 °C for DENV typing.

Reverse transcriptase-polymerase chain reaction (RT-PCR)

Conventional RT-PCR was performed as described by Lanciotti et al. [22] for DENV detection and typing from acute phase samples.

RT-PCR amplification and sequencing of the gene E

For genotyping and phylogenetic analysis, representative samples were selected from the 3 years of epidemic and from distinct regions within the state of Rio de Janeiro. Those DENV-4 isolates (n = 12) were partially sequenced (C/prM/M/E genes), Table 1. Five microliters of the extracted RNA was reverse transcribed into cDNA and amplified for sequencing using AccessQuick™ RT-PCR System (Promega Corporation, Wisconsin, USA). The thermocycling parameters consisted of one cycle of reverse transcription (42 C/60 min), followed by 40 cycles of denaturation (94 C/35 s), annealing (59 C/1 min) and extension (72 C/2 min), ending with a final extension cycle (72 C/10 min), in a GeneAmpPCR System 9700 (Applied Biosystems, California, USA). The cDNA fragments amplified by RT-PCR were directly sequenced in both directions using the BigDye Terminator Cycle Sequencing Ready Reaction Kit (Applied Biosystems, Foster City, CA) version 3.1 and analyzed in an automatic sequencer 3100 (Applied Biosystems, Foster City, CA). Alignments were performed using CLUSTALW2 (http://www.ebi.ac.uk/Tools/msa/clustalw2/). Phylogenetic trees were constructed using the MEGA 7 (http://www.megasoftware.net/), by the "Neighbor-joining" method, according to the Tamura-Nei 93 model and Gamma distribution (TN93 + G), with a bootstrap of 1000 replications.

Real time RT-PCR assay for viremia quantitation

For the viremia quantification of DENV-4 cases (n = 16 [8 dengue and 8 severe dengue]), the TaqMan assay was performed as described previously by Johnson [23]. Due to the small number of severe cases, viremia was randomly analyzed only in 8 samples of each group, for comparison purposes.

NS1 antigen capture ELISA

For the NS1 antigen capture, the Platelia™ Dengue NS1 Ag-ELISA kit (Biorad Laboratories, Marnes-La-Coquette, France) was used according to the manufacturer's protocol. All samples were tested between 1 and 12 days after disease onset. For a better sensitivity for the NS1 capture test, an antigen-antibody complex dissociation protocol performed as previously described by our group [24]. Briefly, the heat-mediated dissociation method was used by boiling 50 μL of serum at 100^0 C in a water bath for five minutes.

The NS1 antigenemia quantification was performed using a standard synthetic antigen curve, based on an equation (y = 1,321× + 0.1271) with R^2 = 0.9542. The standard curve was established using synthetic NS1 protein based on the DENV-4 Dominica 814,669/1981 strain (Native Antigen Company, Oxforshire, United Kingdom) with a 10 fold-dilution. All samples were tested between 1 and 12 days after disease onset.

Statistical analysis

The chi-square and/or Fisher exact tests were used to assess the significance between categorical variables by using Epi Info 7.0.9.34 (Center for Disease Control and Prevention, Atlanta).

Results

A total of 3727 dengue suspected cases from the state of RJ was analyzed from January 2011 to December 2013. After the confirmatory laboratorial diagnosis, 1593 cases were

Table 1 DENV-4 strains (n = 12) isolated in Rio de Janeiro, from 2011 to 2013 used in this study for partial genome sequencing and genotyping

ID/state/year of isolation	Origin of strain (cell line)	Case classification (WHO, 2009)	Genbank accession number
487_11/RJ/2011	Isolated (C6/36)	Dengue	KY084510
5338_11/RJ/2011	Isolated (C6/36)	Dengue	KY084511
1128_12/RJ/2012	Isolated (C6/36)	Dengue	KY084512
3178_12/RJ/2012	Isolated (C6/36)	Dengue	KY084513
3603_12/RJ/2012	Isolated (C6/36)	Dengue	KY084514
5340_12/RJ/2012	Isolated (C6/36)	Dengue	KY084515
408_13/RJ/2013	Isolated (C6/36)	Dengue	KY084516
2663_13/RJ/2013	Isolated (C6/36)	Dengue	KY084517
2848_13/RJ/2013	Isolated (C6/36)	Dengue	KY084518
2960_13/RJ/2013	Isolated (C6/36)	Severe Dengue (Fatal)	KY084519
3248_13/RJ/2013	Isolated (C6/36)	Dengue	KY084520
3602_13/RJ/2013	Isolated (C6/36)	Dengue	KY084521

ID Identification, *RJ* Rio de Janeiro, *WHO* World Health Organization confirmed as dengue positive, and 705 (44.2%) due to DENV-4 infections. Not all analysis, such as those by gender, age, immune response and disease severity were performed in all 705 DENV-4 due to the lack of information in some cases.

The highest percentage of the cases received and confirmed in this study were from the Metropolitan Region of RJ (89.9%; 634/705), and the most affected municipalities by DENV-4 in 2011–2013 were Niterói and Rio de Janeiro, followed by Campos dos Goytacazes, located in the North region of the state, where 44.9% (317/705), 36.8% (260/705) and 7.5% (53/705) of infections by this serotype were confirmed, respectively.

The RT-PCR failed to identified DENV-4 in only one sample (Table 2), which was confirmed by virus isolation, that identified the serotype in 48.7% (298/612) of the samples tested. The detection of anti-DENV IgM, considering both acute and convalescent samples, was possible in 39.4% (104/264) of the cases. However, considering cases with ≥4 days of illness, this marker was detected in 57.0% of the cases. DENV NS1 antigen was identified in 41.5% (231/557) of the DENV-4 cases by using the NS1 antigen capture ELISA according to the manufacturer's instructions, however, after the addition of an antigen-antibody complex dissociation step, the assay sensitivity significantly increased and confirmed 87.6% (488/557; $p = 0.001$) of the samples tested, Table 2.

DENV-4 cases were more frequently observed in females (n = 396) than males (n = 305), and a higher number of cases were observed on children aged 11–15 year old, and was no significant differences were observed between age groups (Fig. 1).

The patient's immune response characterization in primary or secondary infections was possible in 508 DENV-4 cases, due to the lack of information in some cases allowing this analysis. Overall, primary cases were more frequently observed (259/508; 51.0%) than secondary ones (249/508; 49.0%), and despite the lower number of cases in 2011, no significant differences were observed, Table 3. DENV-4 cases (n = 668) were also characterized according to the disease severity. Most of the cases were classified as dengue cases (n = 560; 83.8%), 12.8% (n = 86) as DWAS and 3.2% (n = 22) as severe dengue according to the 2009 WHO criteria, Fig. 2. The clinical manifestations observed in most cases were fever (n = 640; 95.8%), followed by headache (n = 574; 85.9%), independent of the disease severity. Among the most common symptoms observed on dengue, no differences were observed in relation to the disease severity (Fig. 3a). When observing the warning symptoms, a higher proportion of abdominal pain in DWAS cases was observed (n = 75; 87.2%). Despite this, the proportion of abdominal pain in severe dengue cases was considerably lower (n = 3; 13.6%), Fig. 3b.

The NS1 antigenemia on DENV-4 cases (n = 138) showed no differences between NS1 levels from dengue, DWAS or severe dengue cases (Fig. 4a). The same was observed on DENV-4 cases previoulsy negative by NS1 ELISA capture and that resulted positive after heat-mediated immune complex dissociation (Fig. 4b). Viremia was also quantified on dengue (n = 8) and severe dengue (n = 8) cases, however no differences were observed (5.95 log10 RNA copies/mL and 5.83 log10 RNA copies/mL, respectively (p = 0,001).

A relationship between the disease severity and the type of infection (primary or secondary) was shown. There was a greater proportion of a more severe disease among individuals 65 years old and older, however a paired analysis by age showed no significant difference in risk of more severe disease ($p > 0.05$) nor for secondary infections ($p > 0.05$), Table 4.

Fatal cases due to DENV-4 (n = 14) were received and analyzed during the studied period, 42.8% (6/14) occurred in 2012 and 57.1% (8/14) in 2013. Immune response was characterized on 7 cases and, 42.8% (3/7) occurred during a primary infection and 57.1% (4/4), due to secondary ones. Age information was available on 12 cases and, 7 occurred on patients' 16 to 65 years old, Table 5.

The phylogeny based on the partial genome sequencing of representative DENV-4 strains (n = 12) isolated in State of Rio de Janeiro, represented by dengue and one fatal case, demonstrated the circulation of DENV-4 Genotype II (Fig. 5).

Table 2 Distribution of DENV-4 cases analyzed in the State of Rio de Janeiro, Brazil, from 2011 to 2013 and confirmed according to the routine laboratorial diagnosis methodologies used

Methodology/Year	Positive cases/ Total analyzed (%)	*p* value
Virus isolation	298/612 (48.7)	
RT-PCR	704/705 (99.8)	
MAC-ELISA	104/264 (39.4)	
NS1 Capture ELISA	231/557 (41.5)	0.001
NS1 Capture ELISA after dissociation	488/557 (87.6)	

Discussion

The introduction of DENV-4 in the state of Roraima, North Brazil in 2010 warned for the possibility of a new dengue epidemics in Brazil [16], as the main vector, *Aedes aegypti* is widespread in the country. In the disease surveillance, the identification of the vectors has important implications for the disease outbreak control, especially with the rapid disease spread when a new serotype is introduced.

In 2011, the first isolation of DENV- 4 in RJ from cases occurred in the city of Niteroi resulted in the emergence of this serotype in the state in 2012, characterized by isolation of this serotype in 48.7% of confirmed cases. That same year showed for, the first time, the co-circulation of the four DENV serotypes in the state. However, in 2013, DENV-4 was responsible for the largest number of cases in the state.

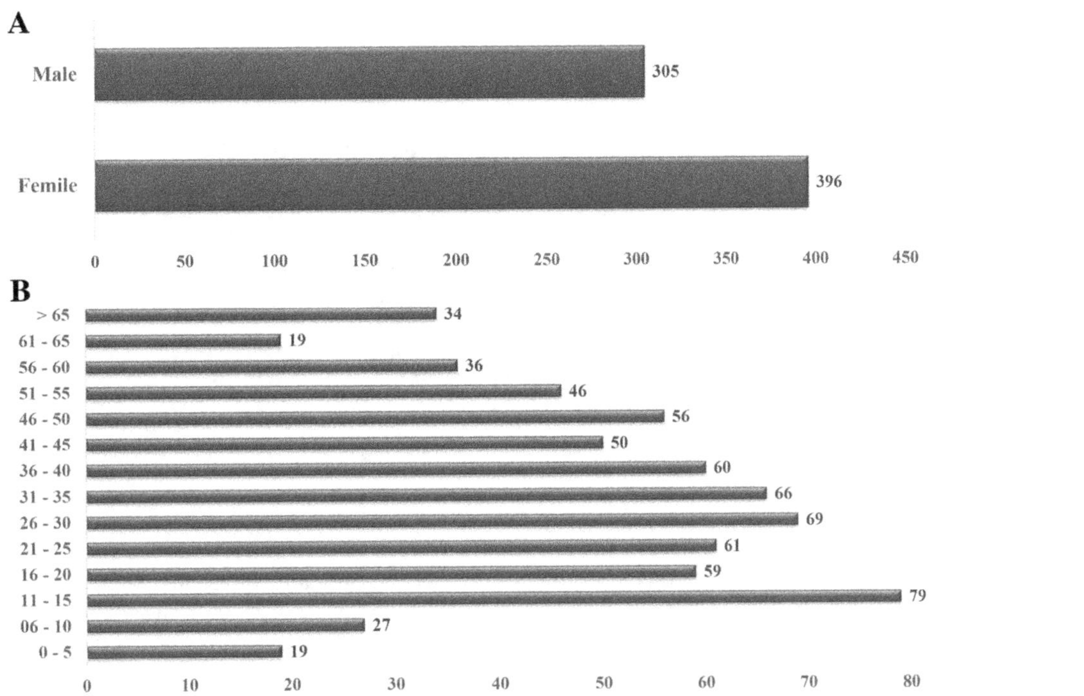

Fig. 1 Distribution of DENV-4 cases by gender (**a**) and age group (**b**), during the epidemic occurred in Rio de Janeiro, Brazil from 2011 to 2013

The Metropolitan region of the state was responsible for most cases occurred during the studied period, mainly in the municipalities of RJ and Niterói. This region has a high population density and high-traffic, which partly explains the concentration of the cases studied [12]. Furthermore, as the Flavivirus Laboratory, FIOCRUZ acts as a Regional Reference Laboratory for dengue diagnosis in Brazil, samples from other municipalities were also received and analyzed.

Although viral isolation is considered the "gold standard" method for dengue viral detection, the sensitivity of the molecular methods in detecting the viral genome offers a great advantage during an epidemic period, as shown by the results presented here. However, it is noteworthy that the high percentage of positive results obtained in RT-PCR may be the result of the selection criteria for the analysis in this study, as known DENV-4 cases were selected. Despite this, previous studies have demonstrated the usefulness of RT-PCR to confirm the cases and identification of the infecting serotype, when the virus isolation was not possible [25, 26].

Serological methods are still the most useful tool for the diagnosis of the disease during epidemics, as observed since its establishment in 1986 in Rio de Janeiro [27]. In this study, the low detection rate of anti-DENV IgM by ELISA (39.4%) was probably due to the acute nature of the cases selected for analysis, as previously described. When it has been described that patients with a primary infection have evidently undetectable IgM antibody titers and there is an increase in detection from a paired sample in the later disease [9]. Usually, higher anti-DENV IgM detection rates are observed after the sixth day after the onset of symptoms. Therefore, considering cases with ≥4 days of symptoms, the detection rate significantly increases.

Table 3 Immune response characterization of DENV-4 cases occurred in Rio de Janeiro from 2011 to 2013

Type of infection (%)/Year	2011 (*n* = 11)	2012 (*n* = 397)	2013 (*n* = 100)	Total (%) (*n* = 508)
Primary	3 (27.3)	198 (49.9)	58 (58.0)	259 (51.0)
Secondary	8 (72.7)	199 (50.1)	42 (42.0)	249 (49.0)

The usefulness of NS1 Ag capture tests for the early diagnosis of dengue, even in limited resourced setting has been shown [28] and evaluated to confirm primary and secondary acute dengue infections [28–31]. In this study, initially, the NS1 capture ELISA detection rate was 41.5% on previously confirmed DENV-4 cases. However, after using a heat immune complex dissociation step, the NS1 detection rate significantly increased to 87.6%, as previously described.

In this study, hemorrhage, shock, increased transaminases levels and central nervous system involvement were considered for severe cases classification. In the study, 3.2% of DENV-4 confirmed cases were classified as severe dengue and 12.8% as dengue with warning signs. We observed that abdominal pain is an important warning sign regarding the evolution of the disease and which can help in the correct patient management and thus, avoiding increased severity and fatal outcome. However, due to the small

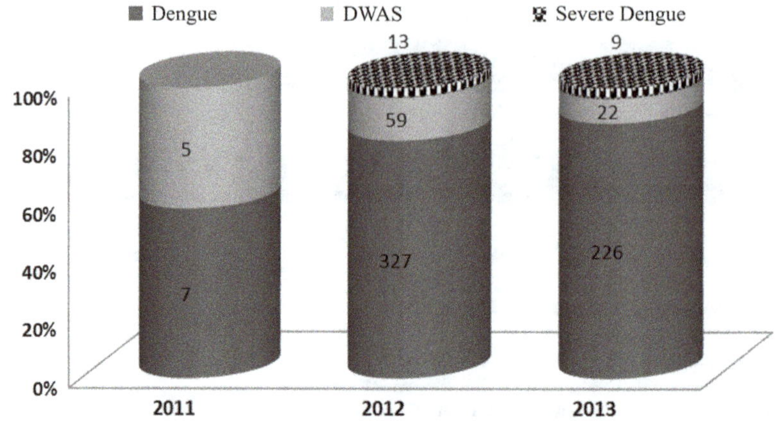

Fig. 2 Yearly distribution of dengue, dengue with warning signs (DWAS) and severe dengue cases by year of occurrence, Rio de Janeiro, Brazil, 2011 to 2013

number of severe cases available in this study, no statistical analysis on the disease severity was performed. Furthermore, during the study period, no increase in the disease severity was observed and this is in agreement with previous observations in the same period in the state of RJ [32]. The lower severity on DENV-4 cases is known [33] and here, 14 deaths due to DENV-4 were confirmed in the period studied.

No significant differences between the viremia on mild dengue and severe cases were observed, which does not corroborate with previous studies analyzing other serotypes [34–36]. However, a limitation of the present study was the small sample size of severe cases. Moreover, the sampling collection represents the patient's first visit to the health unit and the information on their progression to a more severe disease is not available.

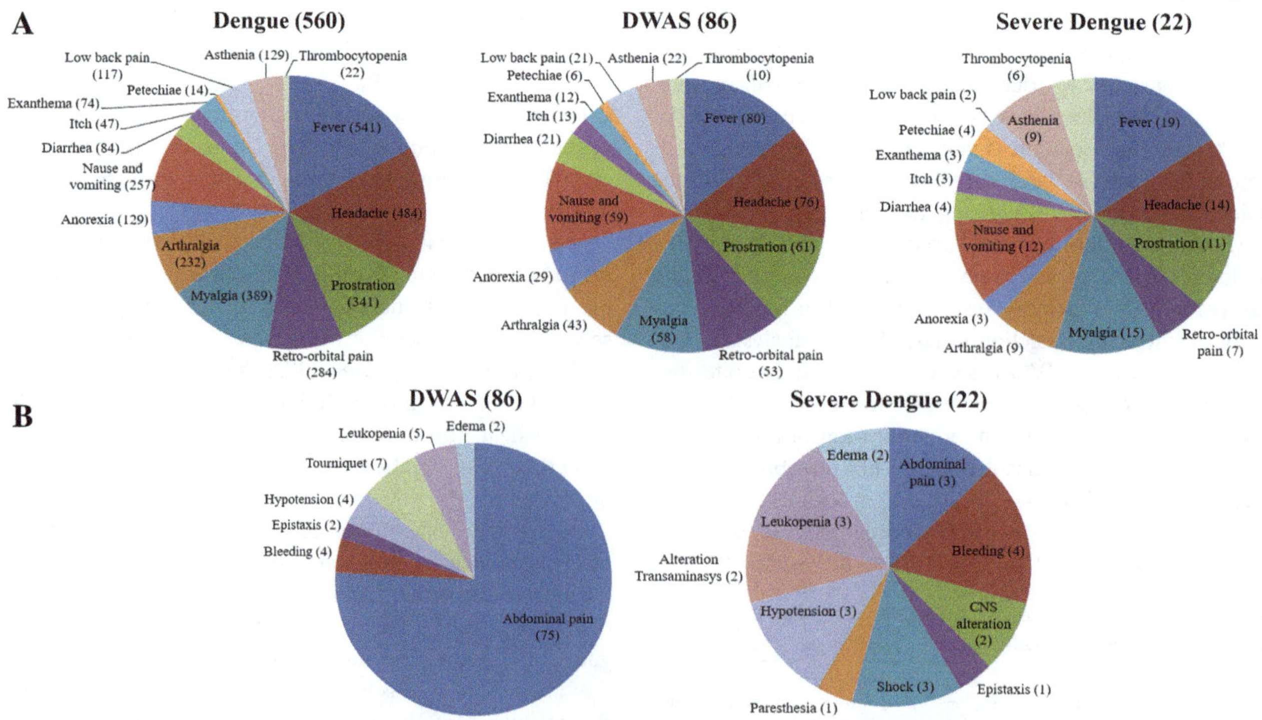

Fig. 3 Distribution of clinical manisfestations from dengue, dengue with warning signs (DWAS) and severe DENV-4 cases occurred in Rio de Janeiro form 2011 to 2013

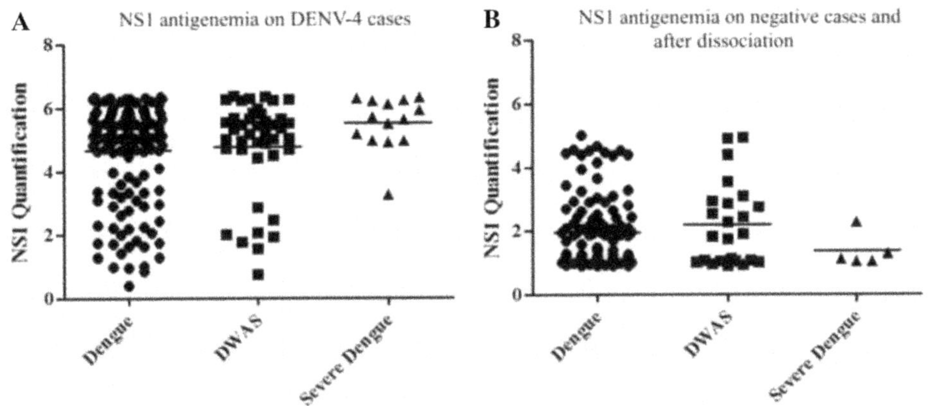

Fig. 4 DENV-4 NS1 antigenemia according to the disease severity. **a** NS1 antigenemia on DENV-4 cases positive for NS1 ELISA; (**b**) NS1 antigenemia on DENV-4 cases previoulsy negative by NS1 ELISA and positive after heat-mediated immune-complex dissociation

DENV-4 strains isolated from 2011 to 2013, following this serotype introduction and spread in RJ were partially sequenced and the phylogenetic analysis demonstrated that those belong to genotype II. Moreover, based on previous studies, the sampling size sequenced here is reliable for this analysis considering the epidemic duration, site and the low-mutation characteristic of DENV [16, 37]. The strains of genotype II first isolated during the outbreak of 1982 in Roraima, North Brazil [38] did not spread to other states at that time. However, this genotype was once again detected in Roraima in 2010, being circulated through Central America, Northeastern South America and the Caribbean [39]. According to Temporão et al. (2011) [16], these strains of genotype II were genetically different from those isolated in the 1980s in Roraima and demonstrated a probable origin from Venezuela and Colombia. However, Nunes et al. [40] complete and partial DENV-4 sequences isolated in Brazil identified the circulation of two genotypes (I and II). Genotype II is the most commonly one observed circulating in South America and the Caribbean. Genotype I, one the other hand is represented by a strain isolated in the Northeast of Brazil (Bahia), which may have some evolutionary relationship with Asian strains, according to phylogenetic analysis performed by Campos et al. [41].

Conclusions

After the DENV-4 isolation in 2011 in RJ, this serotype spread in the following two years and, the co-circulation of the four DENV was evidenced for the first time in the state. The DENV-4 diagnosis by NS1 ELISA was significantly improved by using an immune complex dissociation step. We observed a low percentage of clinical manifestations related to a more severe disease, and despite the occurrence of secondary infections, immune status and age were not related to a more severe disease. Although two distinct DENV-4 genotypes were already reported circulating in Brazil, in this study, genotype II was the only identified during the period in RJ. The

Table 4 Analysis of factors associated to DENV-4 cases in Rio de Janeiro, Brazil, from January 2011 to December 2013

	Dengue		*p* value*	DWAS		*p* value*	Severe dengue		*p* value*
	n	%		*n*	%		*n*	%	
Age group (years)									
≤ 15	102	85.0		15	12.5		3	2.5	>0.05
16–64	426	83.8	>0.05	67	13.1	>0.05	15	2.9	
> 65	20	83.3		1	4.1		3	12.5	
Type of infection									
Primary	159	48.6	>0.05	43	50.5	>0.05	5	31.2	>0.05
Secondary	168	51.4		42	49.5		11	68.8	

*Statistical analysis performed for the comparison of the disease severity to the distinct age groups and type of infection

Table 5 DENV-4 fatal cases (*n* = 14) occurred from 2011 to 2013 in the State of Rio de Janeiro, Brazil

Year	2012	2013
Type of infection (*n* = 7)	*n*	
Primary (*n* = 3)	2	1
Secondary (*n* = 4)	3	1
Age group (*n* = 12)	*n*	
≤ 15 (*n* = 2)	2	NI
16–65 (*n* = 7)	3	4
> 65 (*n* = 3)	NI	3

NI not identified

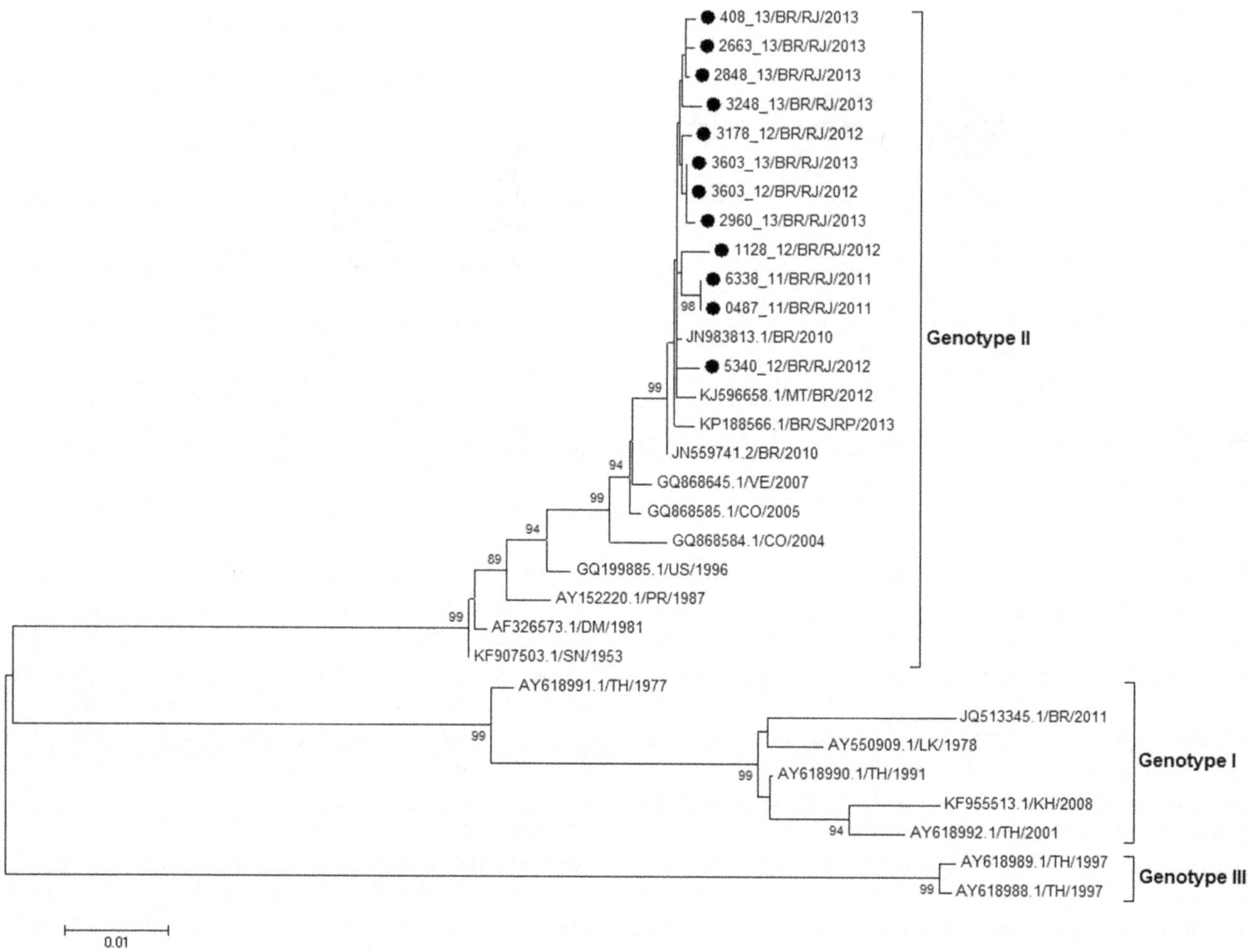

Fig. 5 Phylogenetic analysis based on C/prM/M genes from representative DENV-4 (n = 12) strains isolated from 2011 to 2013, Rio de Janeiro, Brazil. Neighbor-joining method, Tamura-Nei-parameter model (TN93 + G) with gamma parameter 0,23. Bootstrap test (1000 pseudo-replicates) is presented on the basis of the branches. Black circles represent the DENV-4 sequences analyzed. DENV reference strains were named as follows: number of GenBank accession/country/year

impact of the introduction and emergence of DENV-4 in the state of RJ was not well understood and studies accessing a new DENV serotype circulation in an endemic scenario are needed.

Abbreviations

ALT: Alanine transferase; AST: Aspartate aminotransferase; DENV: Dengue Virus; DHF: Dengue hemorrhagic fever; DwWS: Dengue with warning signs; IFAT: Indirect fluorescent antibody test; Ig: Immunoglobulin; RT-PCR: Reverse transcriptase-polymerase chain reaction; SD: Severe dengue; WHO: World Health Organization

Acknowledgements

To Dr. Ana Maria Bispo de Filippis, Eliane Araújo, Simone Sampaio, José da Costa Farias Filho and Leda Maria do Santos for laboratorial and technical support.

Funding

To Conselho Nacional de Desenvolvimento Científico e Tecnológico/CNPq [grant number 303822/2015-5] and Programa Estratégico de Pesquisa em Saúde/PAPES VI-FIOCRUZ [grant number 407690/2012-3], to Coordenação de Aperfeiçoamento de Pessoal de Nível Superior (CAPES), to Fundação de Amparo a Pesquisa do Estado do Rio de Janeiro/FAPERJ [grant number 210.026/2014 to RMR], to FIOCRUZ, and Brazilian Ministry of Health.

Authors' contributions

FBS, RMRN and MH design the study. MH, TMAS, MRQL, PCGN, NRCF, FBN and TCC performed the experiments. MH, TMAS, FBN and FBS wrote the paper. All authors read and approved the final manuscript.

Competing interests

The authors declare that they have no competing interests.

Consent for publication

Not applicable

Author details

[1]Viral Immunology Laboratory, Oswaldo Cruz Institute/FIOCRUZ, Av Brasil 4365, Manguinhos, Rio de Janeiro, RJ 21045-360, Brazil. [2]Flavivirus Laboratory, Oswaldo Cruz Institute, Rio de Janeiro, Brazil.

References

1. Word Health Organization. Sustaining the drive to overcome the global impact of neglected tropical diseases: second WHO report on neglected tropical diseases. Geneva 2013; 25–29.
2. Lindenbach B, et al. Flaviviridae: The viruses and their replication. PH KDaH, ed. Fields Virology. 2001; 991–1041.

3. Lanciotti, et al. Molecular evolution and phylogeny of dengue-4 viruses. Journal of General Virology. 1997;78:2279–84.
4. Weaver SC, Vasilakis N. Molecular evolution of dengue viruses: contributions of phylogenetics to understanding the history and epidemiology of the preeminent arboviral disease. Infections, Genetics and Evolution. 2009;9:523–40.
5. Klungthong C, et al. The molecular epidemiology of dengue virus serotype 4 in Bangkok, Thailand. Virology. 2004; 329:168–179.
6. Claro L, et al. Dengue prevention and control: a review of studies on knowledge, beliefs, and practices. Caderno Saude Publica. 2004;20:1447–57.
7. Schatzmayr HG, et al. An outbreak of dengue virus at Rio de Janeiro. Memórias Instituto Oswaldo Cruz. 1986;81:245–6.
8. Nogueira RM, et al. Isolation of dengue virus type 2 in Rio de Janeiro. Memórias Instituto Oswaldo Cruz. 1990;85:253.
9. Nogueira RM, et al. Dengue epidemic in the stage of Rio de Janeiro, Brazil, 1990-1: co-circulation of dengue 1 and dengue 2 serotypes. Epidemiol Infect. 1993;111:163–70.
10. Nogueira RM, et al. Dengue virus type 3 in Rio de Janeiro. Brazil Memorias Instituto Oswaldo Cruz. 2001;96:925–6.
11. Nogueira RM, et al. Dengue virus type 3, Brazil, 2002. Emerg Infect dis. 2005; 11:1376–81.
12. Teixeira M, et al. Recent shift in age pattern of dengue hemorrhagic fever. Brazil. Emerging Infectious Diseases. 2008;14:1663.
13. Teixeira MG, et al. Dengue: twenty-five years since reemergence in Brazil. Caderno Saude Publica. 2009;25(Suppl 1):S7–18.
14. Secretaria de Vigilancia em Saude, Ministerio da Saude. Dengue. Boletim da semana 48/2008. In. Brasília: Ministério da Saúde, 2008. http://portalsaude.saude.gov.br/index.php/o-ministerio/principal/secretarias/svs/boletim-epidemiologico. Accessed 13 Dec 2016.
15. Secretaria de Vigilancia em Saude, Ministerio da Saude. Informe epidemiológico da dengue: Semanas de 1 a 52 de 2009. In Brasília: Ministério da Saúde, 2009 http://Wwwriorjgovbr/web/Sms Accessed 13 Dec 2016.
16. Temporao JG, et al. Dengue virus serotype 4, Roraima state. Brazil Emerging Infectious Diseases. 2011;17:938–40.
17. Nogueira RM, et al. Dengue virus type 4 arrives in the state of Rio de Janeiro: a challenge for epidemiological surveillance and control. Memorias Instituto Oswaldo Cruz. 2011;106:255–6.
18. Word Health Organization. Dengue: guidelines for diagnosis, treatment, prevention and control. Special Programme for Research and Training in Tropical Diseases. Geneva; 2009. http://www.who.int/tdr/publications/documents/dengue-diagnosis.pdf
19. Igarashi A. Isolation of a Singh's *Aedes albopictus* cell clone sensitive to dengue and chikungunya viruses. Journal General Virology. 1978;40:531–44.
20. Gubler DJ, et al. Mosquito cell cultures and specific monoclonal antibodies in surveillance for dengue viruses. Am J Trop med Hyg. 1984;33:158–65.
21. Miagostovich MP, et al. Evaluation of an IgG enzyme-linked immunosorbent assay for dengue diagnosis. Journal Clinical Virology. 1999;14:183–9.
22. Lanciotti RS, et al. Rapid detection and typing of dengue viruses from clinical samples by using reverse transcriptase-polymerase chain reaction. Journal Clinical Microbiology. 1992;30:545–51.
23. Johnson BW, et al. Serotype-specific detection of dengue viruses in a fourplex real-time reverse transcriptase PCR assay. Journal Clinical Microbiology. 2005;43:4977–83.
24. Lima MRQ, et al. A simple heat dissociation method increases significantly the ELISA detection sensitivity of the nonstructural-1 glycoprotein in patients infected with DENV type-4. J Virol Methods. 2014;204:105–8.
25. Miagostovich MP, et al. Diagnosis of dengue by using reverse transcriptase-polymerase chain reaction. Memórias Instituto Oswaldo Cruz. 1997;92:595–9.
26. Dos Santos FB, et al. A review on dengue diagnosis and epidemiology by a Regional reference laboratory in 25 years, Rio de Janeiro. Brazil Dengue Bulletin. 2013;37:61–76.
27. Andries AC, et al. Field evaluation and impact on clinical management of a rapid diagnostic kit that detects dengue NS1. IgM and IgG PLoS Neglected Tropical Diseases. 2012;6:e1993.
28. Dussart P, et al. Evaluation of an enzyme immunoassay for detection of dengue virus NS1 antigen in human serum. Clin Vaccine Immunol. 2006;13:1185–9.
29. Hang VT, et al. Diagnostic accuracy of NS1 ELISA and lateral flow rapid tests for dengue sensitivity, specificity and relationship to viremia and antibody responses. PLoS Negl Trop dis. 2009;3:e360.
30. Lima Mda R, et al. Comparison of three commercially available dengue NS1 antigen capture assays for acute diagnosis of dengue in Brazil. PLoS Negl Trop dis. 2010;4:738.
31. Huang CH, et al. Laboratory diagnostics of dengue fever: An emphasis on the role of commercial dengue virus nonstructural protein 1 antigen rapid test. Journal Microbiology, Immunology and Infection. 2012; doi: S1684-1182(12)00155-7.
32. Secretaria de Estado de Saúde e Defesa Civil do Rio de Janeiro (SESDEC-RJ). Relatório de casos de dengue. 2009. http://prefeitura.rio/web/sms/dengue-casos-bairro-periodo. Accessed 14 Apr 2013.
33. Amâncio FF, et al. Dengue virus serotype 4 in a highly susceptible population in southeast Brazi. Journal Infection Public Health. 2014;7:547–52.
34. Vaughn DW, et al. Dengue viremia titer, antibody response pattern, and virus serotype correlate with disease severity. J Infect dis. 2000;181:2–9.
35. Endy TP, et al. Relationship of preexisting dengue virus (DV) neutralizing antibody levels to viremia and severity of disease in a prospective cohort study of DV infection in Thailand. J Infect dis. 2004;189:990–1000.
36. de Araújo JM, et al. Quantification of dengue virus type 3 RNA in fatal and non-fatal cases in Brazil, 2002. Trans R Soc Trop med Hyg. 2009;103(9):952–4.
37. Barcelos Figueiredo L, et al. Dengue virus 2 American-Asian genotype identified during the 2006/2007 outbreak in Piauí, Brazil reveals a Caribbean route of introduction and dissemination of dengue virus in Brazil. PLoS One. 2014; 9(11).
38. Osanai CH, et al. Dengue outbreak in boa vista, Roraima. Preliminary report. Revista Instituto de Medicina Tropical. 1983;25:53–4.
39. Acosta et al. Dengue virus serotype 4, Roraima State, Brazil. Emerg Infect Dis. 2011; 17:1979–80.
40. Nunes MR, et al. Phylogeography of dengue virus serotype 4, Brazil, 2010-2011. Emerg Infect dis. 2012;18:1858–64.
41. Campos Rde M, et al. Emergence of dengue virus 4 genotypes II b and I in the city of Rio de Janeiro. J Clin Virol. 2013;56:86–8.

18

A study of clinical, hematological, and biochemical profiles of patients with dengue viral infections in Northwest Ethiopia: implications for patient management

Getachew Ferede[1*], Moges Tiruneh[1], Ebba Abate[2], Yitayih Wondimeneh[1], Endalamaw Gadisa[3], Rawleigh Howe[3], Abraham Aseffa[3] and Belay Tessema[1]

Abstract

Background: Dengue is one of the most common arboviral diseases with increased outbreaks annually in tropical and subtropical areas. In Ethiopia, there are no data regarding clinical, hematological and biochemical parameters which are very important in the clinical management of dengue patients. Hence this study was carried out to provide the first baseline data of clinical, hematological and biochemical profiles of patients infected with dengue virus.

Methods: A cross-sectional study was carried out among febrile patients in northwest Ethiopia from March 2016 to May 2017. Blood samples were collected from dengue presumed cases and tested against dengue specific IgM antibody by enzyme-linked immunosorbent assay (ELISA). Those study participants who fulfilled the inclusion criteria were enrolled in the study. Clinical examination findings were recorded, hematological and biochemical parameters tests were done.

Results: During the study period, a total of 102 dengue cases were included in the study. Of these, there were 16 (15.7%) children and 86 (84.3%) adults between 1 and 76 year age. The most common clinical presentations followed by fever (100%) were a headache 89 (87.3%), myalgia 82 (80.4%), nausea/vomiting 71 (69.6%). The common hematological findings were thrombocytopenia 61 (59.8%), followed by anemia 45 (44.1%) and leucopenia 27 (26.5%) and the elevated levels of biochemical parameters were AST 46 (45.1%) and ALT in 18 (17.6%).

Conclusions: This study highlights the most common clinical and laboratory profiles of dengue viral infections that could alert physicians to the likelihood of dengue virus infections in the study area.

Keywords: Dengue, Clinical features, Hematological tests, Biochemical parameters

Background

Dengue is a mosquito-borne arboviral disease and is a major global public health threat that is prevalent in tropical and sub-tropical regions of the world, mostly in urban and semi-urban areas [1]. The WHO estimates, more than 2.5 billion individuals live at risk of dengue transmission in more than 100 countries and approximately 50-100 million individuals have infected with dengue annually [2]. Of these, 500,000 severe dengue cases are diagnosed each year resulting in 24,000 deaths per year [3–6]. Dengue is endemic in the WHO regions of Africa, the Americas, the Eastern Mediterranean, South-East Asia, and the Western Pacific regions and the Caribbean [7]. In the recent decades, the global incidence of dengue virus (DENV) infection has increased with increasing geographic expansion to new countries [8]. The threat of a possible outbreak of dengue for the

* Correspondence: get29f@gmail.com
[1]Department of Medical Microbiology, School of Biomedical and Laboratory Sciences, College of Medicine and Health Sciences, University of Gondar, Gondar, Ethiopia
Full list of author information is available at the end of the article

first time reported from Ethiopia in 2013 in Dire Dawa. In this outbreak, 11, 409 dengue suspected cases within four months were reported. Fifty (50/88; 56.8%) samples were reported positive for dengue infection and mostly affected age groups were 15-44 year-olds [9]. Dengue cases were also later reported in 2014 from Somali Regional state of Ethiopia, in which 33 (33/57, 57.9%) samples were reported positive for dengue [10].

The leading contributing factors for widespread and increasing dengue incidences are rapid unplanned urbanization and migration of population to urban areas, poor sanitation facilities contributing fertile breeding areas for mosquitoes, lack of vector control and climatic changes [11]. As mosquitoes are widely distributed in Africa and can serve as vectors of dengue virus, when these combined with rapid population growth, unplanned urbanization, and increased international travel, could increase the epidemic risk in African countries [12].

Specific treatment for dengue is not available, but early detection and fluid replacement therapy and use of analgesics and antipyretics with good nursing care ensures marked reduction of the mortality rates 20% to less than 1% due to severe cases [13]. In clinical practice, as it is known, the patient's diagnosis and management are based on clinical manifestations and abnormal laboratory findings [14]. Initial DENV infection may be asymptomatic [15] or may result in a nonspecific febrile illness typically present with the sudden onset of fever, severe headache, bone, joint and muscular pains, mild bleeding manifestation, weakness, myalgia, and rash [16]. All these clinical presentations are similar to many other febrile diseases prevalent in the country; such as malaria, Kala-azar and typhoid fever which pose a diagnostic challenge of dengue [17].

Dengue is caused by infection with any one of the four serotypes of DENV which is an arbovirus single-stranded RNA virus of the genus Flavivirus [18]. Infection with one dengue serotype provides lifelong homotypic immunity to that particular serotype. Different serotypes can be in circulation during an epidemic, and thus, a person can eventually be infected as many as four times, once with each serotype [19]. It is well documented that subsequent infection with different DENV serotypes increases the risk of developing severe dengue [20, 21]. Infection with dengue can be diagnosed by using clinical presentations and laboratory tests. Of the laboratory tests, non-specific tests; like hematological parameters, liver function tests, and serum protein concentration and specific tests; such as viral antigen test, genomic sequence, and serology for antibody detection are used [22, 23].

Dengue was noticed recently in Ethiopia but there is no data concerning clinical and laboratory profiles of the cases with dengue in the country. Physicians should be aware of the most common clinical as well as hematological and biochemical presentations which are important for the clinical management of patients and thus crucial for saving a life. Therefore, this study aimed to highlight the most common clinical features, hematological and biochemical findings of dengue cases.

Methods

Study area and participants

A cross-sectional prospective, hospital-based study was carried out in Metema and Humera Kahsay Abera hospitals, northwest Ethiopia from March 2016 to May 2017.

Inclusion criteria

Febrile patients who were presumed for dengue infection based on 2009 WHO criteria [8] and serologically confirmed with dengue specific IgM antibody. The febrile patient is referred to one whose axillary temperature is ≥ 38 °C.

Exclusion criteria

Cases confirmed as malaria, Kala-azar, typhoid fever, and any other confirmed chronic diseases were excluded in the study.

Data collection

Clinical examinations were performed by a physician on each study participant. Demographic variables, as it has been published in previous work, [24] and clinical profiles of study participants were collected by nurses using the structured questionnaire. The diagnosis of dengue was made based on positive enzyme-linked immunosorbent (ELISA; manufactured by EUROIMMUN diagnostics) [25] assay result for specific IgM antibody for dengue in serum. All the routine investigations such as hematological determination like total leukocyte count (TLC), differential leukocyte count, platelet count; hemoglobin (Hgb) and hematocrit (Hct) were determined by the automated blood analyzer (CELL-DYN 1800, Abbott Laboratories Diagnostics Division, USA). Thick and thin blood smear for malaria parasite, biochemical tests; AST and ALT for liver function tests, creatinine, and BUN for renal function tests and total protein were done by the automated biochemistry analyzer (Vegasys) [26]. The cutoff values of each test results were considered based on reference ranges used by the laboratory. Furthermore, medical charts of all dengue specific IgM positive cases were reviewed for the collection of other information (i.e. Kala-azar, typhoid fever, and any other confirmed chronic cases).

Statistical analysis

Data were entered and analyzed using the SPSS 20.0 statistical software. Descriptive statistic was used to calculate frequency and percentage. Data were presented by using tables and figure.

Results

Clinical profiles of dengue cases during a hospital visit

During the study period, 600 febrile patients who were presumed for dengue viral infections based on 2009 the WHO criteria were tested for dengue-specific IgM antibody. Of these, 114 patients were positive for dengue. Out of positive cases, 102 (89.5%) were included in this study while the remaining 12 (10.5%) were not included in the study due to co-morbidities (Fig. 1). Seventy-eight (78/102; 76.5%) study participants were males. A study participants' age varied from 1 year to 76 years. Eighty sex (86/102; 84.3%) study participants were ≥ 15 years (Table 1). The commonest clinical feature was fever, 102 (100%), followed by headache in 89 (89/102; 87.3%), myalgia 82 (82/102; 80.4%), nausea/vomiting 71 (71/102; 69.6%), abdominal pain 61 (61/102; 59.8%), eye pain and mucosal bleeding 38 (38/102; 37.3%) in each of the cases, conjunctival hemorrhage and hepatomegaly 23 (23/102, 22.5%) in each of the cases. Rashes and tourniquet test in 13 (13/102; 12.7%) and 8 (8/102; 7.8%) of cases were seen, respectively (Table 2).

Hematological profiles of dengue cases during a hospital visit

The most common hematological finding observed was thrombocytopenia (platelet count < 140,000/cumm) in 61 (61/102; 59.8%), followed by anemia (hemoglobin level < 11.5 g/dl) in 45 (45/102; 44.1%) and leucopenia (total leukocyte count < 4,000/cumm) in 27 (27/102; 26.5%) of the cases. Hematocrit > 44% were noted in 10 (10/102; 9.8%) of the cases and it ranged between 9-51%. Neutrophil < 1500 in 16 (16/102; 15.7%) and lymphocyte > 2900 in 2 (2/102; 2%) of the cases were noticed (Table 3).

Biochemical parameters of dengue cases at the time of hospital visit

The results of the biochemical investigation revealed that alanine aminotransferase (ALT) level > 42 IU/L was observed in 18 (18/102; 17.6%) of cases and aspartate aminotransferase (AST) level > 37 IU/L observed in 46 (46/102; 45.1%) of cases. The levels of ALT and AST ranged between 4-347 IU/L and 8-320 IU/L, respectively. Creatinine level > 1.1 mg/dl was observed in 20 (20/102; 19.6%) and BUN > 23.5 mg/dl noted in 15 (15/102; 14.7%) of cases. Hypoproteinaemia (total protein value < 6.6 mg/dl) was observed in 22 (22/102; 21.6%) cases (Table 4).

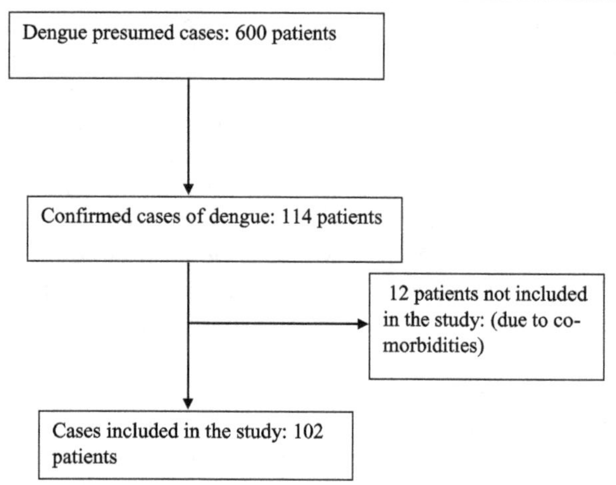

Fig. 1 Flow chart of the study

Table 1 Gender and age of the study participants (N = 102)

Variables	Number of participants	Percentage
Gender		
Male	78	76.5
Female	24	23.5
Age		
< 15 years	16	15.7
≥ 15 years	86	84.3

Discussion

In recent decades, the global prevalence of dengue has increased dramatically due to the limitations of currently available control strategies, such as vaccines and pesticides [27, 28]. Hence early diagnosis and proper medical management are of prime importance. As dengue is a recently known problem in Ethiopia [9, 10], the knowledge regarding its clinical presentations along with laboratory tests is vital for patient management. Hence, this study emphasized to document the first baseline data on clinical manifestations, hematological and biochemical parameters of patients with dengue illness in the country. The evidence generated is crucial for proper management of dengue patients.

In this study, the most frequent clinical presentation was fever, followed by a headache, myalgia, nausea/vomiting and abdominal pain, which is in agreement

Table 2 Clinical presentations of dengue cases at the time of hospital visit (N = 102)

Clinical feature	Number of cases	Percentage
Fever	102	100
Abdominal distention	14	13.7
Headache	89	87.3
Eye pain	38	37.3
Myalgia	82	80.4
Mucosal bleeding	38	37.3
Abdominal pain	61	59.8
Nausea and vomiting	71	69.6
Rash	13	12.7
Tourniquet test	8	7.8
Conjunctival hemorrhage	23	22.5
Hepatomegaly	23	22.5

Table 3 Hematological parameters of dengue cases at the time of hospital visit (N = 102)

Hematological test	No. of patient N (%)	Normal lab value
Platelet count (cells/cumm)		140,000-415,000/cumm
< 140,000	61 (59.8)	
≥140,000	41 (40.2)	
WBC count (cells/cumm)		4,000-10,500/cumm
< 4,000	27 (26.5)	
≥ 4,000	75 (73.5)	
Hemoglobin g/dl		
Male ≤ 13	34 (43.6)	M: 13-16
Female ≤ 12	11 (45.8)	F: 12-15
Sub-total	45 (44.1)	
Hematocrit (%)		
Male > 46	8 (10.3)	M: 38-46
Female > 44	2 (8.3)	F: 35-44
Sub-total	10 (9.8)	
Neutrophil (cells/cumm)		1500-8000
< 1500	16 (15.7)	
≥ 1500	86 (84.3)	
Lymphocyte (cells/cumm)		900-2900
≤ 2900	100 (98)	
> 2900	2 (2)	

Table 4 Biochemical parameters among dengue cases (N = 102)

Parameter	No. of cases N (%)	Normal lab value
ALT (IU/L)		3-42 IU/L
≤ 42	84 (82.4)	
> 42	18 (17.6)	
AST (IU/L)		5-37 IU/L
≤ 37	56 (54.9)	
> 37	46 (45.1)	
Creatinine (mg/dl)		0.6-1.1 mg/dl
≤ 1.1	82 (80.4)	
> 1.1	20 (19.6)	
BUN (mg/dl)		4.7-23.5 mg/dl
≤ 23.5	87 (85.3)	
> 23.5	15 (14.7)	
Total protein (mg/dl)		6.6-8.7mg/dl
< 6.6	22 (21.6)	
≥ 6.6	80 (78.4)	

with the other studies [29, 30]. Rash was seen in 12.7% and hepatomegaly in 22.5% of the cases in our study while in another similar study 28.1% and 12.5% of patients presented with rash and hepatomegaly, respectively [31]. Bleeding diathesis is a common clinical presentation of dengue due to low platelet count and leakage from blood vessels. This is due to the interaction of dengue virus with host cells which cause the release of excess cytokines and stimulation of immunologic mechanism causing vascular endothelial alteration, infiltration of mononuclear cells and perivascular edema [32]. In our study mucosal bleeding was observed in most of the patients, which is in agreement with the other study [33], but in contrast to another study which showed cutaneous bleeding as the most common hemorrhagic manifestation [34]. In another study, hemorrhagic manifestation in the form of petechiae only was reported [31]. The variations in the clinical presentation of different studies might be due to the difference in the strain of the virus and its virulence factor.

Among the hematological profiles, thrombocytopenia was the most common finding in the present study which is consistent with the other studies [35, 36]. Thrombocytopenia might be due to decreased production of platelets due to suppression of the bone marrow by a virus and also due to binding of dengue antigens to platelets and increased antibody mediated immunological destruction of platelets [37, 38]. Leucopenia is one of the hematological parameters which occurs in people who were afflicted with dengue bone marrow suppression [38]. In our study, leucopenia was observed in 26.5% of the cases while in other studies elsewhere leucopenia was observed in 56.9% [39] and in 50% of the cases [40].

Hemoglobin levels less than the cutoff values were observed in 45 (44.1%) of the cases. This could be due to mucosal bleeding in which 38 (37.3%) of the cases had bleeding. This finding is consistent with another study [41]. Increased hematocrit was observed in 6.9% of cases in our study while it is less than the observation of the others studies which was reported 50% [42] and 27% [40] rise in hematocrit value. This might be related to increased severity and is elucidated by the hemoconcentration due to increased intravascular plasma permeability which is the basic pathophysiological changes in dengue.

In this study, higher levels than the normal values of AST in 45.1% and ALT in 17.6% of the cases were observed which showed elevated levels of AST in a greater proportion of cases than ALT. This is in agreement with the other studies elsewhere that reported AST and ALT higher levels in 68.5% and 39.2% of the cases, respectively [43] and similar findings were also reported elevated AST in 72.7% and ALT in 27.3% of cases elsewhere [44]. Dengue virus is hepatotrophic and also damages other organs; hence the observed pattern could be explained due to excess release of AST from damaged muscle cells (nonhepatic source) during infection that leads to more deranged AST than ALT. The ALT is mainly associated with hepatocytes, with the smallest activity in cardiac and skeletal muscle and AST is found in erythrocytes, kidney and brain tissue, cardiac and skeletal muscle and is usually raised because of damage to those sources and response to hepatic damage [45].

The serum creatinine and blood urea (BUN) levels were raised in 19.6% and 14.7% of the cases, respectively. These could be due to a direct viral effect on the glomerular and tubular cells or as a result of tissue injury caused by deregulated host immune response against the viral antigens [46]. Hypoproteinemia was observed in 21.6% of the cases. This could be probable that the complex interaction between virus, host immune response and endothelial cells, may affect the barrier integrity and functions of the vascular endothelial cells leading to plasma leakage causing hypoproteinemia [47].

Although this is the first effort to study clinical, hematological and biochemical profiles of dengue viral infection in Ethiopia, the study has several limitations. Comparisons of those dengue cases with the control group and serial hematological and biochemical changes were not done due to the nature of cross-sectional study design. These could be done in the future for better understanding of dengue viral infection presentation. Regardless of the depicted limitations, this preliminary study ultimately provides the first baseline data on clinical and laboratory profiles of dengue viral infection in the country.

Conclusion

Awareness of clinical features, as well as laboratory findings like hematological and biochemical parameters, are the most important guide to therapy and prognosis of dengue. In this study, fever followed by a headache and myalgia were commonest presenting complaints of dengue patients. Thrombocytopenia, anemia, leucopenia and elevated levels of AST were identified as the most common findings. Thus, these findings should prompt physicians on the probability of dengue infection in the study area.

Abbreviations

ALT: Alanine aminotransferase; AST: Aspartate aminotransferase; BUN: Blood Urea; DENV: Dengue Virus; ELISA: Enzyme-Linked Immunosorbent Assay; HCT: Hematocrit; IgM: Immunoglobulin M

Acknowledgments

We would like to acknowledge the University of Gondar and Armauer Hansen Research Institute for financially supporting this study. The role of the Tropical and Infectious Diseases Research Center at the University of Gondar was an immense contribution to the process. We are very grateful to the patients who provided a sample and also physicians, nurses and laboratory technologists of the Metema and Kahsay Abera hospital for their contribution to data collection.

Funding

This study was funded by the University of Gondar and Armauer Hansen Research Institute. The funders had no role in the design of the study and collection, analysis, and interpretation of data and in writing the manuscript.

Authors' contributions

GF: participated in conception and design of the study, data collection, laboratory analysis, data analysis and interpretations of the findings, drafted the manuscript and write up. MT and EA: participated in the conception and design of the study, data analysis and interpretations of the findings. YW: participated in conception and design of the study, data collection, data analysis and interpretations of the findings. EG, RH, AA: participated in conception and design of the study, interpretations of the findings, BT: participated in conception and design of the study, data collection and laboratory analyses, data analysis and interpretations of the findings. All authors reviewed and approved the final manuscript.

Consent for publication

Not applicable.

Competing interests

The authors declare that they have no competing interests.

Author details

[1]Department of Medical Microbiology, School of Biomedical and Laboratory Sciences, College of Medicine and Health Sciences, University of Gondar, Gondar, Ethiopia. [2]Ethiopian Public Health Institute, Addis Ababa, Ethiopia. [3]Armauer Hansen Research Institute, Addis Ababa, Ethiopia.

References

1. Engelthaler D, Fink T, Levy C, Leslie M. The reemergence of *Aedes aegypti* in Arizona. Emerg Infect Dis. 1997;3:241–2.
2. WHO. dengue and severe dengue. Fact sheet N 117 [cited 2018]. available from: http://www.searo.who.int/thailand/factsheets/fs0008/en/.
3. Gubler D. The global emergence/resurgence of arboviral diseases as public health problems. Arch Med Res. 2002;33:330–42.
4. Shepard D, Coudeville L, Halasa Y, Zambrano B, Dayan G. Economic impact of dengue illness in the Americas. Am J Trop Med Hyg. 2011;84:200–7.
5. Guha-Sapir D, Schimmer B. Dengue fever: new paradigms for a changing epidemiology. Emerg Themes Epidemiol. 2005;2. https://doi.org/10.1186/742-7622-2-1.
6. Natasha A, Mikkel B, Wilder-Smith A. Epidemiology of dengue: past, present and future prospects. Cl in Epidemiol. 2013;5:299–309.
7. Khan A, Hayat A, Masood N, Solangi N, Shaikh T. Frequency and clinical presentation of dengue fever at tertiary care hospital of Hyderabad/ Jamshoro. JLUMHS. 2010;9:88–94.
8. WHO-TDR. Dengue: guidelines for diagnosis, treatment, prevention and control- New Edition. Geneva: World Health Organisation; 2009.
9. Abyot BW, Mesfin M, Wubayehu K, Esayas K, Milliyon W, Abiy G, et al. The first acute febrile illness investigation associated with dengue fever in Ethiopia, 2013: A descriptive analysis. Ethiop J Health Dev. 2014;28:155–61.
10. Yusuf M, Salah A. Epidemiology of Dengue Fever in Ethiopian Somali Region: Retrospective Health Facility Based Study. Central African Journal of Public Health. 2016;2:51–6.
11. Dash A, Bhatia R, Sunyoto T, Mourya D. Emerging and re-emerging arboviral diseases in Southeast Asia. J Vector Borne Dis. 2013;50:77–84.
12. Gubler D. The changing epidemiology of yellow fever and dengue, 1900 to 2003. Immunol Microbiol Infect Dis. 2004;27:319–30.
13. WHO report on global surveillance of epidemic prone infectious diseases. World Health Organization, Geneva. 2005.
14. Kalayanarooj S, Vaughn D, Nimmannitya S, Green S, Suntayakorn S, Kunentrasai N, et al. Early clinical and laboratory indicators of acute dengue illness. J Infect Dis. 1997;176:313 21.

15. Sabin A. Research on dengue during World War II. Am J Trop Med Hyg. 1952;1:30.
16. Karabatsos N. International catalogue of arthropod-borne viruses. 3rd ed. American Society for Tropical Medicine and Hygiene 1985
17. Ananda A, Joel N, Kuritsky G, William L, Harold S, Margolis H. Dengue virus infection in Africa. Emerg Infect Dis. 2011;17:1349–54.
18. Nisalak A, Endy T, Nimmannitya S, Kalayanarooj S, Thisayakorn U, Scott R, et al. Serotype specific Dengue Virus Circulation and Dengue disease in Bangkok, Thailand from 1973 - 1999. Am J Trop Med Hyg. 2003;68:191–202.
19. CDC. Imported Dengue--United States, 1998 and 1998. Morb MortalWkly Rep. 2000;49:248–5.
20. Narayanan M, Aravind M, Thilothammal N, Prema R, Sargunam C, Ramamurty N. Dengue fever epidemic in Chennai - A study of clinical profile and outcome. Indian Pediatr. 2002;39:1027–33.
21. Malavige G, Fernando S, Fernando D, Seneviratne S. Dengue viral infections. Postgrad Med J. 2004;80:588–601.
22. DePaula S, Fonseca B. Dengue: A review of the laboratory tests a clinician must know to achieve a correct diagnosis. Braz J Infect Dis. 2004;8:390–8.
23. Srichaikul T, Nimmannita S. Haematology in dengue and dengue haemorrhagic. Baillieres Best Pract Res Clin Haematol. 2000;13:261–76.
24. Getachew F, Moges T, Ebba A, Yitayih W, Demekech D, Endalamaw G, et al. A serologic study of dengue in northwest Ethiopia: Suggesting preventive and control measures. PLoS Negl Trop Dis. 2018;12:e0006430.
25. EUROIMMUN. Medizinische Labordiagnostika AG, Lübeck, Germany. Available from: http://www.euroimmun.com/products/techniken/mikrototer-elisa-beschreibung.html. Cited 2018.
26. Vegasys. Biochemistry analyzer. Available from: www.amsalliance.com/product/vegasys . Cited 2018.
27. Kyle J, Harris E. Global spread and persistence of dengue. Annu Rev Microbiol. 2008;62:71–92.
28. World Health Organization. Global Strategy for dengue prevention and control, 2012-2020. France: World Health Orgainzation; 2012. ISBN: 9789241504034
29. Rajesh D, MdIshaque Q, Raj S. Clinical and laboratory profile in seropositive dengue cases at a tertiary care hospital, South India. WJPPS. 2017;6:1571–81.
30. Niloy C, Vithyavathi S, Sankar K. Clinical and laboratory profile of different dengue sub types in dengue virus infection. Int J Res Med Sci. 2016;4:743–8.
31. Badawy A, Sharaf H, AdelMahmoud A. Clinical and Hematological Effects of Dengue Viruses Infection. Am J Infect Dis Microbiol. 2016;4:74–8.
32. Nadia A, Malik M, Jamil A, Jahangir M, Tirmiz N, Majid A, et al. Cutaneous manifestations in patients of dengue fever. J Pak Assoc Dermatologists. 2012;22:320–4.
33. Siddiqui F, Haider S, Bhutta Z. Endemic dengue fever: A seldom recognized hazard for Pakistani children. J Infect Dev Ctries. 2009;3:306–12.
34. Adarsh E, Subramanian V. Clinical profile of dengue infection in a tertiary care hospital. Indian J Child Health. 2015;2:68–71.
35. Syed R, Musarrat R, Farhat A. Characteristics and outcome of dengue infection; clinical perspective from a secondary care hospital of Karachi. Pak J Med Sci. 2013;29:115–8.
36. Ahmed S, Ali N, Ashraf S, Ilyas M, Tariq W, Chotani R. Dengue fever outbreak: a clinical management experience. J Coll Physicians Surg Pak. 2008;18:8–12.
37. Lin C, Lei H, Liu C, Liu H, Yeh T, Wang S. Generation of IgM anti-platelet autoamibody in dengue patients. J Med Virol. 2001;63:143–9.
38. Jameel T, Mehmood K, Mujaba G, Choudhry N, Afzal N, Paul R. Changing haematological parameters in dengue viral infections. J Ayub Med Coll Abbottabad. 2012;24:3–6.
39. Kinjal P, Dipanki P, Hematological Parameters DV. ItsUtility in Dengue Fever: A Prospective Study. Int J Sci Res. 2016;5:1077–9.
40. Mohd Y, Shamim A. Evaluation of clinico-hematological and biochemical changes in dengue fever at CIMSH Lucknow. ijcmr. 2017;4:1527–9.
41. Mohamed M, Kalavathi G, Mehul R, Karthik M, Asfiya A, Vagesh S, et al. A Study of Clinical and Laboratory Profile of Dengue Fever in Tertiary Care Hospital in Central Karnataka, India. Glob J Med Res. 2014;14:7–12.
42. Achalkar G. Dengue: a clinic-pathological study of 50 cases. J Evol Med Den Sci. 2013;2:9380–5.
43. Mariappan T. Current emerging situation of dengue in India. Trop Doct. 2013;43:116–9.
44. Spoorti V, Yugandhar R, Prabhakar K. Study of clinical and laboratory profile of dengue fever patients. Eur J Pharm Med Res. 2016;3:613–6.
45. Wahid S, Sanusi S, Zawawi M. A comparison of the pattern of liver involvement in dengue hemorrhagic fever with classic dengue fever. Southeast Asian j trop med public health. 2000;31:259–63.
46. Glassock R. Immune complex-induced glomerular injury in viral diseases: an overview. Kidney Int Suppl. 1991;35:S5–7.
47. Uday G, Jaya kS, Jnaneshwari M. Study of serum aminotransferase levels in dengue fever. Jemds. 2014;3:2445–55.

Evaluation of creatine kinase and liver enzymes in identification of severe dengue

Saiful Safuan Md Sani[1*], Winn Hui Han[1], Mohamad Adam Bujang[2*], Hui Jen Ding[1], Kiah Loon Ng[1] and Mohd Azizuddin Amir Shariffuddin[3]

Abstract

Background: Existing biomarkers such as AST, ALT and hematocrit have been associated with severe dengue but evidence are mixed. Recently, interests in creatine kinase as a dengue biomarker have risen. These biomarkers represent several underlying pathophysiological processes in dengue. Hence, we aimed to assess AST, ALT, CK and hematocrit in identification of severe dengue and to assess the correlational relationship amongst common biomarkers of dengue.

Methods: This was a retrospective cohort study of confirmed dengue patients who were warded in Kuala Lumpur Hospital between December 2014 and January 2015. CK, AST, ALT, hematocrit, platelet count, WBC and serum albumin were taken upon ward admission and repeated at timed intervals. Composite indices based on admission AST and ALT were analyzed. Correlation coefficients and coefficients of determination were computed.

Results: Among the 365 cases reviewed, twenty-two (6%) patients had severe dengue. AST and ALT were found to be good at identification of severe dengue. The AST^2/ALT composite index was the most accurate (AUC 0.83; 95% CI 0.73 - 0.93). Optimal cutoff was 402 with a sensitivity of 59.1% (95% CI: 36.4 - 79.3%) and specificity of 92.4% (95% CI: 89.1 - 95.0%). Modified cutoff of 653 had a sensitivity of 40.9% (95% CI: 20.7 - 63.7%) and specificity of 97.4% (95% CI: 95.1 - 98.8%). Our analyses also suggested that several underlying biological processes represented by biomarkers tested were unrelated despite occurring in the same disease entity. Also, markers of plasma leakage were discordant and AST was likely hepatic in origin.

Conclusions: The composite index AST^2/ALT may be used as a marker for identification of severe dengue based on admission AST and ALT, with two choices of cutoff values, 402 and 653. AST is most likely of liver origin and CK does not provide additional value.

Keywords: Severe dengue, Creatine kinase, AST, ALT, Identification, Sensitivity, Specificity

What is already known about this topic?

It is already known that elevations of both AST and ALT levels are associated with bleeding and dengue hemorrhagic fever. Literature on creatine kinase in dengue is inadequate. Hematocrit and serum albumin are considered as markers of plasma leakage.

* Correspondence: dcicantab5@gmail.com; adam@crc.gov.my
[1]Department of Medicine, Hospital Kuala Lumpur, Jalan Pahang, 50586 Kuala Lumpur, Malaysia
[2]Biostatistic Unit, National Clinical Research Centre, 1st Floor, MMA Building, 124 Jalan Pahang, 53000 Kuala Lumpur, Malaysia
Full list of author information is available at the end of the article

What does this article add?

This study provides evidence that AST and ALT taken upon admission, through composite index AST^2/ALT, are good parameters in identifying severe dengue regardless of types of severe dengue. AST is most likely of liver origin and CK does not provide additional value as a severity marker. Additionally, two markers of plasma leakage (hematocrit and serum albumin), do not correlate with each other.

Background

Dengue infection is endemic to the tropical and subtropical regions of the world and is predicted to worsen and spread to wider latitudes [1]. In 2014, for the first time in history, the number of confirmed dengue cases in Malaysia breached the 50,000-case mark [2].

Like any other disease, dengue has biomarkers which are used to identify dengue infection, act as surrogates for underlying pathological process or identifying severity of infection. Current established biomarkers in clinical practice are hematocrit (Hct), platelet count, white blood cell (WBC), serum albumin and alanine aminotransferase (ALT). Recent studies and the 'breakbone' feature of dengue have sparked an interest in creatine kinase (CK). It has been shown in a small cohort study involving adult dengue patients (n = 39) that CK can be elevated, median 837 (range 194-3832 U/L) [3]. It has been further documented that any level of elevated CK taken after 48-96 h from onset of illness, was indeed associated with a more severe disease (ie. dengue haemorrhagic fever, DHF) by Cox proportional hazard regression analysis, HR 6.98, 95% CI 2.34 - 20.85, $p < 0.001$ [4].

Hepatitis, represented by elevated levels of aspartate aminotransferase (AST) and ALT, has a specific pattern. It is well-documented that AST is elevated to a higher level [5–9] and in a larger proportion [10–13] of patients as compared to ALT. It has also been shown that AST rises and reduces before ALT [8]. Although AST has been found to be elevated greater than ALT, its origin, musculoskeletal or hepatic, has not been proven [8, 11]. The association of transaminitis with disease severity has been found to be inconsistent. One group of investigators in Thailand [9] showed that AST but not ALT was associated with DHF, whilst another group showed both liver enzymes were significantly associated with severe cases (AST $p < 0.001$, ALT $p = 0.003$) [14]. Both AST and ALT have been claimed to be significantly correlated with clinical plasma leakage but the strengths of correlation were not reported [12]. A later study in Vietnam showed that both AST and ALT were associated with shock [8]. They found that AST and ALT levels during the critical phase were significantly higher in dengue patients who experienced shock compared to those without shock ($p < 0.01$). They also found that transaminitis correlated weakly with the nadir thrombocytopenia (Spearman r – 0.2 to −0.3; both $p < 0.05$). One study in Singapore showed no association between transaminases and fatality, (logistic regression analysis (fatal outcome), AST $p = 0.14$, ALT $p = 0.11$) [15], and another showed transaminases lacked the discriminatory function to classify dengue according to severity by the WHO 2009 classification (AST AUROC 0.62 (95% CI:0.57 – 0.67) and ALT AUROC 0.60 (95% CI: 0.54 – 0.64) [11]).

Widely available and practical biomarkers (elevated CK [4], liver transaminases [10–12, 14–17], Hct [17] and low serum albumin [4, 14, 17] and platelet count [12, 14, 16, 17]) have been shown to be associated with more severe disease. These biomarkers each represent a specific underlying pathophysiological process. Hct and serum albumin have long been believed to be representative of plasma leakage [18]. Platelet count and WBC have been shown to be good at reflecting disease course [19]. CK reflects muscle involvement and ALT the liver. Pathophysiological processes occurring in a single disease ought to correlate with each other. Furthermore, as these biomarkers have been shown to be associated with severe disease, a certain degree of correlation is expected amongst them. However, in our clinical observation, we have found them to be discordant with each other. Quantifying their correlation coefficients which measure the strength of those relationships, if any, may clarify their associations with each other.

Hence we endeavoured to evaluate the function of elevated CK, AST and ALT in the early identification of severe dengue. Secondly, we looked to clarify and quantify correlations amongst biomarkers: CK, AST, ALT, Hct, serum albumin, platelet count and WBC. This in turn will clarify whether AST is predominantly liver or muscle in origin.

Methods

Ethical considerations

The study was approved by the Malaysian Research Ethics Committee, Ministry of Health of Malaysia (Research ID NMRR-14-1543-23635). Our report is based on the Standards for Reporting of Diagnostic Accuracy (STARD) 2015 guideline [20].

Study design

This was a retrospective cohort study of adult patients with confirmed dengue infection who were admitted to Kuala Lumpur Hospital. Sample recruitment was conducted from December 2014 until January 2015. Sampling was universal. Inclusion criteria were patients ≥18 years old and presentation which satisfied the WHO 2009 criteria [21] for suspected dengue. In Malaysia, patients with dengue infection are admitted when they manifest severe dengue characteristics, warning signs, have underlying co-morbidities or have healthcare accessibility issues. Our centre adopts these based on recommendations of our own national clinical practice guidelines which in turn have absorbed many of WHO 2009 clinical guidelines recommendations and adopted fully WHO

2009 criteria. In addition, cases selected were required to have the presence of acute dengue viral infection confirmed via presence of NS1 antigen and/or high-titre level of IgG from an admission serum sample. Cases were excluded if they: 1) had underlying liver diseases, or 2) had received recent (within 5 days) intramuscular injections. Cases were subsequently classified into severe and non-severe dengue.

Case notes were reviewed and data, including baseline characteristics, clinical parameters and laboratory findings, were collected using a pre-defined data collection form. All patients received standard management adhering to the 2010 Malaysian Clinical Practice Guideline on Management of Dengue Infection in Adults [22] and the 2009 WHO clinical practice guideline for dengue [21]. CK, AST, ALT, Hct, platelet count, WBC and serum albumin were taken upon ward admission. As per the recommendations in the guidelines, full blood count was repeated at 8-hourly or 6-hourly intervals. Other blood investigations were repeated at least daily or more frequently as required.

Case definitions for dengue

Case definitions for the diagnosis of dengue infection and classification of disease severity were based on the 2009 WHO guidelines. According to that system, a suspected dengue case is defined by the presence of fever plus any two of 1) aches and pain, 2) nausea and/or vomiting, 3) rash, 4) leucopenia, or 5) presence of any warning signs. Warning signs are defined as any one of: 1) abdominal pain or tenderness; 2) persistent vomiting (defined as vomiting a minimum of 3 times within 24 h); 3) non-physiological or supraphysiological bleeding; 4) lethargy; 5) clinical fluid accumulation that manifest as pleural effusion, ascites 6) a palpable liver 2 cm below the costal margin; and 7) an elevated hematocrit to >40% in female and >46% in male, which correspond to an increase of at least 20% in hematocrit from a gender-specific mean population baseline.

Severe dengue was defined by any of: 1) decompensated shock due to severe plasma leakage (defined as systolic blood pressure of <90 mmHg, a fall of ≥40 mmHg from a previous known baseline, or mean arterial blood pressure < 65 mmHg), 2) compensated shock due to severe plasma leakage (defined as clinical manifestations of reduced perfusion in presence of systolic blood pressure of ≥90 mmHg), 3) respiratory compromise due to severe plasma leakage, 4) severe hepatitis (defined as AST level > 1000 IU/L, or ALT level > 1000 IU/L), 5) severe bleeding that required intervention, or 6) severe organ involvement such as acute kidney injury defined by elevated serum creatinine, myocarditis or encephalopathy.

Serology for dengue viral infection

All sera were tested for the presence of NS1 antigen and high-titre serum IgG. These were processed using the ELISA method (PanBio reagents). Our IgG is a high-titre IgG that is positive at titre >1:2560. IgM was not used in our study for 2 reasons. Firstly, it may remain positive weeks beyond an acute infection hence yielding a false-positive in a non-dengue infection, and secondly, to avoid false positive cases due to detection of cross-reacting antibodies.

Measurement of biomarkers

As per standard practice at our centre, biomarkers were collected into appropriate Vacutainers®. CK samples were analyzed using the ultraviolet method, liver transaminases analyzed with International Federation of Clinical Chemistry method (without pyridoxal phosphate activation) and serum albumin were analyzed with bromocresol green (Roche Diagnostics, Malaysia). Platelets were analyzed with hydrodynamic focusing or direct current method, white blood count by flow cytometry and hemoglobin by photometrics (Sysmex, Malaysia).

Composite indices

We formulated and tested several composite indices based on admission AST and admission ALT values in the search for a marker/model with good performance parameters that could help to better identify severe dengue. Composite indices, like body mass index and shock index [23], have been well-established in clinical use. We utilized simple and common mathematical operators e.g. squaring, division and multiplication in the formation of the indices. Simplicity was the core criterion in formulating these indices to allow for ease of clinical use. Fourteen indices were tested but only one, based on ease of calculation by the bedside, was further scrutinized. Though it is known that liver enzymes would vary along the course of illness, we made no attempt to adjust for this variation as it would only complicate deploying its use to the bedside.

Statistical analysis

In a previous study [11], when investigators classified dengue into severe and non-severe dengue according to WHO 2009 classification, AUC of ROC curve obtained for AST was 0.62 (95% CI 0.57 - 0.67). Based on this information, we calculated that a sample size of 19 severe cases was needed for this study, estimating AUC of 72%, confidence level of 95% and power of 80%. No similar information was available for creatine kinase.

All data were analyzed using SPSS software (version 18.0; SPSS Inc., Chicago, IL). Continuous variables were tested for uniformity using the Kolmogorov-Smirnov test and normality with the Shapiro-Wilk test. Categorical variables were expressed as frequencies and percentages, and comparisons analyzed using the Chi-square test or Fisher's exact test, as appropriate. As our data were mostly non-parametric, we used non-parametric analyses for data interrogation. Continuous variables with non-normal distribution were summarized as median and inter-quartile range (IQR) and comparisons were made using the Mann–Whitney U test. Correlation analyses to assess strengths of relationships between biomarkers were made by computing Spearman *r*. Predictive associations between biomarkers were analyzed using regression methods. The method yielding the highest R^2 was then reported.

Areas under curve of receiver-operating characteristic curves (AUROC) of all models (the composite indices, AST, ALT, CK and Hct) to identify at admission the occurrence of severe dengue, with their 95% confidence interval, were computed. As an alternative to validation using a second sample in assessing these models to identify severe dengue upon admission, we used the cross-validation technique. Cross-validation will avoid over-fitting of the models thus ensuring accuracy and validity.

The most accurate marker was then assessed further for its performance at four different cut-off values to achieve: 1) screening (cut-off 1), 2) optimal performance/Youden index (cut-off 2), 3) modified Youden to achieve higher specificity but maintain sensitivity >40% (cut-off 3), and 4) best diagnostic accuracy (cut-off 4). We assumed that these cut-offs would bear clinical relevance. Sensitivity, specificity, positive predictive value (PPV), negative predictive value (NPV), positive likelihood ratio (LR+), negative likelihood ratio (LR-) and diagnostic accuracy, with their 95% confidence intervals were calculated for that best marker. All tests of significance were 2-sided, and we took *p*-value <0.05 to indicate statistical significance.

Results

Patient characteristics

A total of 643 patients with suspected dengue who were admitted to the Department of Medicine, Kuala Lumpur Hospital between December 2014 and January 2015 were identified. Of this, patients were excluded for being NS1 antigen and high-titre IgG negative (169 patients) and younger than 18 years old (109 patients). The final number of eligible patients for final analysis was 365. The admission and in-ward characteristics of the patients are as shown in Tables 1 and 2. Among the patients, 28.9% were obese (BMI ≥27.5 kg/m^2). Elevated admission levels of CK, AST, ALT and Hct occurred in 57.1%, 82.7%, 57.5% and 21.6% of patients, respectively. Elevated peak levels of CK, AST and ALT occurred in 80.6%, 92.2% and 81.9% of patients, respectively.

Severe vs non-severe dengue

In our cohort, 22 (6%) patients had severe dengue, including 1 (4.5%) patient with decompensated shock, 11 (50%) with compensated shock, 2 (9.1%) with respiratory compromise, 8 (36.4%) with severe hepatitis, 2 (9.1%) with acute kidney injury and 1 (4.5%) with encephalitis.

There were some differences in the characteristics of patients with severe and non-severe dengue (see Tables 1 and 2). Patients with severe dengue were significantly more likely to be female, 72.7% vs 39.1%, p = 0.003. These patients were also more likely to have co-morbidities, 36.4% vs. 13.7%, p = 0.009, and were more likely to have diabetes mellitus 13.6% vs. 2.6%, p = 0.03. Patients with severe dengue were more likely to have at least 1 co-morbidity (p = 0.003) but there was no significant difference in terms of presence of multiple co-morbidities (p = 0.06). Patients with severe dengue had significantly higher admission and peak levels of AST and ALT, with peak levels being higher than admission levels. Nadir levels of platelet and serum albumin were also lower in patients with severe dengue.

Diagnostic value of CK, AST and ALT for identifying severe dengue

We evaluated the diagnostic value of CK, AST, ALT, Hct and the 14 formulated composite indices for identifying severe dengue at admission. Overall, the composite index AST^2/ALT was the best performing marker in identifying severe dengue on admission. The AUROC for liver enzymes were moderate, with AST being better than ALT, whilst the AUROC for CK and Hct were poor (Table 3). The four cut-off values for AST^2/ALT were: 98.1 (screening/highest sensitivity cut-off), 402.5 (optimal/Youden index), 653.2 (modified Youden index) and 1193 (highest diagnostic accuracy) (Table 4).

Correlation and predictive associations between markers

Strength of relationships between markers as determined by Spearman *r* and their respective predictive associations as represented by R^2 are shown in Table 5. AST and ALT showed excellent correlation with each

Table 1 Baseline characteristics and clinical parameter of 365 patients hospitalized with dengue

	All		Severe Dengue		Non-severe Dengue		*p*-value
	n	No. (% or IQR)	*n*	No. (% or IQR)	*n*	No. (% or IQR)	
Gender	365						0.003[a]
Male		215 (58.90%)	22	6 (2.80%)	343	209 (97.20%)	
Female		150 (41.10%)	22	16 (10.70%)	343	134 (89.30%)	
Age *(y), median (IQR)*	364	28 (23 - 36)	22	31 (23 - 36)	342	28 (23 - 36)	0.660[b]
BMI, *median (IQR)*	353	24 (21 - 28)	18	25 (21 - 29)	335	24 (21 - 28)	0.700[b]
Co-morbids present	365	55 (15.10%)	22	8 (36.40%)	343	47 (13.70%)	0.009[a]
DM	365	12 (3.30%)	22	3 (13.60%)	343	9 (2.60%)	0.003[a]
Hypertension	365	16 (4.40%)	22	3 (13.60%)	343	13 (3.80%)	0.006[a]
Other co-morbids	365	49 (13.40%)	22	6 (27.30%)	343	43 (12.50%)	0.100[a]
Number of co-morbids	365		22		343		0.003[c]
0		308 (84.40%)	22	14 (63.60%)	343	294 (85.70%)	
1		41 (11.20%)	22	5 (22.70%)	343	36 (10.50%)	
2		12 (3.30%)	22	2 (9.10%)	343	10 (2.90%)	
3		4 (1.10%)	22	1 (4.50%)	343	3 (0.90%)	
More than 1 co-morbids present	365	16 (4.40%)	22	3 (13.60%)	343	13 (3.80%)	0.006[a]

[a]*Fisher's exact test or Chi-square test, as appropriate*
[b]*Mann-Whitney U test*
[c]*Chi-square for trend*
IQR interquartile range, *BMI* body mass index, *DM* diabetes mellitus

other, at admission and at peak values. In addition, admission AST showed a good predictive association with admission ALT (R^2 0.79) but the association weakened at peak values (R^2 0.66) despite better correlation. The correlation between liver enzymes and plasma leakage markers, hematocrit and serum albumin were weak to negligible, $r < 0.10$ and < -0.40. Liver enzymes also showed very poor predictive associations with nadir platelet and nadir serum albumin, R^2 0.003 - 0.09.

CK showed a weak to negligible correlation with liver enzymes at both admission and peak values (r 0.11 - 0.37) (Table 5). The correlations between CK and plasma leakage markers, hematocrit and serum albumin were negligible ($r < 0.30$ and < -0.30). Similarly, the correlations between CK and disease course marker, platelet count, were also negligible ($r < -0.30$). CK showed very poor predictive associations with liver enzymes, leakage markers and disease course marker (R^2 0.001 - 0.13).

Interestingly, we also found that there was a negligible correlation (r 0.19 (95% CI: 0.08 - 0.29), p = 0.001) and a non-existent predictive association (R^2 0.03) between admission Hct and nadir serum albumin (Table 5).

Discussions

Our analysis showed that admission CK was not helpful in identifying severe dengue and does not correlate with any of the biomarkers which represent hepatitis (ALT), plasma leakage (hematocrit and serum albumin) and disease course (platelet count). Musculoskeletal involvement in dengue takes the form of myalgia and arthralgia. It was demonstrated in a cohort of 1716 patients in Latin America that this occurred in 94.3% of their patients [24]. We emphasize again that our study focused on biomarkers at admission - when it would be most relevant time to predict development of severe dengue. Also, as mentioned, our case definitions used the current WHO 2009 guidelines. In Villar-Centeno et al. (2008), the values of CK in the dengue haemorrhagic fever (DHF, WHO 1997) group were mean (95% CI): 549.6 (267.5–831.6) U/L taken 2-4 days into the illness. Our study showed admission CK in the severe dengue group are median(IQR): 212 (116 - 300) U/L taken 3-5 days into the illness. The peak CK values in our study were 404 (171 - 766) U/L. The difference between non-severe and severe groups were not significant (p = 0.43). It seems therefore that although musculoskeletal involvement occurred in almost all dengue patients, its significance beyond symptomatology is unclear. Further studies are needed to demonstrate the clinical relevance of monitoring CK.

However, our study revealed that, at admission, the identification of severe dengue was best using the composite index, AST^2/ALT, based on AST and ALT readings taken at admission. The AUROC was 0.83, which makes it to date one of the two markers with

Table 2 Laboratory parameters of 365 patients hospitalized with dengue

	All		Severe Dengue		Non-severe Dengue		*p*-value
	n	No. (% or IQR)	*n*	No. (% or IQR)	*n*	No. (% or IQR)	
Duration of febrile phase *(d)*	360	4.8 (3.8 - 5.8)	21	5 (4.1 - 7.3)	339	4.8 (3.8 - 5.8)	0.170[b]
Phase at admission, febrile	360	230 (63.90%)	21	16 (76.20%)	339	214 (63.10%)	0.250[a]
Day of presentation *(d)*	361	4.3 (3.2 - 5.3)	22	4.2 (3.1 - 5.1)	339	4.3 (3.2 - 5.4)	0.570[b]
NS1 Ag	356	288 (80.90%)	22	20 (90.90%)	334	268 (80.20%)	0.270[a]
High-titre IgG	360	160 (44.40%)	22	11 (50.00%)	338	149 (44.10%)	0.660[a]
Admission Hct, median (IQR), %	365	42 (39 - 46)	22	41 (37 - 43)	343	42 (39 - 46)	0.160[b]
Admission CK, median (IQR), IU/L	354	208 (103 - 409)	19	212 (116 - 300)	335	207 (103 - 424)	0.760[b]
Admission AST, median (IQR), IU/L	364	79 (47 - 135)	22	231 (97 - 564)	342	75 (47 - 128)	< 0.001[b]
Admission ALT, median (IQR), IU/L	365	51 (29 - 100)	22	122 (49 - 230)	343	49 (28 - 91)	0.003[b]
Nadir WBC, median (IQR), $\times 10^3/\mu L$	364	2.5 (1.9 - 3.6)	22	2.8 (2 - 3.8)	342	2.5 (1.9 - 3.6)	0.540[b]
Nadir Platelet, median (IQR), $\times 10^3/\mu L$	364	41 (21 - 67)	22	27 (10 - 49)	342	42 (22 - 67)	0.020[b]
Nadir Serum Albumin, median (IQR), g/L	326	32 (30 - 36)	21	27 (23 - 29)	305	33 (30 - 36)	< 0.001[b]
Peak CK, median (IQR), IU/L	103	429 (199 - 1044)	10	404 (171 - 766)	93	431 (206 - 1118)	0.430[b]
Peak AST, median (IQR), IU/L	338	123 (74 - 243)	21	585 (144 - 1098)	37	116 (73 - 223)	< 0.001[b]
Peak ALT, median (IQR), IU/L	340	86 (41 - 175)	22	225 (107 - 403)	318	81 (39 - 162)	< 0.001[b]

[a]*Fisher's exact test or Chi square test, as appropriate*
[b]*Mann-Whitney U test*
[c]*Chi-square for trend*
IQR interquartile range, *CK* creatine kinase, *AST* aspartate transaminase, *ALT* alanine transaminase, *WBC* white blood cell count, *AKI* acute kidney injury

Table 3 Area under curve (AUC) of CK, AST, ALT, Hct, AST^2/ALT and 13 other composite indices

Markers	AUC (95% CI)
CK	0.52 (0.40 - 0.64)
AST	0.78 (0.68 - 0.89)
ALT	0.69 (0.56 - 0.81)
Hct	0.59 (0.47 - 0.71)
AST^2/ALT	0.83 (0.73 - 0.92)
AST/ALT	0.77 (0.67 - 0.87)
AST x ALT	0.74 (0.62 - 0.86)
AST^2 x ALT	0.76 (0.64 - 0.87)
AST x √ALT	0.76 (0.64 - 0.87)
√AST x ALT	0.72 (0.60 - 0.84)
AST/√ALT	0.83 (0.73 - 0.92)
√AST/ALT	0.42 (0.30 - 0.55)
$AST^2/\sqrt{ALT}$	0.81 (0.71 - 0.90)
AST^2/ALT^3	0.52 (0.41 - 0.63)
AST^3/ALT	0.81 (0.72 - 0.91)
$AST^3/\sqrt{ALT}$	0.80 (0.69 - 0.90)
AST^3/ALT^2	0.83 (0.73 - 0.93)
AST^4/ALT^3	0.82 (0.73 - 0.92)

AUC area under curve; *AST* aspartate transaminase; *ALT* alanine transaminase; *Hct* hematocrit; *CK* creatine kinase; *CI* confidence interval

highest diagnostic performance. Our composite index requires, however, the performance of liver function tests and AST. At our hospital liver function tests and AST are available on an urgent basis with a short turnaround time. The simplicity of the formula allows for ease of clinical use. We propose 2 cut-offs, 402 and 653, that will help to delineate severe dengue. Such suspicion may arise in those who have, for example, isolated tachycardia in the presence of high grade fever, isolated single manifestation of peripheral sign of shock, a remarkable isolated derangement of hematocrit or isolated mild metabolic acidosis. Choice of cut-off will also depend on clinical resources available, with the higher value more suitable if resources are limited.

In addition, our correlational analysis suggests that AST originates from the liver rather than muscles. AST has been showed to rise earlier and to a higher level than ALT in almost all dengue patients [12]. This makes AST a better marker to monitor the liver and identify severe hepatitis earlier. Its levels also decline earlier than ALT [8], making it well-suited in monitoring the course of hepatitis. In comparison to other biomarkers and composite indices studied, the diagnostic performance of AST was second only to AST^2/ALT, with AUROC of 0.78. Thus, it is better than the traditional ALT in monitoring hepatitis in dengue. Our results of the diagnostic performances of the liver enzymes are better than a previous study [11] because we included severe hepatitis as part of the outcome of severe dengue. We believe it is important to be able to identify the development of severe hepatitis at an earlier stage albeit without the patient manifesting other features of severe dengue.

Our correlational analysis found that the pathophysiological processes that occur in dengue, represented by the different biomarkers studied, do not correlate with each other, confirming our anecdotal observation. This suggests that these processes occur independently of one another in dengue. Adding to the puzzle is our findings that markers of plasma leakage, Hct and serum albumin, do not correlate with each other. The sampling time points of these biomarkers in our study were different. Nonetheless, two markers representing the same disease process ought to have a better degree of correlation. Furthermore, the sampling time points chosen in our analysis were appropriate for each hematocrit and serum albumin. Admission Hct would not be influenced by the later clinical administration of fluid and may be assumed to be the highest before intervention was instituted. Similarly, we used nadir serum albumin which may reflect peak leakage and is unaffected by fluid administration. This paradox needs further evaluation.

The main limitation of our study was that it was retrospective. However, data accuracy was reasonable as management of patients followed standard local management guidelines for dengue with clear specifications of timing of blood investigations. Our second limitation was that we did not perform serotyping. The dominant serotypes during the time of this study were Den-1 at approximately 55% of national surveillance cases and Den-2 at approximately 35%. Den-3 and Den-4 each contributed to less than 10% of cases. Since mid-2013 Den-1 and Den-2 have been the predominant serotypes in Malaysia [25]. Third, although we suggested that AST was of liver origin based on the strong correlation with ALT and negligible correlation with CK, we did not test for other sources of AST such as brain, red blood cells and kidney. However, none of our patient had hemolysis, only 2 patients had increments in serum creatinine and only one had encephalitis. Fourth, we did not perform multivariate analysis on our composite indices. A multivariate analysis would require a larger number of patients with severe dengue, which in turn would be determined by the number of covariates included. Finally, we did not adjust for the usage of paracetamol and traditional medication which is prevalent in our population, which could

Table 4 Diagnostic value of AST^2/ALT to identify severe dengue based on AST & ALT upon admission

Cutoff	Sensitivity % (95% CI)	Specificity% (95% CI)	PPV (95% CI)	NPV (95% CI)	Diagnostic accuracy (95% CI)	LR+ (95% CI)	LR− (95% CI)
> 98.1	95.5 (77.2 - 99.9)	40.5 (35.3 - 45.9)	9.3 (6.2 - 13.9)	99.3 (96.1 - 99.9)	43.8 (38.8 - 49.0)	1.6 (1.6 - 1.6)	0.1 (0.02 - 0.8)
> 402.5	59.1 (36.4 - 79.3)	92.4 (89.1 - 95.0)	33.3 (20.6 - 49.0)	97.2 (94.8 - 98.5)	90.4 (87.0 - 93.0)	7.8 (6.5 - 9.3)	0.4 (0.4 - 0.6)
> 653.2	40.9 (20.7 - 63.7)	97.4 (95.1 - 98.8)	50.0 (29.0 - 71.0)	96.3 (93.7 - 97.8)	94.0 (91.0 - 96.0)	15.6 (9.2 - 26.6)	0.6 (0.5 - 0.7)
> 1193	31.8 (13.9 - 54.9)	99.4 (97.9 - 99.9)	77.8 (45.3 - 93.7)	95.8 (93.2 - 97.4)	95.3 (92.7 - 97.1)	54.6 (11.2 - 264.9)	0.7 (0.6 - 0.8)

AST aspartate transaminase, *ALT* alanine transaminase, *CI* confidence interval, *PPV* positive predictive value, *NPV* negative predictive value, *LR+* positive likelihood ratio, *LR−* negative likelihood ratio

Table 5 Correlation coefficients and coefficients of determination for CK, AST, ALT, markers of plasma leakage and platelet count

	n	Spearman *r* (95% CI)	*p*	R^2
Admission CK - Admission AST	364	0.37 (0.27 - 0.46)	<0.001	0.13[a]
Admission CK - Peak AST	206	0.28 (0.15 - 0.41)	<0.001	0.07[a]
Peak CK - Admission AST	104	0.29 (0.09 - 0.46)	0.003	0.06[a]
Peak CK - Peak AST	92	0.22 (0.03 - 0.39)	0.020	0.06[a]
Admission CK - Admission ALT	364	0.26 (0.16 - 0.35)	<0.001	0.02[b]
Admission CK - Peak ALT	216	0.11 (−0.02 - 0.24)	0.110	0.01[b]
Peak CK - Admission ALT	217	0.25 (0.06 - 0.42)	0.010	0.05[c]
Peak CK - Peak ALT	217	0.12 (−0.08 - 0.32)	0.240	0.02[c]
Admission CK - Admission Hct	364	0.24 (0.14 - 0.33)	<0.001	0.01[c]
Admission CK - Nadir Platelet	363	−0.22 (−0.32 - -0.12)	<0.001	0.01[c]
Admission CK - Nadir Serum Albumin	326	−0.04 (−0.15 - 0.07)	0.500	0.001[c]
Peak CK - Admission Hct	104	0.03 (−0.17 - 0.22)	0.800	0.004[c]
Peak CK - Nadir Platelet	104	−0.10 (−0.29 - 0.09)	0.300	0.01[c]
Peak CK - Nadir Serum Albumin	104	0.06 (−0.13 - 0.25)	0.540	0.01[c]
Admission AST - Admission ALT	365	0.86 (0.82 - 0.88)	<0.001	0.79[b]
Admission AST - Peak ALT	217	0.68 (0.60 - 0.75)	<0.001	0.54[b]
Peak AST - Admission ALT	206	0.66 (0.57 - 0.73)	<0.001	0.45[a]
Peak AST - Peak ALT	189	0.92 (0.89 - 0.94)	<0.001	0.66[b]
Admission Hct - Nadir Platelet	365	−0.14 (−0.24 - -0.03)	0.009	0.06[c]
Admission Hct - Nadir Serum Albumin	327	0.19 (0.08 - 0.29)	0.001	0.03[c]
Nadir Serum Albumin - Nadir Platelet	327	0.52 (0.43 - 0.60)	<0.001	0.14[b]
Admission AST - Admission Hct	365	0.05 (−0.06 - 0.15)	0.380	0.006[c]
Admission AST - Nadir Platelet	365	−0.34 (−0.43 - -0.25)	<0.001	0.04[b]
Admission AST - Nadir Serum Albumin	327	−0.32 (−0.41 - -0.21)	<0.001	0.09[c]
Peak AST - Admission Hct	206	−0.02 (−0.15 - 0.12)	0.800	0.01[c]
Peak AST - Nadir Platelet	206	−0.38 (−0.49 - -0.26)	<0.001	0.08[c]
Peak AST - Nadir Serum Albumin	200	−0.29 (−0.41 - -0.16)	<0.001	0.09[c]
Admission ALT - Admission Hct	365	0.09 (−0.06 - 0.15)	0.080	0.003[c]
Admission ALT - Nadir Platelet	365	−0.19 (−0.43 - -0.25)	<0.001	0.03[c]
Admission ALT - Nadir Serum Albumin	327	−0.16 (−0.41 - -0.21)	0.003	0.04[c]
Peak ALT - Admission Hct	217	−0.02 (−0.06 - 0.15)	0.810	0.01[c]
Peak ALT - Nadir Platelet	217	−0.17 (−0.43 - -0.25)	0.020	0.01[c]
Peak ALT - Nadir Serum Albumin	209	−0.13 (−0.41 - -0.21)	0.050	0.03[c]

[a]*Power regression*
[b]*Linear regression*
[c]*Polynomial regression;*
CK creatine kinase, *AST* aspartate transaminase, *ALT* alanine transaminase, *Hct* hematocrit

have been one of the causes of elevated transaminases. We have focused and limited our discussion to biomarkers examined in our study as per objective. There are of course many other known risk factors that are known to be associated with development of severe dengue, beyond the scope of our study. A larger study that examines extensively all potential risk factors together would be suited to review these.

Conclusion

We conclude that AST^2/ALT may be used as a marker to identify severe dengue based on admission AST and ALT, with two choices of cut-off values, 402 and 653.

Abbreviations

ALT: Alanine aminotransferase; AST: Aspartate aminotransferase; AUROC: Area under the receiver operating characteristic; CI: Confidence interval; CK: Creatine kinase; ELISA: Enzyme-linked immunosorbent assays; Hct: Hematocrit; IgG: Immunoglobulin G; IgM: Immunoglobulin M; IQR: Interquartile range; LR–: Negative likelihood ratio; LR + : Positive likelihood ratio; NPV: Negative predictive value; NS1: Non-structural protein-1; PPV: Positive predictive value; ROC: Receiver operating characteristic; STARD: Standards for reporting of diagnostic accuracy; WBC: White blood cell count; WHO: World Health Organization.

Acknowledgements
The authors would like to thank all the staff and nurses in the Department of Medicine and the Records Office, Kuala Lumpur Hospital. We would also like to thank Dr. Yen Yew Ngau (Head, Department of Medicine, Kuala Lumpur Hospital), Dr. Noel Thomas Ross (Deputy Head, Department of Medicine, Kuala Lumpur Hospital) and Dr. Fatt Soon Lee for their appraisals and support. We would like to thank Ms. Khairul Bariyyah Mohd Hatta for her assistance in technical editing of the manuscript.

Funding
This research did not receive any specific grants from funding agencies in the public, commercial, or not-for-profit sectors.

Authors' contributions
SSMS contributed to the conception, study design, data analysis, data interpretation and drafting the article; HWH contributed to data collection, data interpretation, drafting the article and management of dengue patients; BMA contributed to the data analysis, data interpretation and drafting the article; DHJ contributed to data interpretation, drafting the article and management of dengue patients; NKL contributed to data collection and management of dengue patients; MAAS contributed to the study design, study registration and ethical approval. All authors read and approved the final manuscript.

Consent for publication
Not applicable.

Competing interests
The authors declare that they have no competing interests.

Author details
[1]Department of Medicine, Hospital Kuala Lumpur, Jalan Pahang, 50586 Kuala Lumpur, Malaysia. [2]Biostatistic Unit, National Clinical Research Centre, 1st Floor, MMA Building, 124 Jalan Pahang, 53000 Kuala Lumpur, Malaysia. [3]Clinical Research Centre, Hospital Kuala Lumpur, Jalan Pahang, 50586 Kuala Lumpur, Malaysia.

References

1. Hales S, de Wet N, Maindonald J, Woodward A. Potential effect of population and climate changes on global distribution of dengue fever: an empirical model. Lancet. 2002;360:830–4. doi:10.1016/S0140-6736(02)09964-6.
2. Kenyataan Akhbar Ketua Pengarah Kesihatan Untuk Denggi Minggu 47/ 2014. http://www.moh.gov.my/index.php/database_stores/store_view_page/17/596. Accessed 2 Dec 2014.
3. Misra UK, Kalita J, Maurya PK, Kumar P, Shankar SK, Mahadevan A. Dengue-associated transient muscle dysfunction: clinical, electromyography and histopathological changes. Infection. 2012;40(2): 125–30. doi:10.1007/s15010-011-0203-8.
4. Villar-Centeno LA, Díaz-Quijano FA, Martínez-Vega RA. Biochemical alterations as markers of dengue hemorrhagic fever. Am J Trop Med Hyg. 2008;78(3):370–4.
5. Souza LJD, Alves JG, Nogueira RMR, Gicovate Neto C, Bastos DA, Siqueira EWDS, et al. Aminotransferase changes and acute hepatitis in patients with dengue fever: analysis of 1,585 cases. Braz J Infect Dis. 2004;8(2):156–63. doi: 10.1590/S1413-86702004000200006.
6. Nguyen TL, Nguyen TH, Tieu NT. The impact of dengue haemorrhagic fever on liver function. Res Virol. 1997;148(4):273–7.
7. Guilarde AO, Turchi MD, Siqueira JB Jr, Feres VC, Rocha B, Levi JE, et al. Dengue and dengue hemorrhagic fever among adults: clinical outcomes related to viremia, serotypes, and antibody response. J Infect Dis. 2008;197(6):817 24. doi:10.1086/528805.
8. Hien TT, Vinh NN, Hien PTD, Chinh NT, Simmons C, Wills B. Liver involvement associated with dengue infection in adults in Vietnam. Am J Trop Med Hyg. 2010;83(4):774–80. doi:10.4269/ajtmh.2010.10-0090.
9. Kalayanarooj S, Vaughn DW, Nimmannitya S, Green S, Suntayakorn S, Kunentrasai N, et al. Early clinical and laboratory indicators of acute dengue illness. J Infect Dis. 1997;176(2):313–21. doi:10.1086/514047.
10. Raza FA, Rehman S, Khalid R, Ahmad J, Ashraf S, Iqbal M, et al. Demographic and Clinico-epidemiological features of dengue fever in Faisalabad, Pakistan. PLoS ONE. 2014;9(3):e89868. doi:10.1371/journal.pone.0089868.
11. Lee LK, Gan VC, Lee VJ, Tan AS, Leo YS, Lye DC. Clinical relevance and discriminatory value of elevated liver Aminotransferase levels for dengue severity. PLoS Negl Trop Dis. 2012;6(6):e1676. doi:10.1371/journal.pntd.0001676.
12. Krishnamurti C, Kalayanarooj S, Cutting MA, Peat RA, Rothwell SW, Reid TJ, et al. Mechanisms of hemorrhage in dengue without circulatory collapse. Am J Trop Med Hyg. 2001;65(6):840–7.
13. Kuo CH, Tai DI, Chang-Chien CS, Lan CK, Chiou SS, Liaw YF. Liver biochemical tests and dengue fever. Am J Trop Med Hyg. 1992;47(3):265–70.
14. Thanachartwet V, Oer-Areemitr N, Chamnanchanunt S, Sahassananda D, Jittmittraphap A, Suwannakudt P, et al. Identification of clinical factors associated with severe dengue among Thai adults: a prospective study. BMC Infect Dis. 2015;15(1):1. doi:10.1186/s12879-015-1150-2.
15. Thein T-L, Leo Y-S, Fisher DA, Low JG, Oh HML, Gan VC, et al. Risk factors for fatality among confirmed adult dengue inpatients in Singapore: a matched case-control study. PLoS One. 2013;8(11):e81060. doi:10.1371/journal.pone.0081060.
16. Jayaratne SD, Atukorale V, Gomes L, Chang T, Wijesinghe T, Fernando S, et al. Evaluation of the WHO revised criteria for classification of clinical disease severity in acute adult dengue infection. BMC Res Notes. 2012;5:645. doi:10.1186/1756-0500-5-645.
17. Huy NT, Van Giang T, Thuy DH, Kikuchi M, Hien TT, Zamora J, et al. Factors associated with dengue shock syndrome: a systematic review and meta-analysis. PLoS Negl Trop Dis. 2013;7(9):e2412. doi:10.1371/journal.pntd.0002412.
18. World Health Organization. Dengue haemorrhagic fever: diagnosis, treatment and control. WHO: Geneva; 1997.
19. Tricou V, Minh NN, Farrar J, Tran HT, Simmons CP. Kinetics of viremia and NS1 antigenemia are shaped by immune status and virus serotype in adults with dengue. PLoS Negl Trop Dis. 2011;5(9):e1309. doi:10.1371/journal.pntd.0001309.
20. Bossuyt PM, Reitsma JB, Bruns DE, Gatsonis CA, Glasziou PP, Irwig L, et al. STARD 2015: an updated list of essential items for reporting diagnostic accuracy studies. Radiology. 2015;277(3):826–32. doi:10.1148/radiol.2015151516.
21. World Health Organization, Special Programme for Research, Training in Tropical Diseases, World Health Organization. Department of Control of neglected tropical diseases, World Health Organization. Epidemic, & pandemic alert. Dengue: guidelines for diagnosis, treatment, prevention and control: World Health Organization; 2009.
22. Health Technology Assessment Section, Medical Development Division, Ministry of Health Malaysia. Clinical practice guidelines on Management of Dengue Infection in adults revised 2nd edition: Ministry of Health Malaysia; 2010.
23. Yussof SJ, Zakaria MI, Mohamed FL, Bujang MA, Lakshmanan S, Asaari AH. Value of shock index in prognosticating the short term outcome of death for patients presenting with severe sepsis and septic shock in the emergency department. Med J Malaysia. 2012;67(4):406–11.
24. Halsey ES, Marks MA, Gotuzzo E, Fiestas V, Suarez L, Vargas J, et al. Correlation of serotype-specific dengue virus infection with clinical manifestations. PLoS Negl Trop Dis. 2012;6(5):e1638. doi:10.1371/journal.pntd.0001638.

A retrospective cohort study to predict severe dengue in Honduran patients

Eduardo Fernández[1], Marek Smieja[1,2], Stephen D. Walter[1] and Mark Loeb[1,2*]

Abstract

Background: An important challenge in the identification of dengue is how to predict which patients will go on to experience severe illness, which is typically characterized by fever, thrombocytopenia, haemorrhagic manifestations, and plasma leakage. Accurate prediction could result in the appropriate hospital triage of high risk patients. The objective of this study was to identify clinical factors observed within the first 24 h of hospital admission that could predict subsequent severe dengue.

Methods: We conducted a retrospective cohort study of 320 patients with febrile illness who had confirmation of dengue within one week of admission, using data from the 2009–2010 Honduras Epidemiological Survey for Dengue. The outcome measure was plasma leakage defined using hemoconcentration ≥15% as determined by serial hematocrit testing. We conducted univariable analysis and multivariable logistic regression analysis to construct a predictive model for severe dengue.

Results: Thirty-four (10.6%) of patients in the 320 patient cohort had hemoconcentration ≥15%. In the final multivariable logistic regression model the presence of ascites, OR 7.29, 95% CI 1.85 to 28.7, and a platelet count <50,000 platelets/mm^3 at admission, OR 3.02, 95% CI 1.42 to 6.42, were significantly associated with plasma leakage, while the presence of petechiae, OR 0.24 95% CI 0.080 to 0.73, and headache, OR 0.38, 95% CI 0.15 to 0.95, were negatively associated with leakage. Using an estimated probability of 7% as a threshold for a person being considered a severe case correctly predicted 26 of the 34 severe cases (sensitivity 76.4%) and 201 of the 286 non-severe cases (specificity of 70.3%) for a percentage correctly classified of 70.9%.

Conclusion: We identified signs and symptoms that can correctly identify a majority of patients who eventually develop severe dengue in Honduras. It will be important to further refine our models and validate them in other populations.

Keywords: Severe dengue, Predictors, Models

Background

Dengue fever is a mosquito-borne disease, with a high incidence in tropical and subtropical regions; most cases are reported in South East Asia, the Americas Region and the Pacific Basin [1]. Treatment for the disease is still in development and one vaccine is currently being marketed in affected countries with several other candidates being tested".

Identifying cases of dengue that are likely to eventually develop severe dengue is an important challenge in endemic regions. Previous studies have had varied success in identifying patients that go on to develop severe illness [2–12]. Limitations of these studies include lack of validation [7], single site study [4, 8–10], lack of adjustment for confounding variables [4], restricted to children [8, 11], and selection bias [12]. Although a diagnosis of dengue can be confirmed within days of clinical presentation, identifying those patients who will go on to develop severe dengue could serve as an important form of triage for hospitals. That is, patients at low risk would not require the intensive follow up of high risk patients and this could help reduce the burden on the healthcare system. Conversely, high risk patients would be monitored more closely and given early supportive

* Correspondence: loebm@mcmaster.ca
[1]Department of Clinical Epidemiology and Biostatistics, McMaster University, Hamilton, ON, Canada
[2]Department of Pathology and Molecular Medicine, Institute for Infectious Disease Research McMaster University, Hamilton, ON, Canada

care as they develop evidence of severe disease. Symptoms and signs are typically recorded for patients with suspected dengue and widely available testing, such as blood platelets and hematocrit, is usually done. Thus, a combination of early symptoms and laboratory tests could help quantify the likelihood of severe dengue disease.

Using data from Honduras, the objective of this study was to identify clinical and laboratory factors found at admission that predict severe dengue, previously known as dengue hemorrhagic fever (DHF) and dengue shock syndrome (DSS), in patients that subsequently had a confirmed diagnosis of dengue.

Methods

Study design

We conducted a retrospective cohort study using clinical and laboratory data from Honduras Ministry of Health to predict severe dengue. Data on signs and symptoms of patients who present with dengue is routinely collected in Honduras and submitted to the Honduran National Classification Committee for classification of cases.

Setting and participants

We first used the Ministry of Health data to identify patients with confirmed dengue. Data was collected between 2009 and 2010 from patients who presented with fever and ≥2 symptoms to one of 5 hospitals and outpatient clinics located in Tegucigalpa and San Pedro Sula (the two largest cities in Honduras) and were confirmed to have dengue by serology or viral isolation. If a patient presented within 5 days of the first symptom onset, samples were processed for viral culture following guidelines from the U.S Centers for Disease Control and Prevention (CDC) [13]. If the blood sample was taken on the sixth or later day of onset of symptoms, a test for antibody detection was done using IgM antibody-capture enzyme-linked immunosorbent (IgM Mac ELISA).

Data sources

Serology and viral isolation were performed at the Honduras National Laboratory of Virology according to CDC guidelines and standardized techniques. General practitioners, nurses, and microbiologists completed a data collection form which included epidemiological and clinical information. Symptoms and signs were collected at first presentation while hematology and biochemical tests recorded were those at presentation and those repeated approximately one week later. Fever was defined as a temperature of >37.5 degrees Celsius. Both objective measurements of fever and self-report of fever were included.

Study size

This cohort consists of confirmed dengue patients who were evaluated for severe dengue in tertiary care hospitals in Tegucigalpa and San Pedro Sula. Of the 320 cases, 315 (98%) were diagnosed with dengue by IgM and five (2%) were diagnosed by viral isolation. The patients in this dataset had at least two consecutive readings of hematocrit and platelets in the first 24 h after their admission to the hospital.

Predictor variables

We considered a number of predictor variables for this analysis including 1) demographics, such as age (considered as a categorical variable where children were defined ≤12 years) and sex, 2) symptoms reported within the first 24 h of admission, including fever, headache, retroocular pain, arthralgia, myalgia, rash, anorexia and vomiting, 3) bleeding manifestations, including petechiae, ecchymosis, hematemesis, melena, positive tourniquet, epistaxis, gingival bleeding, tourniquet test, hematuria, metrorrhagia, 4) symptoms and signs of capillary leakage, including abdominal pain, cold extremities, sweating, pale skin, pericardial and pleural effusions, ascites, as well as reduction of medial arterial pressure (based on blood pressure recorded within the first 24 h of admission).

Laboratory data on leukocyte count, platelet count, hemoglobin, and the hematocrit, collected upon admission and 24 h later, were also used as predictor variables. Thrombocytopenia was defined as a platelet count of 100,000 platelets/mm^3 or less [13]. We considered platelets as a binary variable using a cut-off value of 50,000 platelets/mm^3 at 24 h and a cut-off of 100,000 platelets/mm^3 at 48 h.

Outcome

The outcome or dependent variable was plasma leakage. Although death is the most serious outcome for severe dengue, it is uncommon in the Americas [13, 14]. Plasma leakage is a central event in the pathogenesis of severe dengue, leading to hypovolemia, hypotension, edema, shock, and potentially death [1, 13].

Key elements in the classification of severe dengue include the presence of plasma leakage manifestations and hemorrhagic symptoms. In our study, plasma leakage was measured by hemoconcentration using two consecutive readings of hematocrit, the first hematocrit taken at admission and the second 24 h later. Hemoconcentration gradually increases over the course of severe dengue. Although a threshold of 20% above baseline is frequently used, we selected a threshold of 15% to increase the sensitivity of the analysis [7, 14]. Previous studies in Colombia and Puerto Rico have considered thresholds as low as 10% of hemoconcentration, having found that sensitivity is increased while specificity is not significantly reduced [15, 16]. We reasoned that such an intermediate value would maximize the number of cases identified while maintaining specificity.

Data analysis

We conducted a univariate analysis assessing the relationship between the predictor variables and plasma leakage as defined by a 15% increase in hematocrit, an indicator of severe dengue. Variables with a p value <0.2 were considered for multivariable analysis using logistic regression built using forward step-wise selection [17]. Variables were kept in the final model if there were statistically significant ($p < 0.05$) and if no collinearity was observed among them. We assessed collinearity using the tolerance statistic (values >0.2 were acceptable) and the variance inflation factor (VIF), which was acceptable if values were <5. Goodness of fit was determined using Hosmer-Lemeshow statistics ($p > 0.05$ for the model). The final model was validated internally using the bootstrap technique (by sampling with replacement using 320 individuals and sampling 1000 times) [18].

Using the equation of the final logistic regression model, the frequency distribution of predicted probabilities of severer dengue was assessed in order to create a threshold defining the severe case and non-severe case assignments. We selected a threshold for the probability of being a case so that both sensitivity and specificity were maximized. We created an ROC graph to verify the sensitivity and specificity for the selected threshold.

Additionally, as a sensitivity analysis, we created a dichotomous variable for the type of health care facility where patients had presented to either the social security system (accessible only to the insured employed population) or at public health clinics (open to the general population). This was done to account for potential centre effect, that is, differences between the two patient populations.

The analysis was conducted using SPSS version 18.

Results

Participants and main results

Of the 320 patients in the cohort, 139 (43.4%) were female and the mean age was 22.4 years. Two hundred and forty-four (49.2%) were hospitalized six or more days after the onset of the first symptom. Thirty-four (10.6%) met our definition of plasma leakage, based on a hemoconcentration of ≥15%. In univariable analysis, cases were less likely to have petechiae (odds ratio [OR] 0.27 (0.09 to 0.78)) but were more likely to have ascites (OR 5.31, 95% CI 1.47 to 19.2) and platelets ≤50,000 mm^3, OR 2.95 (95% CI 1.38 to 6.74) (Table 1).

The following variables were considered for multivariable analysis: ascites, petechiae, ecchymosis, headache, skin rash, retro-ocular pain, platelet count on admission. As specified a priori, age and sex were included in the model. The final model included the variables headache OR 0.38, 95% CI 0.15 to 0.95, petechiae OR 0.24 95% CI 0.08 to 0.73, ascites OR 7.29, 95% CI 1.85 to 28.7, and platelets <50,000 platelets/$mm^{3,}$ OR 3.02, 95% CI 1.42 to 6.42 at baseline (Table 2).

For goodness of fit, the Hosmer-Lemeshow test showed that the observed event frequencies matched the expected number of events as given by the model. Using various probability cut-offs, we found that a probability cut-off of 7% (where any probability less than 7% was assigned a value of 0 [non-severe case] and any of 7% and over was assigned a value of 1 [severe case]) correctly classified 26 of the 34 cases (sensitivity 76.4%) and 201 of the 286 non-cases (specificity of 70.3%) and yielded an area under the ROC curve of 0.75 (95% CI: 0.66 to 0.83).

The validation of the model with bootstrapping showed estimates (standard error and bias) with narrow confidence intervals (Table 2). The results of model validation are shown in Table 2.

The centre effect was not significant when included in the logistic regression model, OR 1.8, 95% CI 0.85 to 3.9, comparing social security system to public health, and did not affect the other predictor variables.

Discussion

We found that four variables, ascites, headache, petechiae, and low platelets on admission, were independently associated with severe dengue. Our logistic regression model could correctly classify 71% of patients when we set the threshold probability for a being a case at 7%, as indicated by the ROC curve. The model was internally validated by using a bootstrap approach.

Ascites has been reported to be present in the very early stages of dengue and has frequently been associated with evolution to more a severe disease stage. This has been previously reported by other investigators, including ascites not only being a predictor for severe dengue but as an early predictor for admission to intensive care [10, 19, 20]. Similarly, a reduction in platelet count to values under 100,000/mm3 has also been reported as an early warning sign for severe dengue [1, 21]. We found that platelets <50,000/mm^3 were significantly associated with severe dengue in our regression model. Previous reports have described headache as a symptom more likely to be associated with non-severe dengue and occurring with other symptoms like ocular pain [22, 23], consistent with the negative association found in our study.

The presence of petechiae was negatively associated with severe dengue in our model. One previous study found petechiae to be associated with severe dengue,

Table 1 Results of the univariate and multivariable (adjusted) analysis of predictors for severe dengue in a cohort of 340 patients presenting to hospitals in Honduras

	Cases $N = 34$	Non-cases $N = 286$	Odds ratio (95% CI)	Adjusted Odds ratio (95% CI)
Ascites	4 (11.76%)	7 (2.44%)	5.31 (1.47 to 19.2)	7.29 (1.85 to 28.7)
Headache	26 (76.47%)	252 (88.11%)	0.44 (0.18 to 1.05)	0.38 (0.15 to 0.95)
Skin rash	9 (26.47%)	113 (39.51%)	0.55 (0.25 to 1.22)	
Occular pain	23 (67.64%)	221 (77.27%)	0.62 (0.28 to 1.32)	
Petechiae	4 (11.76%)	95 (33.21%)	0.27 (0.09 to 0.78)	0.24 (0.08 to 0.73)
Ecchymosis	0(1.47%)	35 (12.4%)	0.10(0.006 to 1.76)	
Sex (male)	21 (61.76%)	156 (54.54%)	1.34 (0.65 to 2.80)	
Age (≥12 years)	20 (58.82%)	173 (60.49%)	0.93 (0.45 to 1.96)	
Symptom onset to admission (≤ 3 days)	5 (14.709%)	64 (22.38%)	0.60 (0.20 to 1.53)	
Platelets at admission (≤50,000)	24 (70.58%)	128 (44.76%)	2.95 (1.38 to 6.74)	2.9 (1.42 to 6.42)
Platelets at 48 h (≤100,000)	1 (2.94%)	31 (10.84%)	0.25 (0.01 to 1.39)	
Fever	34 (100%)	282 (98.6%)	0.99(0.97 to 1.00)	
Arthralgia	26 (76.5%)	220 (77.0%)	0.97 (0.42 to 2.25)	
Myalgia	29 (85.3%)	251(87.8%)	0.81 (0.30 to 2.22)	
Anorexia	27 (79.4%)	233 (81.4%)	0.88 (0.36 to 2.12)	
Vomiting	15 (44.1%)	98 (34.3%)	1.50 (0.74 to 3.11)	
Hematemesis	1 (2.9%)	20(7.0%)	0.40 (0.05 to 3.10)	
Melena	2 (5.9%)	7 (2.4%)	2.50 (0.50 to 12.50)	
Tourniquet test	3 (8.8%)	15 (5.2%)	1.75 (0.48 to 6.38)	
Epistaxis	7 (20.6%)	43 (15.0%)	1.46(0.60 to 3.58)	
Gingival bleeding	3 (8.8%)	16 (5.6%)	1.63 (0.45 to 5.90)	
Hematuria	1 (2.9%)	9 (3.2%)	0.93 (0.11 to 7.60)	
Methrorragia	1 (2.9%)	8(2.8%)	1.05 (0.13 to 8.69)	
Abdominal Pain	16 (47.0%)	128 (4.5%)	1.10 (0.54 to 2.29)	
Cold extremity	10 (29.4%)	97 (33.9%)	0.81 (0.37 to 1.77)	
Sweating	14 (41.2%)	137 (47.9%)	0.76 (0.37 to 1.60)	
Pallor (skin)	15 (44.1%)	118 (41.3%)	1.12 (0.55 to 2.30)	
Pericardium effusion	0 (0%)	4 (1.4%)	0.98 (0.97 to 1.00)	
Pleural effusion	2 (5.9%)	8 (2.8%)	2.20 (0.44 to 10.70)	

Table 2 Results of the bootstrap for the final model[a]

Predictor	B[b]	Bias[c]	SE	P	B 95% CI
Ascites	1.99	−.182	−2.49	.001	0.37 to 3.45
Petechiae	−1.42	−.419	2.60	.006	3.22 to 0.57
Platelets at admission	1.09	.007	0.43	.008	0.27 to 1.98
Headache	0.98	0.04	0.55	.041	−1.95 to 0.26

[a]Data on 320 participants; 1000 replications
[b]B refers to average of the bootstrap estimates
[c]The bias estimates were compared to the standard error of values of the predictors of the subsamples

however the comparator was of patients without dengue [8]. Another study found rash to be associated with severe dengue and as well as low platelets (< 30,000/ mm^3) but did not report petechiae [9]. Although there was a high prevalence of petechiae in patients with severe dengue in a third study, there was no comparison made to non-severe dengue cases [12].

Our model differs from previous ones in that we used very few laboratory indicators. Prior models that have been developed for severe dengue have used different combinations of laboratory variables (e.g.white blood cells count, aspartame aminotransferase). However, higher cut-off points for thrombocytopenia have been included in previous studies as well as petechiae as a positive predictor [4, 11, 12]. Our study sample consisted of patients with dengue fever admitted to a health facility. Our study differs from many others in that it included information available in the first few hours of admission, using data being collected as medical personnel were triaging the patients.

A strength of our study is that the model equation was transformed into a score that could be applied to patients to classify them as severe cases or non-severe cases. Validation of the model, preferably in a different study sample, is an integral part of developing a model. Although lack of external validation is a limitation of our model, our use of bootstrapping sampling led to the development of accurate estimators. We acknowledge the fact that death could not be used as an outcome because of the low death rate and so we selected difference of hematocrits in the first two readings after the admission of patients. We acknowledge that using changes in platelet levels would be an alternative approach [3]. We also acknowledge that our use of a positive IgM represents probable and not confirmed dengue and that hydration and volume expansion could have had an effect on hematocrit.

A limitation of our study is that our model yielded a high level of specificity but relatively low sensitivity using a 50% threshold, in a population where the severe cases represented close to 10% of the sample. We reduced the cut-off to 7% for the probability of being a case in order to increase sensitivity, but this inevitably led to a decrease in specificity. Since clinical practice is centered on the identification of cases with high risk, we reasoned that it was important to increase the ability of the model to rule out severe dengue detect, which means that a reduction of the cutoff point may detect a larger number of true cases (about 80%) but also increasing the false positive rate (i.e. reducing specificity). Another potential limitation is that our study was conducted when other viruses, such as Chikungunya and Zika, were not circulating. There is a possibility that this would have affected the predictive value of our model. Since we conducted an analysis using a database on suspected dengue, we did not have access to the final diagnosis of non-dengue cases. Another limitation of our model is that predictive accuracy may have been overestimated. In order to fully validate the model, an external data set would be required and the predictive accuracy tested.

Ideally, our model would best be used in conjunction with other diagnostic methods that add their own accuracy to the model. The use of the model equation and ROC can provide a better sense of the best cut-point, or verification of the adequate selection of this threshold. The development of a score system can provide a way to determine which patients are at higher risk of severe dengue, contributing to a better patients triage in hospitals and their emergency rooms.

The findings in our study are relevant to regions with reduced access to diagnostic tests such as imaging technology to detect fluid extravasation. From a public health perspective, our model can be a valuable tool to screen populations during epidemic periods and in areas with high transmission can assist in the classification of cases.

Acknowledgements
Not applicable.

Funding
There was no specific grant supprt for this work.

Authors' contributions
EF, MS, SW, ML developed the concept and design of the study. EF collected the data. EF, MS, SW, ML contributed to the analysis. EF, MS, SW, ML drafted the manuscript, revised it critically, and gave final approval of the final versión of the manuscript to be published. EF, MS, SW, ML agree to be accountable for all aspects of the work in ensuring that questions related to the accuracy or integrity of any part of the work are appropriately investigated and resolved.

Ethics approval and consent to participate
This study is based on data that is routinely collected by the public health system in Honduras. We did not assemble a cohort and because the data we received is not nominal and does not have any unique identifiers, we received confirmation from the McMaster Research Ethics Board that ethics review was not required. Dr. Fernandez obtained approval from the Ethics Committee of the School of Medical Sciences University of Honduras about using the data, which were national surveillance data on dengue. Approval was obtained on the basis that there would be no contact with human subjects but only use of a governmental database. Institutional authorization was also required, which was obtained from the Director of Health Surveillance and the Chair of the National Laboratory of Virology in Honduras.

Consent for publication
Not applicable.

Competing interests
The authors declare that they have no competing interests.

References

1. Halstead SB. Pathogenesis of dengue: challenges to molecular biology. Science. 1988 Jan 29;239(4839):476–81.
2. Thomas L, Moravie V, Besnier F, Valentino R, Kaidomar S, Coquet LV, et al. Clinical presentation of dengue among patients admitted to the adult emergency department of a tertiary care hospital in Martinique: implications for triage, management, and reporting. Ann Emerg Med. 2012 Jan;59(1):42–50.
3. Lee VJ, Lye DC, Sun Y, Fernandez G, Ong A, Leo YS. Predictive value of simple clinical and laboratory variables for dengue hemorrhagic fever in adults. J Clin Virol. 2008 May;42(1):34–9.
4. Thomas L, Verlaeten O, Cabie A, Kaidomar S, Moravie V, Martial J, et al. Influence of the dengue serotype, previous dengue infection, and plasma viral load on clinical presentation and outcome during a dengue-2 and dengue-4 co-epidemic. Am J Trop Med Hyg. 2008 Jun;78(6):990–8.

5. Teck SL, LW A, Grace SLY, Lee C, Ng JCT, Lyn J, et al. Epidemiological characteristics of the 2005 and 2007 dengue epidemics in Singapore – similarities and distinctions. Western Pac Surveill Response J. 2011;2(2):24–9.
6. Tun Y, Ang LW, Chow A, Chew SK. Seroprevalence study on past and recent dengue virus infection in Singapore. Singapore: Ministry of Health. 2007 July-September;2007
7. Diaz-Quijano FA, Martinez-Vega RA, Villar-Centeno LA. Early indicators of severity in dengue virus infection. Enferm Infecc Microbiol Clin. 2005 Nov;23(9):529–32.
8. Biswas HH, Ortega O, Gordon A, Standish K, Balmaseda A, Kuan G, et al. Early clinical features of dengue virus infection in nicaraguan children: a longitudinal analysis. PLoS Negl Trop Dis. 2012;6(3):e1562.
9. Mena Lora AJ, Fernandez J, Morales A, Soto Y, Feris-Iglesias J, Brito MO. Disease severity and mortality caused by dengue in a Dominican pediatric population. Am J Trop Med Hyg. 2014 Jan;90(1):169–72.
10. Huy NT, Thao NT, Ha TT, Lan NT, Nga PT, Thuy TT, et al. Development of clinical decision rules to predict recurrent shock in dengue. Crit Care. 2013 Dec 2;17(6):R280.
11. Potts JA, Thomas SJ, Srikiatkhachorn A, Supradish PO, Li W, Nisalak A, et al. Classification of dengue illness based on readily available laboratory data. Am J Trop Med Hyg. 2010 Oct;83(4):781–8.
12. Cavalcanti LP, Coelho IC, Vilar DC, Holanda SG, Escossia KN, Souza-Santos R. Clinical and epidemiological characterization of dengue hemorrhagic fever cases in northeastern, Brazil. Rev Soc Bras Med Trop. 2010 Jul-Aug;43(4):355–8.
13. WHO, editor. Dengue hemorrhagic fever: diagnosis, treatment, prevention and control. 3rd ed. Geneva: World Health Organization; 2009.
14. San Martin JL, Brathwaite O, Zambrano B, Solorzano JO, Bouckenooghe A, Dayan GH, et al. The epidemiology of dengue in the americas over the last three decades: a worrisome reality. Am J Trop Med Hyg. 2010 Jan;82(1):128–35.
15. Kuno G, Gomez I, Gubler DJ, An ELISA. Procedure for the diagnosis of dengue infections. J Virol Methods. 1991 Jun;33(1–2):101–13.
16. Rigau-Perez JG, Bonilla GL. An evaluation of modified case definitions for the detection of dengue hemorrhagic fever. Puerto Rico Association of Epidemiologists. P R Health Sci J. 1999 Dec;18(4):347–52.
17. Bewick V, Cheek L, Ball J. Statistics review 14: logistic regression. Crit Care. 2005 Feb;9(1):112–8.
18. Efron B. Bootstrap methods: another look at the Jacknife. The annals of statistics 1979. January 1979;7(1):1–26.
19. Ooi ET, Ganesananthan S, Anil R, Kwok FY, Sinniah M. Gastrointestinal manifestations of dengue infection in adults. Med J Malaysia. 2008 Dec; 63(5):401–5.
20. Srikiatkhachorn A, Krautrachue A, Ratanaprakarn W, Wongtapradit L, Nithipanya N, Kalayanarooj S, et al. Natural history of plasma leakage in dengue hemorrhagic fever: a serial ultrasonographic study. Pediatr Infect Dis J 2007 Apr;26(4):283–290; discussion 91-2.
21. Wiwanitkit V, Manusvanich P. Can hematocrit and platelet determination on admission predict shock in hospitalized children with dengue hemorrhagic fever? A clinical observation from a small outbreak. Clin Appl Thromb Hemost. 2004 Jan;10(1):65–7.
22. Domingues RB, Kuster GW, Onuki de Castro FL, Souza VA, Levi JE, Pannuti CS. Headache features in patients with dengue virus infection. Cephalalgia. 2006 Jul;26(7):879–82.
23. Rivas-Llamas R, Chaín-Castro RA, Murillo-Llanes J, Ramírez-Zepeda MG, Gadea-Alvarez T, López-López E. Haemorrhagic manifestations in dengue. Rev Biomed. 2005;16:87–94.

21

Immunogenicity of the CYD tetravalent dengue vaccine using an accelerated schedule

Judith Kirstein[1], William Douglas[2], Manoj Thakur[3], Mark Boaz[3], Thomas Papa[4], Anna Skipetrova[4] and Eric Plennevaux[4*]

Abstract

Background: The live attenuated tetravalent dengue vaccine (CYD-TDV) is licensed using a 0-, 6- and 12-month schedule in dengue-endemic areas. An effective shorter schedule may provide more rapid, optimal protection of targeted populations during vaccine campaigns in dengue-endemic countries. We compared immune responses to two schedules of CYD-TDV in a non-endemic population. We also evaluated the impact of yellow fever (YF) co-administration.

Methods: This phase II, open-label, multicentre study enrolled 390 healthy 18–45-year-olds in the USA with no prior exposure to dengue. Participants were randomised (4:4:4:1) to four treatment groups stratified by prior YF vaccine status: Group 1, CYD-TDV standard 0–6–12 months schedule; Group 2, CYD-TDV accelerated 0–2–6 months schedule; Group 3, CYD-TDV accelerated schedule with YF co-administered (dose 1); Group 4, YF vaccination only. Neutralising antibody geometric mean titres (GMTs) and percentages of seropositive participants (antibody titres ≥10 [1/dil]) were measured against each dengue serotype using a 50% plaque reduction neutralisation test.

Results: On D28 post-CYD-TDV dose 3, there were no marked differences in seropositivity rates and GMTs between Groups 1 and 2. In Groups 1 and 2 respectively, 73.4 and 82.4% were dengue seropositive for ≥3 serotypes, with 50.0 and 42.6% seropositive against all four serotypes. Flavivirus status (FV+ or FV–) at baseline did not markedly affect GMTs and seropositivity rates with either schedule. In Groups 1 and 2, GMTs measured 6 months after the third dose decreased against all serotypes, except for a small increase in GMT for serotype 4 in Group 1. In addition, dengue seropositivity remained above 70% for serotypes 2, 3 and 4 in Groups 1 and 2. Co-administration with YF did not affect antibody responses against dengue and YF or impact vaccine safety following completion of the compressed schedule, compared to dengue or YF vaccination alone.

Conclusions: The live attenuated CYD-TDV vaccine given in a compressed schedule in a non-endemic setting can elicit similar antibody responses to the licensed CYD-TDV schedule.

Keywords: Dengue, Live attenuated tetravalent dengue vaccine, Yellow fever, Vaccination schedule

* Correspondence: Eric.Plennevaux@sanofipasteur.com
[4]Sanofi Pasteur, Siège Social, 14 Espace Henry Vallée, 69007 Lyon, France
Full list of author information is available at the end of the article

Background

There are an estimated 390 million dengue virus infections worldwide annually, of which around 100 million are associated with clinical manifestations [1, 2]. The majority of infections occur in endemic regions, particularly South East Asia, India, Central and South America, and Africa [1], with dengue also spreading to previously unaffected areas [2].

The live attenuated tetravalent dengue vaccine (CYD-TDV) is approved for use in individuals aged ≥9 years in several endemic countries, administered in 3 doses over a 12-month period (at 0, 6 and 12 months). For endemic populations, an accelerated schedule could provide more rapid protection and increase vaccination compliance in targeted populations. The possibility of using shorter CYD-TDV vaccination schedules therefore needs to be evaluated.

For this study, we elected to describe antibody responses to CYD-TDV in healthy participants in a flavivirus negative, non-endemic setting with the standard vaccination schedule compared to an accelerated, 0–2–6-month schedule. We also evaluated CYD-TDV immunogenicity and safety following concomitant administration with yellow fever (YF) vaccine.

Methods

Study design and participants

This phase II, randomised, open-label, multicentre study was conducted between December 2011 and September 2013 in the United States (NCT01488890; December 8, 2011), in accordance with the Declaration of Helsinki and the International Conference on Harmonisation-Good Clinical Practice. The study protocol was approved by an Institutional Review Board which covered each study site. Written informed consent was obtained from all participants. The study adheres to CONSORT reporting guidelines.

Healthy 18–45-year-olds were enrolled. For those reporting previous YF vaccination, documentation (Vaccination Card/record) was provided. Key exclusion criteria were: participation in another clinical trial during the 4 weeks preceding first vaccination; women who were pregnant or of childbearing potential or breastfeeding; receipt of previous flavivirus (FV) vaccine (with the exception of previous YF vaccination for participants classified as YF+).

Participants were randomised (4:4:4:1) to four treatment groups, using the permuted block method with stratification of prior YF vaccine status, to receive CYD-TDV at 0, 6 and 12 months (Group 1; 'standard' vaccination schedule); 0, 2 and 6 months (Group 2; 'compressed' vaccination schedule); 0, 2 and 6 months with concomitant single YF vaccine dose at month 0 (Group 3); or single YF vaccine dose only (Group 4; not described here). Group 1 and 2 participants were stratified by prior YF vaccination status (YF+ or YF−) in the 3 months to 10 years preceding first study vaccine dose, and randomised such that 50% of Group 1 and 2 participants and no participants in Group 3 had prior reported YF. Equal numbers of YF+ and YF− participants were randomised (n = 40 in each) to subsets for antibody kinetic assessment (subgroups K1 and K2). Participants who were YF+ were ineligible for inclusion in Groups 3 or 4. Treatment was allocated using an interactive voice response system or interactive web response. Study duration was 18 months (Fig. 1).

Vaccines

CYD-TDV was presented as a powder for reconstitution in 0.5 mL saline (NaCl 0.4%) immediately before use. Each 0.5 mL dose contained 5 ± 1 $\log_{10}$ cell-culture infectious dose 50% of each of the four live attenuated recombinant CYD-TDV virus serotypes. YF vaccine (YF-VAX®; Sanofi-Pasteur) was presented as a powder and reconstituted in saline immediately before use. Each 0.5 mL dose contained ≥4.74 $\log_{10}$ plaque forming units of the 17D YF virus strain. Both vaccines were administered subcutaneously into the deltoid region of the upper arm.

Assessment of CYD-TDV immunogenicity

Dengue antibody responses

Dengue neutralising antibody geometric mean titres (GMTs) and seropositivity rates were determined for each dengue serotype at baseline and various intervals following each CYD-TDV dose. Primary endpoints were dengue antibody response at 28 days and 6 months following completion of standard (Group 1) versus compressed (Group 2) vaccination schedules. Secondary immunogenicity endpoints included: dengue antibody responses at 12 months following completion of the compressed schedule in Groups 2 and 3; dengue antibody responses following doses 1 and 2 in Groups 1 and 2 (irrespective of prior YF vaccination); dengue antibody responses by baseline FV seropositivity (defined as seropositivity to dengue or YF, or both) in Groups 1 and 2; and dengue antibody responses in YF− participants from Group 2 versus Group 3 to assess a potential effect of co-administration with YF vaccine.

GMTs were measured for each dengue virus serotype using a dengue 50% plaque reduction neutralisation test ($PRNT_{50}$), performed at Sanofi Pasteur's Global Clinical Immunology Department (GCI), Swiftwater, Pennsylvania, USA. Baseline YF neutralising antibodies were assessed using $PRNT_{80}$ (Focus Diagnostics Inc., Cypress, California, USA) [3]. Serial two-fold dilutions of serum to be tested, previously heat-inactivated, were mixed with a constant challenge dose of YF vaccinal strain 17D. The mixtures were inoculated in duplicate in wells of a microplate of confluent Vero cells. Following

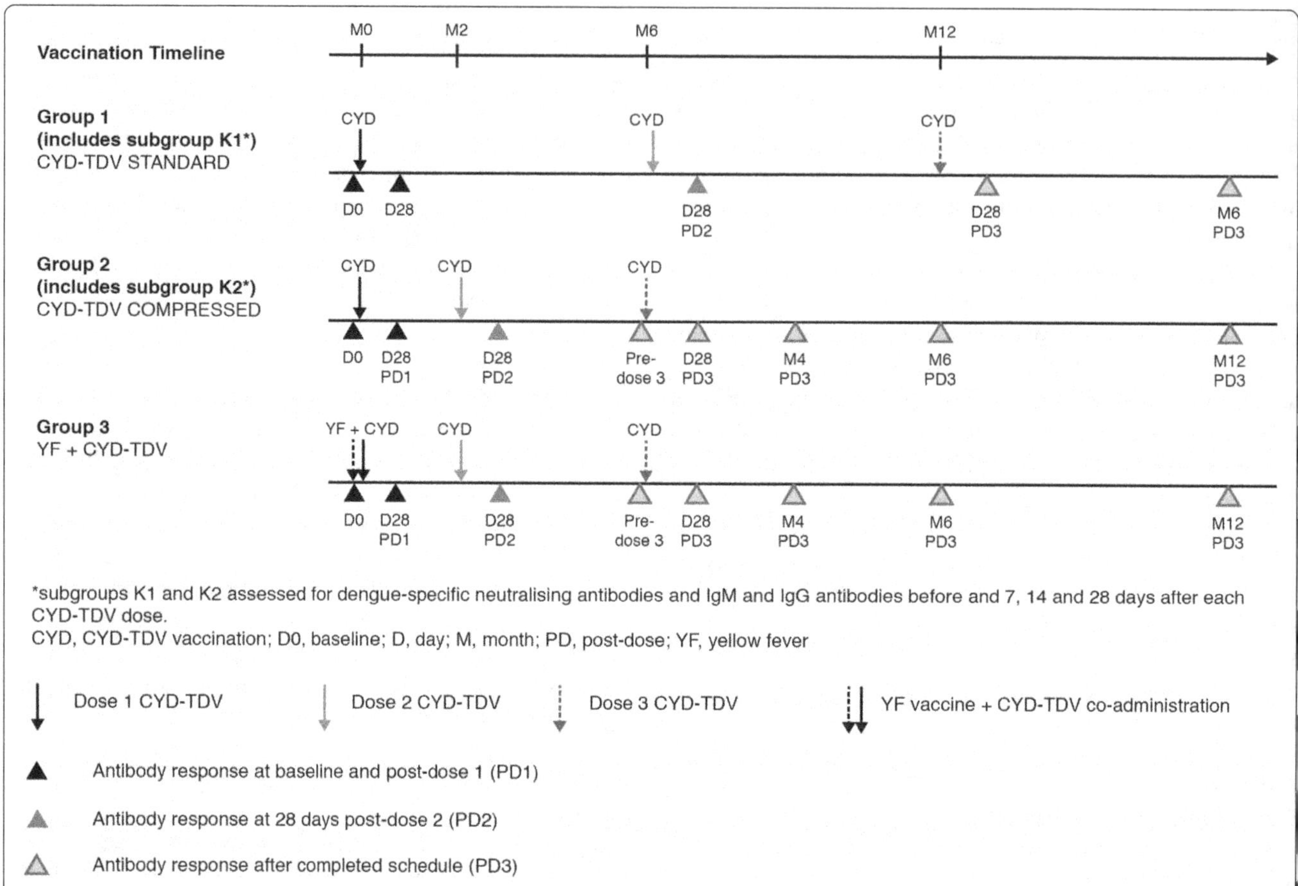

Fig. 1 Study design

adsorption, cell monolayers were overlaid. The presence of dengue virus infected cells was indicated by plaque formation. Neutralizing antibody titers were calculated and expressed as the reciprocal dilution reducing the mean plaque count by 50%. Negative control wells represented 100% viral load. Dengue or YF seropositivity was defined as antibody titres ≥10 (1/dil), as previously utilized in the vaccine's clinical development [4] (Additional file 1: Methods).

Antibody kinetics

Subgroups K1 and K2 were assessed for dengue-specific neutralising antibodies and IgM and IgG antibodies before and 7, 14 and 28 days after each CYD-TDV dose. IgM and IgG were measured by enzyme-linked immunosorbent assay (ELISA) using commercially available EL1500M and EL1500G DxSelect kits, respectively (Focus Diagnostics Inc., Cypress, California, USA).

Blood samples

Blood samples (10 mL) were stored at room temperature for 1–2 h following blood draw and refrigerated; samples were centrifuged within 24 h to collect sera. Sera were stored at or below − 20 °C and shipped frozen for analysis.

Safety assessment

Participants were monitored for immediate systemic adverse events (AE) during the first 30 min after each vaccine dose. Solicited injection site reactions (pain, erythema, and swelling) were recorded up to 7 days and solicited systemic reactions (fever, headache, malaise, myalgia, and asthenia) up to 14 days after each dose. Unsolicited AEs were recorded up to 28 days. Serious AEs (SAEs) and AEs of special interest (AESIs) were recorded throughout the study.

An early safety review was planned for the first 25% of total participants 14 (+ 2) days after their first vaccination. Enrolment was to be paused if one of the following was observed in CYD-TDV recipients: an unexpected related SAE, ≥20% incidence rate of Grade 3 fever post-dose 1, a serious AESI. No safety concerns were identified at this review, thus enrolment continued as planned.

Sample size and statistical methods

For Groups 1–3, 120 participants per group gave a probability of 95% for observing at least 1 AE with true incidence of 2.5%, assuming a dropout rate of 15% a total of 102 evaluable participants was anticipated. The sample size was arbitrarily set to 30 participants for Group 4. This was a descriptive study with no formal hypothesis testing. The 95% confidence intervals (CIs) of point estimates were calculated using normal approximation for quantitative data and exact binomial distribution (Clopper-Pearson method) for proportions. It was assumed that neutralising antibody titres were log-normally distributed.

Immunogenicity data were presented for the full analysis dataset, defined as participants who received at least one CYD-TDV or YF vaccine dose and who had at least one blood sample with post-dose serology results. The safety analysis set comprised participants who received at least one CYD-TDV or YF vaccine injection.

Results

Participants

A total of 390 participants were included: 120 in each Group 1–3 and 30 in Group 4; 40 participants (20 YF– and 20 YF+) from Groups 1 and 2 were enrolled into subgroups K1 and K2, respectively. Overall, 298 (76.4%) participants completed the study (Fig. 2).

Baseline participant characteristics are summarised in Table 1. Dengue seropositivity at baseline (those with ≥10 [1/dil] for ≥1 serotype) ranged from 7.0 to 7.7%. Of participants who reported prior YF vaccination, 97.5% had YF antibody titres ≥10 (1/dil).

CYD-TDV immunogenicity

Impact of compressed CYD-TDV vaccination schedule

Dengue antibody GMTs and percentages of seropositive participants increased for all serotypes following the third CYD-TDV dose of both schedules. There was no marked difference in GMTs by serotype between the two schedules. For both schedules, the highest GMTs were for serotype 4 and the lowest for serotype 1 (Table 2). At 28 days post-dose 3, 73.4% (Group 1) and 82.4% (Group 2) participants were dengue seropositive for ≥3 serotypes, with 50.0 and 42.6% seropositive against all four serotypes.

GMTs, measured 6 months after the third dose, decreased for all serotypes in Groups 1 and 2 with the exception of a small increase in GMT for serotype 4 in Group 1 (Table 2). In addition, dengue seropositivity remained above 70% for serotypes 2, 3 and 4 in Groups 1 and 2.

For the compressed schedule (Groups 2 and 3), no difference in GMTs was observed between 6 and 12 months post-dose 3 for any serotype (Additional file 2: Table S1). Group 1 GMTs were not measured beyond 6 months post-dose 3.

There were no marked differences between compressed and standard schedules in GMTs by serotype 28 days after each of the 3 doses (Additional file 2: Table S2). The 28-day post-dose 2 increase in GMTs was similar for all serotypes irrespective of whether dose 2 was given 2 (Group 2) or 6 months (Group 1) after the first dose (Additional file 2: Table S2). GMTs declined to

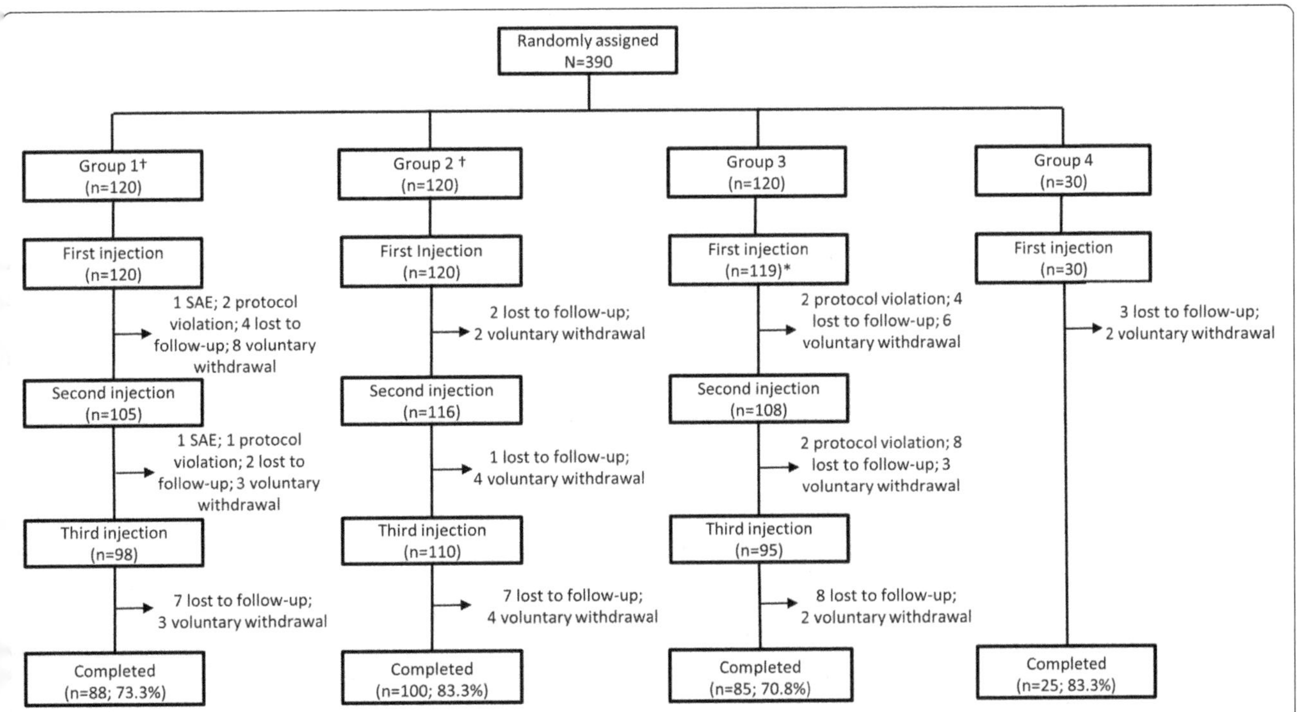

Fig. 2 Participant flow through the study (total randomised participants) *Participant presented with Hodgkin's lymphoma and was discontinued from the study before receiving any vaccine dose †Groups 1 and 2 were further randomised to subgroups K1 (n = 40) and K2 (n = 40)

Table 1 Participant characteristics at baseline (full analysis set)

	Group 1 (N = 117)	Group 2 (N = 119)	Group 3 (N = 114)
Sex, n (%)			
Female	57 (48.7)	61 (51.3)	58 (50.9)
Age, years			
Mean (SD)	31.8 (7.7)	32.6 (7.3)	32.8 (7.6)
Racial origin			
White Caucasian	88 (75.2)	103 (86.6)	88 (77.2)
Black or African American	21 (17.9)	14 (11.8)	19 (16.7)
Other	8 (6.8)	2 (1.7)	7 (6.1)
Seropositivity status, n (%)[a]			
Dengue seropositive	9 (7.7)	9 (7.6)	8 (7.0)
Yellow fever seropositive[b]	59 (50.4)	61 (51.3)	6 (5.3)
Flavivirus seropositive	63 (53.8)	65 (54.6)	11 (9.6)

n number of participants with the specified characteristic, *N* total number of participants in the study group, *SD* standard deviation

[a]Participants were defined as dengue or YF seropositive if they had neutralising antibody titres > 10 1/dilution (for at least one serotype for dengue seropositivity); participants were considered FV seropositive if they were seropositive for dengue of YF, or both

[b]Participants were randomised to treatment groups with stratification on prior reported YF vaccination (in the 3 months to 10 years preceding first study vaccine dose), such that 50% of Group 1 and 2 participants and no participants in Group 3 had prior reported YF. Laboratory confirmation of YF seropositive status according to protocol revealed discrepancies between the YF $PRNT_{50}$ assay and the reported YF vaccination history; the YF seropositive status of participants at baseline was thus re-calculated using YF $PRNT_{80}$, a more stringent assay compared to YF $PRNT_{50}$. Results based on $PRNT_{80}$ are shown for YF and FV seropositive status

similar levels pre-dose 3 for both the compressed and standard schedules (Additional file 2: Table S2).

Impact of baseline flavivirus status

FV status (FV+ or FV−) did not markedly affect GMTs against serotypes 1, 2 or 3 in Group 1 or for any serotype in Group 2 while serotype 4 GMTs tended to be lower in FV+ than FV− participants in Group 1 (51.7 versus 91.8, 28 days post-dose 3; Table 3). Seropositivity rates were comparable between FV+ and FV− participants in Group 1 for serotypes 1–3 and in Group 2 for serotype 4. However, they tended to be lower in FV+ than FV− participants for serotype 4 in Group 1 (82.7% versus 95.3%) and higher in FV+ participants for serotypes 1–3 in Group 2 (range, 51.0% among FV− to 94.9% among FV+ post-dose 3; Table 3).

Impact of YF vaccine co-administration

Dengue antibody response following co-administration with YF versus one dose of CYD-TDV alone is shown in Table 4 for YF− participants. Post CYD-TDV dose 1, GMTs and dengue seropositivity were similar for serotypes 1 and 2 between pooled YF− from Groups 1 and 2 and Group 3 (YF vaccine co-administration), but were higher for serotypes 3 and 4 in Groups 1 and 2 than Group 3 (Table 4).

The same trends in GMTs and dengue seropositivity were observed 28 days post-dose 2 (data not shown), but were no longer apparent 28 days post-dose 3. GMTs [95% CI] for Group 2 YF− participants versus Group 3: serotype 3, 47.3 [32.5–69.0] versus 30.2 [22.8–40.1] and serotype 4, 89.2 [53.3–149] versus 71.2 [52.0–97.7]; seropositivity [95% CI]: serotype 3, 85.4% [72.2–93.9] versus 73.5% [62.7–82.6] and serotype 4, 83.3% [69.8–92.5] versus 84.3% [74.7–91.4].

Antibody kinetics For subgroups K1 and K2, dengue IgM levels peaked at 28 days post-dose 1, then declined to the study end (Additional file 2: Figure S1A). The percentage of IgM-positive participants rose from 5.0% pre-dose 1 (both subgroups) to peak values of 72.5% (subgroup K1) and 92.5% (subgroup K2) at 28 days post-dose 1. These percentages dropped to 71.1% at month 2 and 45.7% pre-dose 2 (month 6) for subgroup K1, and 87.5% pre-dose 2 (month 2) for subgroup K2. No substantial increases were observed following doses 2 or 3. Over 50% of participants were IgM-positive up to 14 months post-dose 1 in both subgroups (Additional file 2: Figure S1B).

Dengue IgG levels increased up to 2 months post-dose 1 in both subgroups, and increased further following subsequent doses (Additional file 2: Figure S1A). For both subgroups, the percentage of IgG-positive participants reached at least 70% by 2 months post-dose 1 and 90% by day 14 post-dose 2, remaining above 80% in both subgroups to the study end (Additional file 2: Figure S1B). A limited number of participants (1–2 per subgroup) had a ≥ 4-fold increase in IgG levels post-dose 2 or 3.

Safety and reactogenicity of CYD-TDV The safety profile of CYD-TDV was similar for Groups 1 and 2. No safety concerns were observed following CYD-TDV co-administration with YF (Group 3; Table 5) compared to CYD-TDV alone (Groups 1 and 2) or YF alone (Group 4, Additional file 2: Table S3).

One participant (Group 3) reported an AE within 30 min after the first CYD-TDV dose (mild [grade 1] dizziness). The percentage of participants reporting solicited reactions was higher following co-administration of CYD-TDV and YF vaccines (Group 3, 75.7%) than following the first CYD-TDV dose (Groups 1 [63.6%] and 2 [64.7%]). In Groups 1–3, solicited reactions were reported less frequently after doses 2 and 3 than after dose 1 and were mostly of grade 1 intensity, started within 3 days after vaccine injection, and resolved spontaneously by day 6. Pain was the most frequently reported injection site reaction after any CYD-TDV dose and was mostly grade 1 intensity, ranging from 28.0% (Group 1) to 34.8% (Group 3) post-dose 1; headache, malaise, and myalgia were the most frequently reported solicited systemic reactions after each dose (29.4% [Group 2, myalgia] to 51.3% [Group 3, headache] post-dose 1).

Table 2 Dengue antibody GMTs and seropositivity status in the "standard" dengue vaccination schedule (Group 1) versus the "compressed" dengue vaccination schedule (Group 2)

Time point	Group 1 (*N* = 117)			Group 2 (*N* = 119)		
	n	GMT (95% CI)	Seropositive, % (95% CI)	n	GMT (95% CI)	Seropositive, % (95% CI)
Serotype 1						
Baseline	117	5.38 (4.85–5.96)	1.7 (0.2–6.0)	119	5.13 (4.98–5.28)	2.5 (0.5–7.2)
28 days post-dose 3	93	14.8 (11.3–19.4)	52.7 (42.1–63.1)	108	15.9 (12.6–20.0)	56.5 (46.6–66.0)
6 months post-dose 3	88	13.3 (10.2–17.4)	47.7 (37.0–58.6)	104	9.01 (7.54–10.8)	32.7 (23.8–42.6)
Serotype 2						
Baseline	117	5.19 (4.82–5.58)	0.9 (0.0–4.7)	119	5.22 (4.96–5.50)	2.5 (0.5–7.2)
28 days post-dose 3	94	51.2 (38.2–68.6)	84.0 (75.0–90.8)	108	59.9 (45.8–78.4)	88.0 (80.3–93.4)
6 months post-dose 3	88	45.6 (31.6–65.6)	75.0 (64.6–83.6)	104	38.7 (29.5–50.8)	80.8 (71.9–87.8)
Serotype 3						
Baseline	117	5.32 (4.94–5.73)	2.6 (0.5–7.3)	119	5.28 (5.03–5.55)	4.2 (1.4–9.5)
28 days post-dose 3	94	45.7 (35.0–59.8)	85.1 (76.3–91.6)	107	59.3 (47.0–74.7)	90.7 (83.5–95.4)
6 months post-dose 3	88	30.2 (22.8–40.2)	79.5 (69.6–87.4)	104	34.5 (27.5–43.3)	80.8 (71.9–87.8)
Serotype 4						
Baseline	117	5.78 (5.16–6.48)	6.8 (3.0–13.0)	119	5.11 (4.90–5.33)	0.8 (0.0–4.6)
28 days post-dose 3	94	66.8 (50.9–87.8)	88.3 (80.0–94.0)	107	83.1 (61.4–112.0)	86.0 (77.9–91.9)
6-months post-dose 3	88	74.8 (54.9–102.0)	86.4 (77.4–92.8)	104	41.7 (31.2–55.9)	74.0 (64.5–82.1)
≥ 3 serotypes						
Baseline	117	NA	0.9 (0.0–4.7)	119	NA	0.8 (0.0–4.6)
28 days post-dose 3	94	NA	73.4 (63.3–82.0)	108	NA	82.4 (73.9–89.1)
6-months post-dose 3	88	NA	64.8 (53.9–74.7)	104	NA	58.7 (48.6–68.2)
All 4 serotypes						
Baseline	117	NA	0.9 (0.0–4.7)	119	NA	0.8 (0.0–4.6)
Post-dose 3	94	NA	50.0 (39.5–60.5)	108	NA	42.6 (33.1–52.5)
6-months post-dose 3	88	NA	43.2 (32.7–54.2)	104	NA	26.9 (18.7–36.5)

Seropositive defined as antibody titres ≥10 (1/dil) against each serotype, and against at least 3 or all 4 serotypes with the parental dengue virus strain
GMT geometric mean titre, *n* number of participants with available data for endpoint, *NA* not applicable

Unsolicited AEs within 28 days following any injection were reported at similar frequencies for Groups 1, 2, and 3 (13.7–28.3%). Non-serious AEs were mostly systemic, grade 1 or 2 intensity and mostly assessed as not related to vaccination. The percentage of participants reporting an unsolicited adverse reaction (AR) was low across Groups 1–3 (0–7.6%) (Table 5). No AE led to study discontinuation in any group in the 28 days following injection. Three participants reported SAEs within 28 days, none of which were considered related to vaccination. During the trial, 13 participants experienced SAEs: 4 (3.3%) in Groups 1 and 2, and 5 (4.2%) in Group 3. One SAE was reported by the investigator as related to vaccination: a blighted ovum was detected 7 weeks after inadvertent vaccination of a woman during early pregnancy (Group 1; details provided in Additional file 2: Results). Three non-serious AESIs were reported by three participants within 7 days following the first injection; two (flushing of the face [Group 2] and asthma [Group 3]) were assessed as related to vaccination.

Discussion

This phase II study in healthy adults in a non-endemic area shows that an accelerated 0–2–6-month CYD-TDV vaccination schedule elicits a similar immune response to the licensed 0–6–12-month schedule. More rapid protection would be beneficial in the setting of public health programmes where a shorter schedule may allow potentially better compliance in dengue-endemic populations. Our study also supports that dengue antibody responses to the second CYD-TDV dose can be elicited when given 2 months after the first dose in a non-endemic setting. Notably, two other live attenuated tetravalent dengue vaccines, administered as a single dose [5] or 2 doses 90 days apart [6], are currently in phase III development.

Table 3 Dengue antibody response post-dose 3 by baseline FV status

	Group 1 ($N = 117$)						Group 2 ($N = 119$)					
	FV Seropositive[a] ($N = 63$)			FV Seronegative[b] ($N = 54$)			FV Seropositive[a] ($N = 65$)			FV Seronegative[b] ($N = 54$)		
	n	GMT (95% CI)	Seropositive %	n	GMT (95% CI)	Seropositive %	n	GMT (95% CI)	Seropositive %	n	GMT (95% CI)	Seropositive %
Serotype 1												
Baseline	63	5.73 (4.72–6.94)	3.2 (0.4–11.0)	54	5.00 (NC)	0.0 (0.0–6.6)	65	5.23 (4.96–5.53)	4.6 (1.0–12.9)	54	5.00 (NC)	0.0 (0.0–6.6)
28 days post-dose 3	51	15.6 (10.6–23.0)	54.9 (40.3–68.9)	42	13.9 (9.49–20.4)	50.0 (34.2–65.8)	59	17.2 (12.7–23.3)	61.0 (47.4–73.5)	49	14.4 (10.1–20.7)	51.0 (36.3–65.6)
6 months post-dose 3	49	14.8 (10.0–21.7)	53.1 (38.3–67.5)	39	11.7 (8.04–17.1)	41.0 (25.6–57.9)	58	10.3 (7.85–13.4)	36.2 (24.0–49.9)	46	7.63 (6.16–9.46)	28.3 (16.0–43.5)
12 months post-dose 3		NA			NA		55	9.35 (7.50–11.7)	40.0 (27.0–54.1)	44	7.45 (5.87–9.47)	25.0 (13.2–40.3)
Serotype 2												
Baseline	63	5.35 (4.67–6.13)	1.6 (0.0–8.5)	54	5.00 (NC)	0.0 (0.0–6.6)	65	5.42 (4.93–5.96)	4.6 (1.0–12.9)	54	5.00 (NC)	0.0 (0.0–6.6)
28 days post-dose 3	52	60.0 (39.4–91.4)	84.6 (71.9–93.1)	42	42.1 (27.9–63.4)	83.3 (68.6–93.0)	59	68.1 (48.9–94.7)	94.9 (85.9–98.9)	49	51.4 (32.8–80.6)	79.6 (65.7–89.8)
6 months post-dose 3	49	52.5 (32.1–85.8)	79.6 (65.7–89.8)	39	38.1 (21.7–67.0)	69.2 (52.4–83.0)	58	53.0 (37.4–75.2)	91.4 (81.0–97.1)	46	26.0 (17.2–39.3)	67.4 (52.0–80.5)
12 months post-dose 3		NA			NA		56	32.7 (22.6–47.4)	82.1 (69.6–91.1)	44	22.9 (15.5–33.7)	68.2 (52.4–81.4)
Serotype 3												
Baseline	63	5.61 (4.89–6.45)	4.8 (1.0–13.3)	54	5.00 (NC)	0.0 (0.0–6.6)	65	5.53 (5.06–6.05)	7.7 (2.5–17.0)	54	5.00 (NC)	0.0 (0.0–6.6)
28 days post-dose 3	52	44.8 (31.3–64.3)	84.6 (71.9–93.1)	42	46.9 (30.9–71.2)	85.7 (71.5–94.6)	59	71.2 (53.4–94.8)	94.9 (85.9–98.9)	48	47.3 (32.5–69.0)	85.4 (72.2–93.9)
6 months post-dose 3	49	33.0 (23.4–46.5)	85.7 (72.8–94.1)	39	27.1 (16.6–44.3)	71.8 (55.1–85.0)	58	48.5 (36.0–65.3)	87.9 (76.7–95.0)	46	22.5 (16.3–31.0)	71.7 (56.5–84.0)
12 months post-dose 3		NA			NA		56	24.1 (17.6–33.0)	73.2 (59.7–84.2)	44	15.4 (11.1–21.2)	61.4 (45.5–75.6)
Serotype 4												
Baseline	63	6.55 (5.32–8.07)	12.7 (5.6–23.5)	54	5.00 (NC)	0.0 (0.0–6.6)	65	5.20 (4.81–5.63)	1.5 (0.0–8.3)	54	5.00 (NC)	0.0 (0.0–6.6)
28 days post-dose 3	52	51.7 (35.1–76.2)	82.7 (69.7–91.8)	42	91.8 (63.3–133)	95.2 (83.8–99.4)	59	78.5 (54.3–114)	88.1 (77.1–95.1)	48	89.2 (53.3–149)	83.3 (69.8–92.5)
6 months post-dose 3	49	60.0 (38.4–93.8)	81.6 (68.0–91.2)	39	98.7 (64.8–150)	92.3 (79.1–98.4)	58	39.8 (26.9–59.0)	70.7 (57.3–81.9)	46	44.3 (28.3–69.5)	78.3 (63.6–89.1)
12 months post-dose 3		NA			NA		56	46.9 (32.2–68.4)	80.4 (67.6–89.8)	44	48.7 (30.5–77.5)	81.8 (67.3–91.8)

GMT geometric mean titre, *n* number of participants with available data for endpoint, *NA* not applicable, *NC* not calculated

[a]FV seropositive participants at baseline defined as: participants with ≥10 1/dil for at least 1 dengue serotype (sera tested by PRNT) or for YF virus (sera with $PRNT_{80}$)

[b]FV seronegative participants are defined as those participants with < 10 1/dil for all dengue serotypes and for YF virus (using sera with $PRNT_{80}$)

Table 4 Dengue antibody GMTs and seropositivity status, in YF non-immune participants following CYD-TDV alone (Groups 1 and 2 pooled) or CYD-TDV co-administered with YF vaccine (Group 3)

Time point	Group 1 and 2 pooled, YF− (*n* = 116)			Group 3, YF− (*n* = 108)		
	n	GMT (95% CI)	Seropositive, % (95% CI)	n	GMT (95% CI)	Seropositive, % (95% CI)
Serotype 1						
Baseline	116	5.19 (4.87–5.53)	1.7 (0.2–6.1)	108	5.00 (NC)	0 (0.0–3.4)
Post-dose 1	116	8.71 (7.04–10.8)	23.3 (15.9–32.0)	108	7.68 (6.46–9.14)	20.4 (13.2–29.2)
Serotype 2						
Baseline	116	5.06 (4.94–5.19)	0.9 (0.0–4.7)	108	5.06 (4.94–5.20)	0.9 (0.0–5.1)
Post-dose 1	116	18.8 (13.9–25.3)	46.6 (37.2–56.0)	108	10.8 (8.63–13.4)	35.2 (26.2–45.0)
Serotype 3						
Baseline	116	5.21 (4.97–5.47)	2.6 (0.5–7.4)	108	5.28 (4.90–5.69)	2.8 (0.6–7.9)
Post-dose 1	114	28.5 (20.4–39.7)	57.9 (48.3–67.1)	108	8.88 (7.23–10.9)	25.0 (17.2–34.3)
Serotype 4						
Baseline	116	5.43 (4.99–5.92)	3.4 (0.9–8.6)	108	5.26 (4.90–5.65)	1.9 (0.2–6.5)
Post-dose 1	114	229 (139–378)	74.6 (65.6–82.3)	107	22.6 (15.9–32.3)	48.6 (38.8–58.5)

YF seronegative participants at baseline are defined as those participants with YF baseline titre < 10 1/dil using $PRNT_{80}$. Dengue seropositive defined as dengue antibody titres ≥10 (1/dil) against each serotype, and against at least 3 or all 4 serotypes with the parental dengue virus strain
GMT geometric mean titre, *n* number of participants with available data for endpoint, *YF* yellow fever

Dengue neutralising antibody GMTs and seropositivity rates after a CYD-TDV vaccination course were lower in our study than in trials undertaken in endemic settings, among adults [7–10] and children [11–13]. Previous large scale studies have demonstrated that a significant proportion of study participants living in endemic areas are FV− prior to vaccination. When dengue antibody responses from FV− participants are compared to the results from this study, the GMTs are very similar: 31.2–75.5 among 2–45-year-olds in Vietnam [10]; 53.4–255 among children in Brazil [14], and 37.6–174 in children in other Latin American countries [12]. Similarly, in adults (18–45 years old) from Singapore, a region of low endemicity, among whom baseline FV seropositivity levels were low, dengue GMTs following vaccination were of a similar magnitude, or only slightly higher depending on serotype, as compared to GMTs observed in the current study [15]. Our findings suggest that the dengue antibody responses elicited following an accelerated vaccine schedule for CYD-TDV are comparable to those elicited by the licensed schedule among adults from non-endemic areas, and appear to be of a similar magnitude to those observed in previous studies among FV-naïve individuals from endemic countries. Further investigation is warranted to determine whether a shorter schedule may be effective in eliciting comparable dengue antibody responses in previously exposed populations from endemic areas.

In our study, a proportion of participants were recruited on the basis of previous YF vaccination; as such, overall baseline FV serostatus can be considered to be driven by baseline YF serostatus. We cannot rule out their exposure to other untested flaviviruses potentially in circulation at the time; the proportion of these previously exposed participants was low and thus unlikely to impact the data. Although some differences in dengue antibody response were observed between FV+ and FV− participants, the differences were inconsistent between serotypes and the number in each sub-group was small, limiting the interpretation of these results. Furthermore, it cannot be excluded that an impact might be observed in a population previously exposed to dengue, YF or another FV. Recent long-term safety data have shown there was an increased risk of hospitalized and severe virologically-confirmed dengue in dengue vaccinated participants who were seronegative; this onset was approximately 3 years after first vaccine dose in 9–16-year-olds [16]. Based on these results, the WHO Strategic Advisory Group of Experts has issued new guidance on the administration of CYD-TDV, with vaccination recommended in seropositive individuals only [17].

As a threshold of protection has not yet been established for dengue using the PRNT assay results, conclusions cannot be drawn on the potential implications of these findings regarding protection against occurrence of symptomatic dengue in these participants. In two pivotal phase III studies, it was suggested that higher post-dose 3 titers were predictive of high vaccine efficacy across all serotypes and age groups [18]. However, protective $PRNT_{50}$ titers may vary by serotype, age and endemicity, as shown in an integrated immunogenicity analysis of CYD-TDV up to 4 years after vaccination [19]. Another limitation of this study is that the PRNT assay does not allow us to differentiate between homotypic antibody responses (believed to confer long term immunity), and heterotypic (cross-reactive) antibody responses (conferring short term cross-protection) [20].

Table 5 Safety overview after each CYD-TDV dose – safety analysis set

	Group 1 (*N* = 120)		Group 2 (*N* = 120)		Group 3 (*N* = 119)	
	n/M	% (95% CI)	n/M	% (95% CI)	n/M	% (95% CI)
First CYD-TDV dose						
Solicited reaction	75/118	63.6 (54.2–72.2)	77/119	64.7 (55.4–73.2)	87/115	75.7 (66.8–83.2)
Solicited injection site reaction[a]	34/118	28.8 (20.8–37.9)	42/118	35.3 (26.8–44.6)	40/115	34.8 (26.1–44.2)
Solicited systemic reaction	65/118	55.1 (45.7–64.3)	68/118	57.1 (47.7–66.2)	77/115	67.0 (57.6–75.4)
Unsolicited non-serious AE	34/120	28.3 (20.5–37.3)	32/120	26.7 (19.0–35.5)	27/119	22.7 (15.5–31.3)
Unsolicited non-serious AR	7/120	5.8 (2.4–11.6)	4/120	3.3 (0.9–8.3)	9/119	7.6 (3.5–13.9)
Unsolicited non-serious injection site AR[a]	4/120	3.3 (0.9–8.3)	3/120	2.5 (0.5–7.1)	0/119	0.0 (0.0–3.1)
Unsolicited non-serious systemic AE	31/120	25.8 (18.3–34.6)	30/120	25.0 (17.5–33.7)	25/119	21.0 (14.1–29.4)
Unsolicited non-serious systemic AR	3/120	2.5 (0.5–7.1)	2/120	1.7 (0.2–5.9)	7/119	5.9 (2.4–11.7)
Second CYD-TDV dose						
Solicited reaction	44/101	43.6 (33.7–53.8)	57/114	50.0 (40.5–59.5)	40/96	41.7 (31.7–52.2)
Solicited injection site reaction	21/101	20.8 (13.4–30.0)	32/114	28.1 (20.1–37.3)	24/96	25.0 (16.7–34.9)
Solicited systemic reaction	38/101	37.6 (28.2–47.8)	43/114	37.7 (28.8–47.3)	33/96	34.4 (25.0–44.8)
Unsolicited non-serious AE	15/105	14.3 (8.2–22.5)	18/116	15.5 (9.5–23.4)	15/108	13.9 (8.0–21.9)
Unsolicited non-serious AR	3/105	2.9 (0.6–8.1)	2/116	1.7 (0.2–6.1)	0/108	0.0 (0.0–3.4)
Unsolicited non-serious injection site AR	1/105	1.0 (0.0–5.2)	1/116	0.9 (0.0–4.7)	0/108	0.0 (0.0–3.4)
Unsolicited non-serious systemic AE	15/105	14.3 (8.2–22.5)	18/116	15.5 (9.5–23.4)	15/108	13.9 (8.0–21.9)
Unsolicited non-serious systemic AR	2/105	1.9 (0.2–6.7)	1/116	0.9 (0.0–4.7)	0/108	0.0 (0.0–3.4)
Third CYD-TDV dose						
Solicited reaction	36/91	39.6 (29.5–50.4)	47/107	43.9 (34.3–53.9)	37/89	41.6 (31.2–52.5)
Solicited injection site reaction	19/91	20.9 (13.1–30.7)	29/106	27.4 (19.1–36.9)	21/89	23.6 (15.2–33.8)
Solicited systemic reaction	32/91	35.2 (25.4–45.9)	39/107	36.4 (27.4–46.3)	32/89	36.0 (26.1–46.8)
Unsolicited non-serious AE	19/98	19.4 (12.1–28.6)	17/110	15.5 (9.3–23.6)	13/95	13.7 (7.5–22.3)
Unsolicited non-serious AR	2/98	2.0 (0.2–7.2)	0/110	0.0 (0.0–3.3)	1/95	1.1 (0.0–5.7)
Unsolicited non-serious injection site AR	2/98	2.0 (0.2–7.2)	0/110	0.0 (0.0–3.3)	0/95	0.0 (0.0–3.8)
Unsolicited non-serious systemic AE	17/98	17.3 (10.4–26.3)	17/110	15.5 (9.3–23.6)	13/95	13.7 (7.5–22.3)
Unsolicited non-serious systemic AR	0/98	0.0 (0.0–3.7)	0/110	0.0 (0.0–3.3)	1/95	1.1 (0.0–5.7)

AE adverse event, *AR* adverse reaction, *CI* confidence interval, *M* number of participants evaluable for the specified endpoint, *n* number of participants with the specified event

[a]For CYD-TDV injection only; YF safety data not presented here

We also observed a lower post-dose 1 dengue antibody response, for serotypes 3 and 4, following co-administration of YF and CYD-TDV vaccines compared to CYD-TDV alone. This potential effect was rectified following the complete vaccination schedule. Further research on the impact of co-administration of FV vaccines is warranted.

The evaluation of IgM antibody kinetics demonstrated that an IgM response may be detected up to several months after vaccination in this study population. IgG levels also increased throughout the vaccination schedule, with > 80% of participants IgG-positive at study end. While these findings are based on a small numbers of participants (40 per group), they suggest that CYD-TDV induces long-lasting dengue neutralising antibody responses and IgM and IgG responses (6–12 months post-dose 1) in this population. This highlights the potential for vaccine-induced false positives in the diagnosis of dengue based on IgM and IgG serological assays, as previously described [21].

The CYD-TDV safety profile in our study was acceptable for both vaccination schedules, and in-line with previous studies [7, 10, 12, 22, 23].

Conclusions

In conclusion, in a non-endemic setting, CYD-TDV given in a compressed 0–2–6-month schedule can elicit similar antibody responses to the standard 0–6–12-month schedule. Further studies would be needed to evaluate whether this proposed schedule may also apply in endemic populations.

Additional files

Additional file 1: Methods. PRNT assay. Additional information on the methods for the PRNT assay and serostatus at baseline.

Additional file 2: Results. SAEs during the trial considered related to vaccination**.** Additional information on the SAEs during the trial considered related to vaccination. **Table S1.** Dengue antibody GMTs in the "compressed" dengue vaccination schedule by FV status (Groups 2 and 3) and with YF co-administration (Group 3). **Table S2.** Dengue antibody GMTs in the "standard" dengue vaccination schedule (Group 1) versus the "compressed" dengue vaccination schedule (Group 2) pre-dose and 28 days post-dose during the study. **Table S3.** Safety overview after a single dose of YF vaccine – safety analysis set. **Figure S1.** A. Kinetics of dengue IgG and IgM responses (GMTs [measured by ELISA]; full analysis set). B. Kinetics of dengue IgG and IgM responses (percentage of participants positive for IgM/IgG; full analysis set).

Abbreviations

AE: Adverse event; AESI: Adverse event of special interest; CYD-TDV: Live attenuated tetravalent dengue vaccine; ELISA: Enzyme-linked immunosorbent assay; FV: Flavivirus; GMT: Geometric mean titres; IgG: Immunoglobulin G; IgM: Immunoglobulin M; PRNT: Plaque reduction neutralisation test; SAE: Serious adverse event; YF: Yellow fever

Acknowledgements

The authors would like to thank all the participants who participated in the trial, and the following investigators for their contributions to data collection: Jeffry Jacqmein, Steven Folkerth, Ivan Rarick, Donald Birkindine, Carol Johnson, and Andrew Tak. The Authors also thank the following individuals from Sanofi Pasteur for their contributions to the design and data collection or interpretation of the data: Jennifer Kasztejna, Jose Rivera, Béatrice Roy, Lydie Michaudet, Julien Bertrand, Marie Philibert, Margaret Buenzli and Nona Ghazanfari, and personnel at Sanofi Pasteur's Global Clinical Immunology Department (Swiftwater, Pennsylvania, USA) for performing PRNT assays. Jo-Ann West (Sanofi Pasteur) provided manuscript coordination support on behalf of Sanofi Pasteur. Editorial assistance with the preparation of the manuscript was provided by a professional medical writer, Juliette Gray of inScience Communications, Springer Healthcare, funded by Sanofi Pasteur.

Funding

This study was sponsored by Sanofi Pasteur. The sponsor participated in the trial design and managed all operational aspects of the study, including monitoring data collection, statistical analyses, and writing of the report.

Authors' contributions

MB, TP, AS and EP were involved in the design and operational management of the study. MT was the lead study statistician. JK and WD were principal investigators in this study. All authors (JK, WD, MT, MB, TP, AS, and EP) contributed to the interpretation of the data, contributed to this publication and approved the final manuscript for submission. All authors (JK, WD, MT, MB, TP, AS, and EP) had access to the study data and are responsible for the veracity and completeness of the data reported.

Consent for publication

Not applicable.

Competing interests

MT, MB, TP, AS and EP were all employees of Sanofi Pasteur at the time of the study. MB holds stocks in Sanofi Pasteur. JK and WD have no conflicts of interest to declare.

Author details

[1]Advanced Clinical Research, West Jordan, UT, USA. [2]Benchmark Research, Sacramento, CA, USA. [3]Sanofi Pasteur, Global Clinical Immunology, Discovery Drive, Swiftwater, PA 18370, USA. [4]Sanofi Pasteur, Siège Social, 14 Espace Henry Vallée, 69007 Lyon, France.

References

1. Bhatt S, Gething PW, Brady OJ, Messina JP, Farlow AW, Moyes CL, Drake JM, Brownstein JS, Hoen AG, Sankoh O, et al. The global distribution and burden of dengue. Nature. 2013;496(7446):504–7.
2. World Health Organization: Global strategy for dengue prevention and control: 2012–2020. 2012. Avilable from: http://www.who.int/denguecontrol/9789241504034/en/. Accessed 18 Sept 2018.
3. Thomas SJ, Nisalak A, Anderson KB, Libraty DH, Kalayanarooj S, Vaughn DW, Putnak R, Gibbons RV, Jarman R, Endy TP. Dengue plaque reduction neutralization test (PRNT) in primary and secondary dengue virus infections: how alterations in assay conditions impact performance. Am J Trop Med Hyg. 2009;81(5):825–33.
4. L'Azou M, Assoukpa J, Fanouillere K, Plennevaux E, Bonaparte M, Bouckenooghe A, Frago C, Noriega F, Zambrano B, Ochiai RL, et al. Dengue seroprevalence: data from the clinical development of a tetravalent dengue vaccine in 14 countries (2005–2014). Trans R Soc Trop Med Hyg. 2018; 112(4):158–68.
5. Durbin AP, Kirkpatrick BD, Pierce KK, Carmolli MP, Tibery CM, Grier PL, Hynes N, Opert K, Jarvis AP, Sabundayo BP, et al. A 12-month-interval dosing study in adults indicates that a single dose of the National Institute of Allergy and Infectious Diseases tetravalent dengue vaccine induces a robust neutralizing antibody response. J Infect Dis. 2016;214(6):832–5.
6. Rupp R, Luckasen GJ, Kirstein JL, Osorio JE, Santangelo JD, Raanan M, Smith MK, Wallace D, Gordon GS, Stinchcomb DT. Safety and immunogenicity of different doses and schedules of a live attenuated tetravalent dengue vaccine (TDV) in healthy adults: a phase 1b randomized study. Vaccine. 2015;33(46):6351–9.
7. Dayan GH, Thakur M, Boaz M, Johnson C. Safety and immunogenicity of three tetravalent dengue vaccine formulations in healthy adults in the USA. Vaccine. 2013;31(44):5047–54.
8. Torresi J, Heron LG, Qiao M, Marjason J, Chambonneau L, Bouckenooghe A, Boaz M, van der Vliet D, Wallace D, Hutagalung Y, et al. Lot-to-lot consistency of a tetravalent dengue vaccine in healthy adults in Australia: a randomised study. Vaccine. 2015;33(39):5127–34.
9. Dubey AP, Agarkhedkar S, Chhatwal J, Narayan A, Ganguly S, Wartel TA, Bouckenooghe A, Menezes J. Immunogenicity and safety of a tetravalent dengue vaccine in healthy adults in India: a randomized, observer-blind, placebo-controlled phase II trial. Hum Vaccin Immunother. 2016;12(2):512–8.
10. Tran N, Luong CQ, Vu TQH, Forrat R, Lang J, Vu QD, Bouckenooghe A, Wartel TA. Safety and immunogenicity of recombinant, live attenuated tetravalent dengue vaccine (CYD- TDV) in healthy Vietnamese adults and children. J Vaccines Vaccination. 2012;3:7.
11. Sabchareon A, Wallace D, Sirivichayakul C, Limkittikul K, Chanthavanich P, Suvannadabba S, Jiwariyavej V, Dulyachai W, Pengsaa K, Wartel TA, et al. Protective efficacy of the recombinant, live-attenuated, CYD tetravalent dengue vaccine in Thai schoolchildren: a randomised, controlled phase 2b trial. Lancet. 2012;380(9853):1559–67.
12. Villar LA, Rivera-Medina DM, Arredondo-Garcia JL, Boaz M, Starr-Spires L, Thakur M, Zambrano B, Miranda MC, Rivas E, Dayan GH. Safety and immunogenicity of a recombinant tetravalent dengue vaccine in 9-16 year olds: a randomized, controlled, phase II trial in Latin America. Pediatr Infect Dis J. 2013;32(10):1102–9.
13. Capeding MR, Tran NH, Hadinegoro SR, Ismail HI, Chotpitayasunondh T, Chua MN, Luong CQ, Rusmil K, Wirawan DN, Nallusamy R, et al. Clinical efficacy and safety of a novel tetravalent dengue vaccine in healthy children in Asia: a phase 3, randomised, observer-masked, placebo-controlled trial. Lancet. 2014;384(9951):1358–65.
14. Dayan GH, Garbes P, Noriega F, Izoton de Sadovsky AD, Rodrigues PM, Giuberti C, Dietze R. Immunogenicity and safety of a recombinant tetravalent dengue vaccine in children and adolescents ages 9-16 years in Brazil. Am J Trop Med Hyg. 2013;89(6):1058–65.

15. Leo YS, Wilder-Smith A, Archuleta S, Shek LP, Chong CY, Leong HN, Low CY, Oh ML, Bouckenooghe A, Wartel TA, et al. Immunogenicity and safety of recombinant tetravalent dengue vaccine (CYD-TDV) in individuals aged 2-45 y: phase II randomized controlled trial in Singapore. Hum Vaccin Immunother. 2012;8(9):1259–71.
16. Sridhar S, Luedtke A, Langevin E, Zhu M, Bonaparte M, Machabert T, et al. Effect of Dengue Serostatus on Dengue Vaccine Safety and Efficacy. N Engl J Med. 2018 Jul 26;379(4):327-340. https://www.ncbi.nlm.nih.gov/pubmed/29897841.
17. WHO Strategic Advisory Group of Experts: Executive summary: CYD-TDV dengue vaccine.
18. Moodie Z, Juraska M, Huang Y, Zhuang Y, Fong Y, Carpp LN, Self SG, Chambonneau L, Small R, Jackson N, et al. Neutralizing antibody correlates analysis of tetravalent dengue vaccine efficacy trials in Asia and Latin America. J Infect Dis. 2018;217(5):742–53.
19. Vigne C, Dupuy M, Richetin A, Guy B, Jackson N, Bonaparte M, Hu B, Saville M, Chansinghakul D, Noriega F, et al. Integrated immunogenicity analysis of a tetravalent dengue vaccine up to 4 y after vaccination. Hum Vaccin Immunother. 2017;13(9):2004–16.
20. Guy B, Jackson N. Dengue vaccine: hypotheses to understand CYD-TDV-induced protection. Nat Rev Microbiol. 2016;14(1):45–54.
21. Plennevaux E, Sabchareon A, Limkittikul K, Chanthavanich P, Sirivichayakul C, Moureau A, Boaz M, Wartel TA, Saville M, Bouckenooghe A. Detection of dengue cases by serological testing in a dengue vaccine efficacy trial: utility for efficacy evaluation and impact of future vaccine introduction. Vaccine. 2016;34(24):2707–12.
22. Poo J, Galan F, Forrat R, Zambrano B, Lang J, Dayan GH. Live-attenuated tetravalent dengue vaccine in dengue-naive children, adolescents, and adults in Mexico City: randomized controlled phase 1 trial of safety and immunogenicity. Pediatr Infect Dis J. 2011;30:e9–e17.
23. Gailhardou S, Skipetrova A, Dayan GH, Jezorwski J, Saville M, Van der Vliet D, Wartel TA. Safety overview of a recombinant live-attenuated tetravalent dengue vaccine: pooled analysis of data from 18 clinical trials. PLoS Negl Trop Dis. 2016;10(7):e0004821.

22

Assessing changes in knowledge, attitude and practices on dengue diagnosis and management among primary care physicians after the largest dengue epidemic in Singapore

Junxiong Pang[1,2*], Zoe Jane-Lara Hildon[2,3,4], Tun Linn Thein[1], Jing Jin[1] and Yee Sin Leo[1,2,5,6]

Abstract

Background: Dengue results in high morbidity and mortality globally. The knowledge, attitude and practices (KAP) of dengue management, including diagnosis, among primary care physicians (PCPs) are important to reduce dengue transmission and burden. However, there is a lack of understanding on the impact of dengue epidemic on dengue management. Hence, the aim of this study is to examine the changes in KAP on dengue management among PCPs before and after the largest dengue epidemic in 2013 in Singapore.

Methods: Surveys were mailed to 2000 and 1514 PCPs registered under the Singapore Medical Council in March of year 2011 and 2014, respectively. Survey data were then collected between April and June of that year. Chi-square or Fisher's exact test was used for comparing categorical variables. A multivariate logistic regression model was implemented to determine independent factors for frequent use of dengue diagnostic tests (DDTs). All tests were conducted at 5% level of significance. Adjusted odds ratio and corresponding 95% confidence intervals were reported, where applicable. Qualitative data were descriptively coded for themes and analysis.

Results: Among PCPs surveyed in 2011 and 2014, 89.9% and 86% had good knowledge on dengue management respectively. The usage of DDTs had increased significantly in 2014 ($N = 164$;56%) as compared to 2011 ($N = 107$;29.5%) in both private and public clinics ($p < 0.001$). Dengue Duo point-of-care test (POCT) kits was independently associated with frequent use of DDTs (adjusted odds ratio = 2.15; 95% confidence interval = 1.25–3.69). There was a significant reduction in referral of dengue patients to hospital (31.4% in 2011; 13.3% in 2014; $p < 0.001$), and a significant increase in frequency of clinic follow-ups (18.4% in 2011; 28.5% in 2014; $p = 0.003$). One key theme highlighted was that dengue management can be improved with availability of POCT kit, better awareness of the disease and any revised clinical guidelines.

Conclusion: The knowledge on dengue management remained high, while the attitude and practices, particularly on the usage of DDTs improved significantly after a large epidemic. Furthermore, PCPs had more confident in managing dengue patients in primary care settings and in educating patients on the importance of vector control and dengue warning signs to reduce dengue transmission and burden.

Keywords: Dengue epidemic, Primary care, Dengue management, Dengue diagnosis, Knowledge, Attitude, Practices

* Correspondence: pangv@hotmail.com
[1]Institute of Infectious Diseases and Epidemiology, Tan Tock Seng Hospital, 144 Moulmein Road, Singapore 308089, Singapore
[2]Saw Swee Hock School of Public Health, National University of Singapore, Singapore, Singapore
Full list of author information is available at the end of the article

Background

Dengue, one of the major global burdens, is estimated to affect at least 50 million people annually [1]. Dengue haemorrhagic fever (DHF) and Dengue shock syndrome (DSS) are severe clinical manifestations for dengue infection in both adult and children. Identifying the disease early and predicting the possible outcomes effectively is a leading concern for Public Health specialists managing the disease [2]

Dengue fever (DF) is endemic in the tropical and subtropical regions, including Singapore [2]. Dengue was first reported in Singapore in the early 1960 [3]. Since 1969, with the implementation of vector control and surveillance, public health education and law enforcement, there has been a general decline in disease incidence, until in 1990 when dengue began to surge again [4]. Since then, Singapore has faced several dengue epidemic. Spikes have been recorded in 2005 and 2007 with 14,209 and 8826 cases respectively [5]. The largest dengue epidemic was experienced in the year 2013 with 22,170 reported dengue cases with eight deaths [6]. In Singapore, the occurrence of DF and DHF are influenced by several factors such as lowered herd immunity and virus transmission outside the home by *Aedes* mosquitoes, which potentially resulted in the resurgence of dengue incidences among adult population [7].

In 1997, the World Health Organization introduced dengue management guidelines for diagnosis, treatment, prevention and control [8]. A revised edition was released in 2009 with updated information for better clinical management, vector management and laboratory diagnosis [9]. Dengue virus infection may be asymptomatic or symptomatic that may lead to unpredictable severe outcomes such as death. In the three largest outbreak clusters in Singapore, it was revealed that 73.2% of residents with recent infection were asymptomatic [5]. Hence, early detection of these dengue cases and monitoring of disease severity are important parts of dengue management to reduce dengue transmission and burden.

Moreover, to avoid over-hospitalization during an epidemic, it is important to have a system not only for early detection but also effective outpatient monitoring. Since the development of Dengue Duo POCT kit [10], there were many clinical validation studies performed such as the SD Dengue Duo POCT kit (Standard Diagnostics, Inc., Gyeonggi-do, Korea) with sensitivities and specificities ranging from 75.5–92.9% and 88.8–100% respectively using frozen serum or plasma samples [11–14]. This commercially available assay uses whole blood to obtain dengue positivity result within 30 min of patient presentation. In 2013, SD Dengue Duo POCT kit was also validated in Singapore with sensitivity and specificity of 93.9% and 92.0% respectively [15], with significant reduction (from estimated four hours to an hour) in the time required from patient presentation to appropriate clinical management in a tertiary hospital. This kit, which includes both dengue NS1 antigen and dengue IgM & IgG antibody detection, is likely to enhance early diagnosis of dengue and reduce dengue burden at the primary healthcare settings. A good understanding of the changes in KAP of the dengue management among the PCPs will be important to reduce dengue burden. Even though there were two cross-sectional KAP studies focusing on the dengue management of PCPs in Southern Vietnam [16] and Southern Taiwan [17], there is still a lack of understanding on the changes of KAP after a large dengue epidemic.

Therefore the aims of this study were to (1) Examine changes in primary care physicians knowledge, attitude and practices, in particular on the usage of dengue diagnostic tests and related clinical practices; (2) Enquire about their experience on using the POCT kit; (3) Gather recommendations for improved service delivery in patient diagnostics and clinical care management to facilitate reduction in dengue burden.

Methods

Study design

Surveys were mailed to 2000 and 1514 PCPs registered under the Singapore Medical Council in March of year 2011 [18] and 2014, respectively. Survey data were then collected back between April and June of that year. The survey form was developed by clinical researchers and was piloted prior to the actual survey. A total of 364 (18.3%) and 293 (19.4%) surveys were mailed back in 2011 and 2014, respectively. We compared survey data using baseline data collected in 2011 [18] and a follow-up survey in 2014. The survey included open-ended questions enquiring about the usage experience and/or perception of the new POCT kit introduced in 2014 to facilitate dengue diagnosis.

Survey questionnaire

The questionnaire was designed with four parts. They were (1) practitioner demographics (gender, age, type of practice and qualification), (2) dengue management – including related knowledge, dengue diagnostic practices, and clinical care; (3) attitudes toward POCT and (4) responses to the dengue epidemic in 2013. The baseline survey included 25 multiple-choice questionnaires [18]. However, only 18 of these questions were retained in the 2014 survey so that meaningful comparisons focusing on dengue management can be performed (Additional file 1).

In relation to repertoires of disease management, participants were asked about their preferred method of dengue diagnosis, the level clinical care of confirmed patients, and their knowledge on dengue clinical guidelines. The dengue warning signs recommended by the World Health Organization used to classify Dengue into levels of severity was assessed [1]. These warning signs include: abdominal pain or tenderness, persistent vomiting, clinical fluid accumulation, bleeding/mucosal bleeding, drowsiness, fatigue, lethargy, breathlessness, increase in haematocrit concurrent with rapid decrease in platelet count and hepatomegaly. Participants were asked about their awareness of the warning signs and to list down three common ones.

In the follow-up survey in 2014, participants were asked about their awareness on rapid Dengue POCT, their level of interest in using it and any perceived challenges/benefits if they have experience using it. Two open-ended questions were designed to seek participants' opinion and experience about surge management, and how participants had managed the 2013 epidemic and the changes in dengue management after these dengue epidemics.

Analytic methods

Analysis was performed with consideration of both the quantitative and qualitative data gathered in the survey. For the quantitative analyses, the data were stratified by type of practice, i.e. government subsidized polyclinic, private practice. Chi-square or Fisher's exact test was used for comparing categorical variables. A multivariate logistic regression model was implemented to determine independent factors for frequent use of DDTs. All tests were conducted at 5% level of significance. We reported adjusted odds ratio and corresponding 95% confidence intervals where applicable. All statistical analyses were performed using SPSS Version 16 (SPSS Inc., Chicago, IL). Qualitative data were descriptively coded for themes on the topics of the experience of using the POCT kit, the management of dengue epidemics and changes in dengue management after dengue epidemic. NVivo 10 software Version 10, 2012 (QSR International Pty Ltd.) was used to manage the textual data.

Results

Demographics characteristics of PCPs surveyed in 2011 and 2014

A total of 364 PCPs participated (18.3% response rate) in the survey in 2011 [18]. A total of 293 PCPs participated (19.4% response rate) in the survey in 2014 (Table 1). Among these, majority were male (N = 157; 53.6%), and were pre-dominantly in the age-group of 41–60 years old (N = 185; 63.1%) and from the private sector (N = 206; 70.3%). There was significantly lesser male PCPs (p = 0.046) in year 2014 (N = 157; 53.6%) than year 2011 (N = 223; 61.3%). There were significantly more PCPs in the 41–60 years old group, but lesser in the above 60 years old group ($p < 0.0001$) in the survey year 2014 (N = 185; 63.1% & N = 26; 8.9% respectively) than year 2011 (N = 185; 50.8% & N = 67; 18.4% respectively). The proportion of PCPs with post-graduate degree qualifications was significantly higher in survey year 2014 (N = 158; 53.9%) than in 2011 (N = 124; 34.1%; $p < 0.001$; Table 1).

Table 1 Demographics of primary care physicians

Years	2011 N = 364 (%)	2014 N = 293 (%)	P value	CFPS 2011[a] N = 1400 (%)
Gender				
Male	223 (61.3)	157 (53.6)	**0.046**	(60)
D.N.P.	3 (0.8)	1 (0.3)		
Age				
21–40 years	111 (30.5)	82 (28.0)		(58) for <45 yrs
41–60 years	185 (50.8)	185 (63.1)		
61 years or above	67 (18.4)	26 (8.9)	**<0.001**	(42) for ≥45 yrs
D.N.P.	1 (0.3)	0		
Highest Qualifications				
M.B.,B.S. (or equivalent) only	231 (63.5)	133 (45.4)		N.A.
Post-graduate degrees	124 (34.1)	158 (53.9)	**<0.001**	N.A.
D.N.P.	9 (2.4)	2 (0.7)		
Practice				
Private	253 (69.5)	206 (70.3)		(55.9)
Polyclinic	105 (28.8)	87 (29.7)	0.931	(44.1)
D.N.P.	6 (1.7)	0		

Post-graduate degrees- Graduate Diploma in Family Medicine, Master in Medicine (Family Medicine), Membership of Royal College of Physicians

P values calculated by Fisher's exact test. P value in bold represents a statistical significant difference

D.N.P. Data not provided by participants, *M.B.B.S.* Bachelor of Medicine and Bachelor of Surgery, *N.A.* Not available

[a]*CFPS* College of Family Physicians Singapore (As of June 2011) [24]

Knowledge on dengue warning signs and clinical management

Majority of PCPs ($N = 250$; 86%) knew at least one of the World Health Organization-guided dengue warning signs in survey year 2014, which is significantly higher than in year 2011 survey ($N = 285$; 78.3%; $p = 0.024$) (Table 2). The top three responses in survey year of 2014 include the bleeding/mucosal bleeding ($N = 139$; 55.6%) followed by abdominal pain or tenderness ($N = 97$; 38.8%) and drowsiness, fatigue, lethargy, breathlessness ($N = 44$; 17.6%) (Additional file 2). Based on the three clinical scenarios designed to assess the level of clinical management, the majority of PCPs (75.7%) gave the preferred responses in at least 2 questions (Additional file 3). In overall, 89.9% and 86% of the PCPs surveyed had good knowledge on dengue management in 2011 and 2014 ($p > 0.05$), respectively.

Attitude and practices on dengue diagnostic tests

The proportion of the PCPs who always use DDTs, instead of relying only on clinical diagnosis, increased significantly in survey year 2014 ($N = 164$; 56%) compared to 2011 ($N = 107$; 29.5%; $p < 0.001$; Table 2). The proportion of public PCPs who always use DDTs increased significantly in survey year 2014 ($N = 53$; 60.9%) compared to 2011 ($N = 9$; 7.9%; $p < 0.001$). Moreover, the proportion of public (0% in 2014 and 36.8% in 2011; $p < 0.001$) and private (8.3% in 2014 and 17% in 2011; $p = 0.008$) PCPs who had never used diagnostic testing decreased significantly in survey year 2014 compared to survey year 2011. A significantly higher proportion of PCPs ($N = 236$; 80.5%) used DDTs in more than 50% of their consultations for suspected dengue in survey year 2014 compared to year 2011 ($N = 176$; 48.5%; $p < 0.001$).

In 2011, about 74.8% ($N = 211$) of the PCPs relied on Dengue serology (IgM/IgG) test in the laboratory as Dengue Duo POCT kit was not available in the market then. In 2014, after the introduction of Dengue Duo POCT kit, about 37.7% ($N = 104$) of the PCPs used the Dengue Duo POCT kit. Besides the Dengue Duo kit, Dengue serology (IgM/IgG) test and Dengue non-structural antigen 1 assay test were frequently used in 2014 ($N = 91$, 33% and $N = 62$, 22.5% respectively). The proportion of PCPs who used dengue reverse transcription- polymerase chain reaction assay was significantly reduced in survey year 2014 ($N = 9$, 3.3%) compared to survey year 2011 ($N = 37$, 13.1%; $p < 0.001$). These trends are similar in both private and public polyclinics (Table 2).

Using data from 2014 survey, a multivariate logistic regression was performed to identify factors associated with frequent behaviour (comparing between 'Always' and 'Sometimes/Never' groups) of DDTs utilization. After adjusting for confounding factors (gender, age, place of

Table 2 Dengue diagnostic practices among primary care physicians

	Overall		*P* value	Private practice		*P* value	Polyclinic practice		*P* value
	2011 *N* = 364 (%)	2014 *N* = 293 (%)		2011 *N* = 253 (%)	2014 *N* = 206 (%)		2011 *N* = 105 (%)	2014 *N* = 87 (%)	
WHO warning signs									
Yes	285 (78.3)	250 (85.3)	**0.024**	N.A.	171 (83.4)	N.A.	N.A.	79 (91.9)	N.A.
D.N.P.	3 (0.8)	2 (0.7)			2 (1)			1 (1.1)	
Dengue Diagnostic Test (DDT)									
Always (100%)	107 (29.4)	164 (56.0)	**<0.001**	98 (38.7)	111 (53.9)	**0.001**	7 (6.7)	53 (60.9)	**<0.001**
Often (51–99%)	69 (19.0)	72 (24.5)	0.086	51 (20.2)	52 (25.2)	0.216	17 (16.2)	20 (23.0)	0.274
Sometimes (1–50%)	105 (28.8)	40 (13.7)	**<0.001**	61 (24.1)	26 (12.6)	**0.002**	41 (39)	14 (16.1)	**<0.001**
Never (0%)	82 (22.5)	17 (5.8)	**<0.001**	43 (17.0)	17 (8.3)	**0.008**	39 (37.1)	0	**<0.001**
D.N.P.	1 (0.3)	0		0	0		1 (1)	0	
Dengue Diagnostic Test (DDT)									
> 50% of the time	176 (48.4)	236 (80.5)	**<0.001**	149 (58.9)	163 (79.1)	**<0.001**	24 (22.9)	73 (83.9)	**<0.001**
D.N.P.	1 (0.3)	0		0	0		1 (1)	0	
Most Frequently Used DDT Among Those Who Reported Usage of DDT									
Dengue serology (IgM/IgG)	211 (74.8)	91 (33)	**<0.001**	144 (68.6)	59 (31.2)	**<0.001**	62 (93.9)	32 (36.8)	**<0.001**
Dengue non-structural antigen 1 (NS1) assay	31 (11)	62 (22.5)	**<0.001**	29 (13.8)	47 (24.9)	**0.003**	1 (1.5)	15 (17.2)	**0.002**
Dengue RT-PCR	37 (13.1)	9 (3.3)	**<0.001**	36 (17.1)	7 (3.7)	**<0.001**	1 (1.5)	2 (2.3)	>0.999
Dengue duo POCT kit	0 (0.0)	104 (37.7)	**<0.001**	0	67 (35.4)	**<0.001**	0	37 (42.5)	**<0.001**
D.N.P.	3 (1.1)	10 (3.5)		1 (0.5)	9 (4.8)		2 (3)	1 (1.2)	

D.N.P. Data not provided by participants, *RT-PCR* Reverse-transcription polymerase chain reaction, *N.A.* Not available
P value in bold represents a statistical significant difference

practice and qualifications), only Dengue duo POCT kits was found to be independently associated with frequent use of DDTs (adjusted odds ratio = 2.15, 95% confidence interval = 1.25–3.69) (Table 3).

Clinical care and practices for dengue

Compared with survey year 2011, significantly smaller proportion of PCPs referred more than 50% of their dengue patients to hospital in survey year 2014 (N = 114, 31.4% in 2011 vs. N = 39, 13.3% in 2014; $p < 0.001$; Table 4). About 45.4% of the PCPs set the platelet count of ≤80,000/mm^3 as cut off point for referral to hospital, although a significant increase was also seen in proportion of PCPs who uses the platelet count of ≤50,000/mm^3 (N = 83, 22.8% in 2011 vs N = 115, 39.2% in 2014; $p < 0.001$). Moreover, there was a significant increase in proportion of PCPs who reviewed dengue patients on average 5–6 times as part of the dengue management in survey year 2014 (N = 83, 28.3%) as compared to survey year 2011 (N = 66, 18.1%; $p = 0.003$). This trend is similar among private and public PCPs. About 57–59% of the PCPs monitored the fluid intake/urine output more than 50% of their time during patient management in both survey years. Within the public polyclinics, there was a significant increase in proportion of PCPs in survey year 2014 (N = 59, 67.8%) who monitored the fluid intake/urine output more than 50% of their time during patient management compared to survey year 2011 (N = 61, 58.1%; $p < 0.001$). There was not much difference in the proportion of PCPs who performed postural blood pressure monitoring more than 50% of their time during patient management in general. However, there was a significant increase (N = 61, 58.1% in 2011 vs N = 59, 67.8% in 2014; $p < 0.001$) in proportion of PCPs who performed postural blood pressure monitoring more than 50% of their time during patient management in the public PCPs, but a significant reduction among private PCPs (N = 126, 49.8% in 2011 vs N = 82, 39.8% in 2014; $p = 0.038$; Table 4).

Table 3 Factors associated with 'always' versus 'often/sometimes' behaviour of using Dengue diagnostic test in survey year 2014[a]

Variables in equation	Adjusted Odds Ratio (95% confidence interval)	*P* value
Type of Dengue diagnostic test		
Other tests	Referent	
Dengue duo POCT kit	**2.15 (1.25–3.69)**	**0.01**
Gender		
Male	Referent	
Female	1.16 (0.69–1.96)	0.57
Age		
21–40 years	Referent	
41–60 years	0.71 (0.38–1.32)	0.27
61 years or above	0.72 (0.24–2.14)	0.56
Place of practice		
Private	Referent	
Polyclinic	0.79 (0.42–1.46)	0.45
Qualifications		
M.B.,B.S. (or equivalent)	Referent	
GDFM	1.05 (0.56–1.95)	0.88
M.Med (Fam. Med.)	1.08 (0.56–2.10)	0.81
MRCP	2.81 (0.30–26.62)	0.37

P values calculated by binary logistic regression. *P* value in bold represents a statistical significant association

GDFM Graduate Diploma in Family Medicine, *M.Med (Fam. Med.)* Master in Medicine (Family Medicine), *MRCP* Membership of Royal College of Physicians

[a]2014 study only

Knowledge, attitude and experience toward POCT kits

About 68.9% (N = 202) of the PCPs in survey year 2014 heard about POCT, and 88.1% (N = 258) of the PCPs were interested to know more about POCT (Table 5). The top three preferred methods of gaining more information was through postal information (N = 76, 31.5%), website with video (N = 70, 29%) and through email and written documentation (N = 68, 28.2%).

Only 41 (20.3%) out of 202 PCPs who have heard about POCT had personally experienced using POCT (Table 6), even though 104 PCPs (Table 2) had reported using POCT as their preferred method for diagnosis of dengue. The top three perceived benefits in using POCT in their clinic were saving patient's waiting time (N = 203, 84.2%), helping case management (N = 195, 80.9%) and more accurate diagnosis (N = 137, 56.8). In addition, the top three perceived challenges in using POCT in their clinic were "not cost-effective" (N = 61, 25.3%), "existing heavy workload" (N = 41, 17%) and "no time for training" (N = 32, 13.3%).

The attitude and perception of PCPs were sought in a qualitatively method on their current usage and implementation of POCT in the clinic using open ended questions. Based on the responses received among those PCPs who are currently using POCT, the common reasons for usage included "the availability of Dengue duo POCT kit in their clinic" and "it is a standard test in their clinic" (Table 7). Other advantages that were highlighted were "the flexibility to diagnose in both early and late phase of fever", "easy to use" and "having accurate result". In general, they felt that POCT is useful and two of the PCPs who responded also highlighted that "patients really appreciate a quick diagnosis". However, there was also some PCPs who expressed concerns, despite the current usage of POCT. They expressed concern about the cost and accuracy in using POCT as well as the fact that laboratory tests are likely more accurate than POCT kit.

Among PCPs who have not used POCT in the clinic, they had the perception that POCT has "very little improvement

Table 4 Dengue clinical management practices among primary care physicians

	Overall		P value	Private practice		P value	Polyclinic practice		P value
	2011 N = 364 (%)	2014 N = 293 (%)		2011 N = 253 (%)	2014 N = 206 (%)		2011 N = 105 (%)	2014 N = 87 (%)	
Referral to hospital									
> 50%	114 (31.4)	39 (13.3)	**<0.001**	99 (39.1)	36 (17.5)	**<0.001**	14 (13.3)	3 (3.4)	**0.020**
D.N.P.	1 (0.3)	0		1 (0.4)	0		0	0	
Usage of platelet count									
≤ 100,000/mm3	88 (24.2)	30 (10.2)	**<0.001**	79 (31.2)	29 (14.1)	**<0.001**	8 (7.6)	1 (1.1)	**0.042**
≤ 80,000/mm3	190 (52.2)	133 (45.4)	0.085	117 (46.2)	101 (49.0)	0.574	70 (66.7)	32 (36.8)	**<0.001**
≤ 50,000/mm3	83 (22.8)	115 (39.2)	**<0.001**	54 (21.3)	66 (32.0)	**0.010**	27 (25.7)	49 (56.3)	**<0.001**
Platelet count is not an indicator	3 (0.8)	15 (5.1)	**0.001**	3 (1.2)	10 (4.9)	0.230	0 (0.0)	5 (5.7)	**0.018**
Average number of clinical review per patient									
1–2	64 (17.6)	29 (9.9)	**0.005**	49 (19.4)	20 (9.7)	**0.004**	14 (13.3)	9 (10.3)	0.656
3–4	217 (59.6)	171 (58.4)	0.688	140 (55.3)	118 (57.3)	0.775	74 (70.5)	53 (61)	0.172
5–6	66 (18.1)	83 (28.3)	**0.003**	48 (19)	59 (28.6)	**0.020**	16 (15.2)	24 (27.6)	**0.049**
> 6	12 (3.3)	8 (2.7)	0.820	11 (4.3)	7 (3.4)	0.637	1 (1)	1 (1.1)	1.000
D.N.P.	5 (1.4)	2 (0.7)		5 (2)	2 (1)		0	0	
Fluid Intake/Urine Output Test									
> 50% of the time	208 (57.1)	172 (58.7)	0.751	142 (56.1)	113 (54.9)	0.777	61 (58.1)	59 (67.8)	**<0.001**
D.N.P.	1 (0.3)	0		0	0		1 (1)	0	
Use of postural blood pressure									
> 50% of the time	179 (49.2)	121 (41.3)	**0.049**	126 (49.8)	82 (39.8)	**0.038**	61 (58.1)	59 (67.8)	**<0.001**

D.N.P. Data not provided by participants, *RT-PCR* reverse-transcription polymerase chain reaction, *NA* not applicable
P value in bold represents a statistical significant difference

Table 5 Knowledge on point of care rapid Dengue test based on survey performed in year 2014 (*N* = 293)

	N (%)
Heard about point of care rapid Dengue test	
Yes	202 (68.9)
No, Not sure	89 (30.4)
D.N.P.	2 (0.7)
Wish to know more about point of care rapid Dengue test	
Yes	258 (88.1)
No	31 (10.6)
D.N.P.	4 (1.3)
Preferred mode of information[a]	
Postal written information	76 (31.5)
Website with video	70 (29.0)
Email and written demonstration	68 (28.2)
Seminar through demo	41 (17.0)
Public posters	8 (3.3)
Other	4 (1.7)

D.N.P. Data not provided by participants
[a]Multiple answered allowed

in patients' management", and the current overwhelming workload of their staffs actually deterred them from using (Additional file 4: Table S1). A major concern for private PCPs was the cost of expired kits. For instance, expired kits will be a loss for their business if there are not enough suspected dengue patients for testing. The lack of an official test report for their patients' assurance is also one of the reason of not using POCT. Moreover, it was highlighted that the Environmental Health Institute in Singapore provides free laboratory dengue testing for interested PCPs who are keen to participate in their dengue surveillance program so there is no urgency in trying out these POCTs. Despite these concerns, some PCPs anticipated improvements in efficiency of patient diagnosis after implementing POCT, so they were keen to use POCT in the near future.

Perception of surge management during dengue largest spike in 2013

There were two final open-ended questions that focused on the experience of PCPs during the largest dengue spike in 2013 (Additional file 4: Table S2) as well as the changes in disease management since the outbreaks in 2005 and 2007 (Additional file 4: Table S3). In general, physicians claimed to be more vigilant, ordered full blood count and dengue diagnosis tests for suspected patients more

Table 6 Usage on point of care rapid dengue test

	N (%)
Usage of point of care rapid dengue test in clinic among PCPs who knows about it (*N* = 202)	
Yes	41 (20.3)
No	157 (77.7)
D.N.P.	4 (2)
Duration of using point of care rapid dengue test (*N* = 41)	
< 1 month	4 (9.8)
1–3 months	3 (7.2)
> 3 months	30 (73.2)
D.N.P.	4 (9.8)
Benefits perceived by PCPs in using POCT in their clinic[a]	
Saves waiting time	203 (84.2)
Helps case management	195 (80.9)
More accurate diagnosis	137 (56.8)
Minimum usage of resources	91 (37.8)
Manage surge in Dengue	87 (36.1)
Don't know about it	44 (18.3)
Others (benefits)	8 (3.3)
Challenges perceived by PCPs in using POCT in their clinic[a]	
Not cost effective	61 (25.3)
Too much workload	41 (17.0)
Too much time for training	32 (13.3)
Not accurate	27 (11.2)
No challenges	26 (10.)
No comment	1 (0.4)
Others (Challenges)	49 (20.3)

D.N.P. Data not provided by participants
[a]Multiple answered allowed

frequently than before. Although there was a dengue spike in 2013, 38 of the PCPs reflected that the situation was still manageable in their clinics. For confirmed cases, they did close monitoring on full blood count and other symptoms more frequently. They also played a more active role in educating patients on dengue warning signs and the importance of vector control (Additional file 4: Table S2).

There were 187 PCPs who had practiced during the earlier smaller dengue spikes in 2004 and 2007. The majority of them felt that case management has since improved. Majority attributed to the availability of better dengue diagnosis tests, as well as better awareness of the disease among the community and doctors. Moreover, clearer clinical guidelines were also made more available and accessible to PCPs since then. The PCPs also highlighted that doctors were more confident in managing dengue patients as outpatients and so fewer patients were referred to hospital (Additional file 4: Table S3).

Discussion

Primary care physicians (PCPs) play very important role in early diagnosis and notification of dengue cases to reduce dengue transmission and burden [1]. The right knowledge, attitude and practices on dengue management among PCPs are critical for dengue control and public education [16, 17]. Since 2011, there have been advances in providing better dengue management for suspected dengue patients in Singapore. Gan et al. in 2014 reported the high performance of point-of-care diagnostic Dengue duo test in detecting dengue infection in a clinic setting in Singapore [15]. Leo et al. in 2013 reported the validation of the new World Health Organization guideline in Singapore. The study reported that dengue patients without any of the seven warning signs as stated in the guideline may be managed as outpatients, while referral of patients who presented with any of these warning signs may lead to over-hospitalization [19].

Over the years between year 2011 and 2014, the proportion of PCPs who always diagnosed dengue using diagnostic test had increased by about two folds, and those who never used diagnostic test to confirm dengue fell by about three folds (Table 3). Compared to private PCPs, all of PCPs from polyclinics had higher preference to perform diagnostic test for patients with suspected dengue in 2014. Although Dengue duo POCT kit was only introduced in 2013, more than one third of PCPs had preference to use the POCT kit based on the survey in 2014. On further assessment, Dengue duo POCT test was independently associated with frequent use of diagnostic test after adjusting for age, gender, level of professional qualification and place of practice. This highlights the impact of POCT in increasing the usage of diagnostic test in primary healthcare setting to confirm dengue for early management of dengue cases as well as for dengue control via notification to Ministry of Health.

The PCPs emphasized that availability of the POCT kit at the place of practice, accuracy of the test, rapidness of results and cost-effectiveness favored its use. The PCPs' preference to receive more information on diagnostic tests was through postal mails or website with video demonstration on its usage. They were also concerns over the use of this new POCT kit. These concerns were the lack of quality control and increased workload in the clinic, which were also highlighted in another study by Pai et al. in 2012 [20]. Our findings suggested that further development of more accurate and user-friendly test kits, as well as having highly accessible training platforms for front line care providers are likely to increase the use of dengue diagnostic test in both public and private primary healthcare settings to enhance patient management.

After the large dengue epidemic, most PCPs felt that dengue case management had improved. This was likely due to the availability of better dengue diagnostic tests, greater awareness of the disease and clearer clinical

Table 7 Positive and negative experiences among PCPs who are using or have used POCT before

Themes	Frequency	Quotes
Positive		
Can be used to diagnose in both early and late phase of fever	36	*"NS1 can detect Dengue before D5 fever. IgM/IgG for fever > D5."*
Available	21	*"Available in our clinic."* *"This is usually what's available at our lab."*
Good/Useful	16	*"Best thing since sliced bread"* *"Useful as a good screening tool when Dengue fever is suspected"*
Free	15	*"Free test via EHI diagnosis"*
Standard test	14	*"Standard protocol."* *"Standard test at commercial lab used."*
Rapid result	10	*"I love using it. Gives rapid diagnosis on Dengue fever suspect"*
Accurate result	5	*"Dengue duo- quite happy with it so far accurate."*
Easy to use	5	*"Using it seems simple enough."*
Diagnosis in early phase of fever	2	*"Very useful for early identification of cases so patients are more likely to agree to do daily blood for monitoring."*
Patient's positive opinion	2	*"Patients really appreciate a quick diagnosis."*
Cost-effective	1	*"I find it useful, fast selective and cost effective."*
Negative		
Concern about cost	9	*"Given free so used it for trial otherwise expensive"*
Concern about accuracy	7	*"After doing 3 cases on suspected Dengue- had 2 false negative- not found!"*
Troublesome to use	2	*"Cumbersome / troublesome to use."*
Trust	2	*"I only use it at night or Sunday... Still trust the lab test for Dengue more than portable kit."*
Other test also used	2	*"Has to supplemented by FBC sent to the lab to have haematocrit/platelet."*
Not had occasion to use it much	2	*"[used] very little [so] not enough suspected cases seen."*
Only used when instructed to	1	*"Have used it during referral to a study in our clinic. But now stopped."*
Lack of official evaluation of it's efficacy	1	*"Lack of official reports."*
Patient's negative opinion	1	*"Patients are still new to the idea of a rapid test kit."*

guidelines. Compared to the 2011 survey, the survey in 2014 showed PCPs referred patients to hospital with a lower platelet cut-off of ≤50,000/mm^3, which is clinically more relevant for close monitoring. Similar platelet cut-off was also reported by Thaver et al. in 2011 amongst the Pakistanis PCPs [21]. We also found that our Singapore PCPs became more confident, and committed to managing the dengue patients as outpatients, with closer monitoring, where possible. This was reflected in the significant reduction in patient referrals to hospital and the increased number of clinical reviews at the primary healthcare setting.

Carrasco et al. in 2011 highlighted that managing dengue cases in hospital incurred 10 times more cost than ambulatory care in Singapore ($600 vs. $60 per day, respectively) [22]. Lee et al. also reported in 2013 that after the implementation of the new admission criteria including dengue outcome calculator which utilizes simple and readily available clinical information, the proportion of dengue cases who were being managed as inpatients fell from 91.9% in 2006 to 53.9% in 2008 with saving of US$ 1.4 million in year 2008 [23]. Similar cost savings to both patients and the government is likely possible with a significant reduction in dengue referrals to hospital with the increasing usage of POCT based on the findings in this study.

We were limited by the fact that there were significant differences in gender, age groups and the highest qualifications attained among the PCPs surveyed in 2011 and 2014. As such, we cannot completely exclude the impact of these demographic differences. However, regardless of the demographic differences, the knowledge level on clinical management remained high, suggesting that the impact on PCPs' attitude and practices of dengue diagnosis should be relatively small. We were also limited by the survey method in collecting more explorative qualitative data. However, open-ended survey questions provided additional in depth information about physicians attitudes and experiences on dengue clinical management and diagnosis. The case management data that was collected was based on three case management scenarios (Additional file 3) with the aim to understand common practices amongst primary care physicians. These data will not be able to capture the optimal case management of a suspected dengue case but only the current preferred case management of a suspected dengue case. In fact, Dengue has many overlapping features with other febrile illnesses. It would be ideal to apply simple, cheap and easy to use diagnostic test at primary care sites for optimal case management. In addition, this study involved only PCPs who were practicing during the 2013 epidemic due to their valid practicing licenses and clinic addresses. As such, this study is not able to conclude if PCPs who were not practicing during 2013 epidemic had the same awareness as those PCPs who were practicing. Last but not least, the low response rate may not provide a complete understanding of the changes in KAP on dengue management after a large dengue epidemic. However, a comparison on the demographics of PCPs between this study and another national study published in 2014 [24], the proportion of PCPs surveyed reflects the general PCPs reasonably well, although there are more older PCPs than younger PCPs (<45 years old) in both 2011 and 2014 surveys (Table 1).

Conclusions

After the largest dengue outbreak in 2013, knowledge on clinical management of dengue remain high, but not higher between year 2011 and 2014. However, there were significant improvements in the diagnosis of dengue, particularly on the importance of using a diagnostic kit such as the dengue Duo POCT kit. There were also significant increase in awareness and practices of the best practices of dengue clinical management between 2011 and 2014. In order to improve acceptance & usage of the POCT kit to facilitate early diagnosis of dengue, it may be worth emphasizing the importance of continuous medical education via web-based video trainings and postal information, the sharing of formal evaluations of the diagnostic tests in local settings through seminars or dialogue sessions, as well as the support of the local government in providing subsidy for the usage of POCT kit in the primary healthcare settings.

Additional files

Additional file 1: Survey on knowledge, attitudes, practice related to dengue management amongst primary care physicians. This provides the questions that were used to assess the KAP of the primary care physicians.

Additional file 2: The awareness of the dengue warning signs among primary care physicians. Data on dengue warning signs recommended by the World Health Organization that the participants are aware of.

Additional file 3: The clinical scenarios used to assess the level of clinical management. Data on the three clinical scenarios surveyed to assess the level of clinical management.

Additional file 4: Perceptions of PCPs on POCT and clinical management experience during 2013 outbreak. Data on the perceptions of PCPs who do not have any experience on POCT and the management experience and changes during and after the 2013 outbreak.

Abbreviations

DDTs: Dengue diagnostic tests; DF: Dengue fever; DHF: Dengue haemorrhagic fever; DSS: Dengue shock syndrome; KAP: Knowledge, attitude and practices; PCPs: Primary care physicians; POCT: Point-of-care-test

Acknowledgements

Authors thank Dr. Wong Chia Siong and colleagues from College of Family Physicians for assistance in pre-testing of survey questions, all participants for completing the survey, Diana Tan and Chai Siaw Ching for providing administrative assistance, Nadiah for data entry and Adriana Tan for data management.

Funding

This study was supported by STOP Dengue Translational Clinical Research programme, funded by the National Research Foundation through the National Medical Research Council, Singapore (Grant number NMRC/TCR/005/2008) as well as the National University of Singapore Start-up grant. The funders had no role in study design, data collection and analysis, decision to publish, or preparation of the manuscript.

Authors' contributions

ZJLH and YSL conceived the project and designed the study. TLT and JJ designed the questionnaire and collected the data. JP and TLT analyzed the data and wrote the manuscript. JP, ZJLH and YSL supported the manuscript editing. All authors read and approved the final manuscript.

Competing interests

The authors declare that they have no competing interests

Consent for publication

Not applicable

Author details

[1]Institute of Infectious Diseases and Epidemiology, Tan Tock Seng Hospital, 144 Moulmein Road, Singapore 308089, Singapore. [2]Saw Swee Hock School of Public Health, National University of Singapore, Singapore, Singapore. [3]Johns Hopkins Center for Communication Programs, Johns Hopkins University, Baltimore, USA. [4]Department of Global Health and Development, Faculty of Public Health & Policy, London School of Hygiene and Tropical Medicine, London, UK. [5]Yong Loo Lin School of Medicine, National University of Singapore, Singapore, Singapore. [6]Lee Kong Chian School of Medicine, Nanyang Technological University, Singapore, Singapore.

References

1. WHO: Dengue: Guidelines for Diagnosis, Treatment, Prevention and Control. World Health Organization 2009.
2. Gubler DJ. Dengue and dengue hemorrhagic fever. Clin Microbiol Rev. 1998;11(3):480–96.
3. Chew A, Leng GA, Yuen H, Teik KO, Kiat LY, Hong LC, et al. A haemorrhagic fever in Singapore. Lancet. 1961;1(7172):307–10.
4. Hii YL, Rocklov J, Ng N, Tang CS, Pang FY, Sauerborn R. Climate variability and increase in intensity and magnitude of dengue incidence in Singapore. Glob Health Action. 2009;2
5. Ler TS, Ang LW, Yap GS, Ng LC, Tai JC, James L, et al. Epidemiological characteristics of the 2005 and 2007 dengue epidemics in Singapore - similarities and distinctions. Western Pac Surveill Response J. 2011;2(2):24–9.
6. Hapuarachchi HC, Koo C, Rajarethinam J, Chong CS, Lin C, Yap G, et al. Epidemic resurgence of dengue fever in Singapore in 2013-2014: a virological and entomological perspective. BMC Infect Dis. 2016;16:300.

7. Ooi EE, Goh KT, Gubler DJ. Dengue prevention and 35 years of vector control in Singapore. Emerg Infect Dis. 2006;12(6):887–93.
8. WHO: Dengue haemorrhagic fever: diagnosis, treatment, prevention and control. 2nd edition. Geneva. In: World Health Organisation. 1997.
9. WHO: Dengue: Guidelines for Diagnosis, Treatment, Prevention, and Control. New edn. Geneva. *World Health Organisation* 2009.
10. Peeling RW, Artsob H, Pelegrino JL, Buchy P, Cardosa MJ, Devi S, et al. Evaluation of diagnostic tests: dengue. Nat Rev Microbiol. 2010;8(12 Suppl):S30–8.
11. Wang SM, Sekaran SD. Early diagnosis of dengue infection using a commercial dengue duo rapid test kit for the detection of NS1, IGM, and IGG. Am J Trop Med Hyg. 2010;83(3):690–5.
12. Nga TT, Thai KT, Phuong HL, Giao PT, Hung le Q, Binh TQ, et al. Evaluation of two rapid immunochromatographic assays for diagnosis of dengue among Vietnamese febrile patients. Clin Vaccine Immunol. 2007;14(6):799–801.
13. Osorio L, Ramirez M, Bonelo A, Villar LA, Parra B. Comparison of the diagnostic accuracy of commercial NS1-based diagnostic tests for early dengue infection. Virol J. 2010;7:361.
14. Blacksell SD, Jarman RG, Bailey MS, Tanganuchitcharnchai A, Jenjaroen K, Gibbons RV, et al. Evaluation of six commercial point-of-care tests for diagnosis of acute dengue infections: the need for combining NS1 antigen and IgM/IgG antibody detection to achieve acceptable levels of accuracy. Clin Vaccine Immunol. 2011;18(12):2095–101.
15. Gan VC, Tan LK, Lye DC, Pok KY, Mok SQ, Chua RC, et al. Diagnosing dengue at the point-of-care: utility of a rapid combined diagnostic kit in Singapore. PLoS One. 2014;9(3):e90037.
16. Nguyen NM, Whitehorn JS, Luong Thi Hue T, Nguyen Thanh T, Mai Xuan T, Vo Xuan H, et al. Physicians, primary caregivers and topical repellent: all under-utilised resources in stopping dengue virus transmission in affected households. PLoS Negl Trop Dis. 2016;10(5):e0004667.
17. Ho TS, Huang MC, Wang SM, Hsu HC, Liu CC. Knowledge, attitude, and practice of dengue disease among healthcare professionals in southern Taiwan. J Formos Med Assoc. 2013;112(1):18–23.
18. Lee LK, Thein TL, Kurukularatne C, Gan V, Lye DC, Leo YS. Dengue knowledge, attitudes, and practices among primary care physicians in Singapore. Ann Acad Med Singap. 2011;40(12):533–8.
19. Leo YS, Gan VC, Ng EL, Hao Y, Ng LC, Pok KY, et al. Utility of warning signs in guiding admission and predicting severe disease in adult dengue. BMC Infect Dis. 2013;13:498.
20. Pai NP, Vadnais C, Denkinger C, Engel N, Pai M. Point-of-care testing for infectious diseases: diversity, complexity, and barriers in low- and middle-income countries. PLoS Med. 2012;9(9):e1001306.
21. Thaver AM, Sobani ZA, Qazi F, Khan M, Zafar A, Beg MA. Assessing the need for training: general practitioners' knowledge, attitude and practice concerning dengue and malaria in Karachi. Pakistan Int Health. 2011;3(2):126–30.
22. Carrasco LR, Lee LK, Lee VJ, Ooi EE, Shepard DS, Thein TL, et al. Economic impact of dengue illness and the cost-effectiveness of future vaccination programs in Singapore. PLoS Negl Trop Dis. 2011;5(12):e1426.
23. Lee LK, Earnest A, Carrasco LR, Thein TL, Gan VC, Lee VJ, et al. Safety and cost savings of reducing adult dengue hospitalization in a tertiary care hospital in Singapore. Trans R Soc Trop Med Hyg. 2013;107(1):37–42.
24. Tan NC, Aw L, Khin LW, Thirumoorthy T, Lim SH, Tai BC, et al. How do primary care physicians in Singapore keep healthy? Singap Med J. 2014; 55(3):155–9.

Series of 10 dengue fever cases with unusual presentations and complications in Sri Lanka: a single centre experience in 2016

S. A. M. Kularatne[1], Udaya Ralapanawa[1*], Chamara Dalugama[1], Jayanika Jayasinghe[1], Sawandika Rupasinghe[1] and Prabashini Kumarihamy[2]

Abstract

Background: Dengue has global importance as a dreaded arboviral infection. It has 4 serotypes of epidemiological imporatnce. The classification denotes two clinical spectrums- dengue fever (DF) and dengue haemorragic fever (DHF). Most cases are stereotype and amenable to fluid resuscitation. However, unusual manifestations cause fatalities and often overlooked. This study describes 10 such dengue cases to fill the knowledge gaps.

Case presentation: All 10 patients presented to the Teaching Hospital, Peradeniya, Sri Lanka during mid-year epidemic of dengue in 2016. The mean age is 27 years (range 12-51 years) comprising 6 females and 4 males. The group had 7 DHF, 3 DF and 2 primary dengue infections who predominantly had severe bleeding into gut. Other potentially life threatening problems were acute severe hepatitis, severe septic shock, myocarditis, erratic rapid plasma leak, intracranial bleeding, diarrhoea and decompenstaed dengue shock due to 3rd space fluid leak. Blood transfusions and other empirical therapeutic methods were used apart from meticulous fluid management to suit issues of each patient. Bedside ultrasound scanning helped early detection of critical phase. All recovered fully.

Conclusions: Dengue is an extremely challenging infection to treat in the globe today. Above unusual presentation and complications could be fatal, if not detected early where therapeutic window period is very short. Clinicians need awareness of these problems which are not uncommon, but underreported and often overlooked. The clinical management of each patient was described for the purpose sharing the experiences.

Keywords: Dengue, Expanded dengue syndrome, Fulminant liver failure, Myocarditis, Septic shock, Dengue shock syndrome, DHF, Sri Lanka

Background

Dengue is the most common arboviral infection in the Southeast Asia. Dengue virus has four related but antigenically distinct serotypes: DENV-1, DENV-2, DENV-3, and DENV-4 [1]. The global burden of dengue has increased in recent decades causing huge impact on both human health and the national economics [1–3] . Dengue infection has a diverse clinical presentation ranging from asymptomatic subclinical infection to severe multi-organ involvement [3]. Although, vascular plasma leak is the commonest manifestation, dengue can manifest in multitude of unusual presentations due to organ dysfunction that can carry high mortality [2, 3]. Early detection of such manifestations and prompt action could avert the adverse outcome where clinicians need knowledge and experience. Aim of this case series is to present 10 such unusual dengue cases managed in a single hospital over 1 year period. These patients presented to Teaching Hospital, Peradeniya (THP), Sri Lanka in

* Correspondence: udayapralapanawa@yahoo.com
[1]Department of Medicine, Faculty of Medicine, University of Peradeniya, Peradeniya, Sri Lanka
Full list of author information is available at the end of the article

2016 and recovered fully following problem based tailored management.

Case 1: (erratic rapid plasma leak during early critical phase)

A 22-year-old female admitted to THP with a one-day history of fever proceeded by frontal headache of 3 days. On admission, she had arthralgia, myalgia, mild postural dizziness and nausea. She has passed urine normal amount. She was hemodynamically stable with a blood pressure of 96/64 mmHg without a postural drop. Abdomen was soft and non-tender. Clinically, she did not have evidence of plasma leak. Her blood test was positive for dengue NS1 antigen. On 3rd day of fever, ultra sound scan of abdomen detected thin rim of free fluid in the hepato-renal pouch and moderate gall bladder wall oedema with mild pericholycystic fluid. She did not have pleural effusion or ascites. Neither she had postural drop of blood pressure, tachycardia or right hypochondrial tenderness. However, her haematocrit has risen from 33 to 38%. In a flash, within the next 6 h, she developed significant ascites (moderate) and bilateral moderate pleural effusions with a reduction of urine output. She had fluctuation of urine output and blood pressure and required several normal saline boluses and Dextran-40 along with frusemide to maintain vital parameters. Sixty percent of her calculated fluid quota was utilized in the 1st 12 h of tentative critical phase. Her clinical status gradually improved within the next 3 days. But, there was delayed resolution of effusion and ascites. Her serum albumin level dropped during the critical phase and took days reverse. Her recovery was uneventful and discharged on day 6 of the hospital stay. She had erratic rapid leaking of plasma into serous cavities during critical phase.

Case 2: (severe hepatitis with increased transaminases and gross ascites after critical phase)

A previously healthy 39-year-old female, admitted to the THP with a history of fever for 4 days. She had nausea, vomiting, arthralgia, myalgia and headache. She did not have any bleeding manifestations or abdominal pain. On examination, she had mild dehydration with low volume pulse. Blood pressure was 100/80 mmHg in supine position and 90/80 mmHg on standing. Right lung base was stony dull on percussion and had absent breath sounds. Ultrasound scan revealed a right sided plural effusion with free fluid in the abdomen. The patient was managed as critical phase of dengue haemorrhagic fever (DHF) with meticulous titration of fluids according to the haematocrit values. She remained hemodynamically stable with a stable haematocrit values during the critical phase. On day 7 of illness, dengue serology showed positive IgM and IgG titers. After completion of critical phase on 7th day of the illness, she complained of abdominal pain and back pain. Clinical examination found s mild icterus and tense ascites. Laboratory investigations revealed a marked rise in liver enzyme levels (ALT 204 to 1391 u/L and AST 505 to 4519 u/L) with an INR of 1.9. Diagnosis of acute hepatitis leading into acute liver failure was made and viral hepatitis was excluded by doing hepatitis A IgM, hepatitis B surface antigen and hepatitis C IgM which were negative. She denied self-medication with high doses of paracetamol. Further, she was treated with intravenous N acetyl cysteine 150 mg/hour infusion as an empirical treatment. Her low albumin level was corrected with intravenous human albumin administration. Antibiotics including oral metronidazole and intravenous ceftriaxone was administered at the same time to cover bacterial infections. She was given intravenous vitamin K for 3 days to prevent clotting factor depletion whilst monitoring liver transaminases and clotting parameters. Finally she was discharged on 12th day of the illness with near normal liver transaminases and normal clotting profile without residual free fluids in her abdomen. Further follow of after 21 days revealed completely normal liver biochemistry.

Case 3: (DEN 2, intracranial Haemorrhage in DHF)

A19- year-old male, previously healthy university student admitted to THP having a febrile illness with arthralgia and myalgia for 5 days duration. On the way to the hospital, the patient had postural dizziness and fainting attack causing impact on the forehead. Soon after admission, he developed a generalized tonic-clonic seizure which lasted for 5 min with post ictal drowsiness. On examination, he was not pale but had conjunctival hemorrhages. He had a contusion over the forehead due to fall. He was hemodynamically stable with a blood pressure of 126/90 mmHg and a pulse rate of 92 beats per minute without clinical evidence of plasma leaking. Ultrasound scan revealed a thin rim of free fluid in the abdomen. Dengue NS 1 antigen and Dengue Ig M and IgG both were positive. Serotype of dengue was identified as DEN 2. Diagnosis of DHF entering into critical phase was made and commenced intense monitoring with administration of intravenous and oral fluid according to guidelines, Meanwhile, the patient was found to be drowsy but arousable without having any lateralizing neurological deficits. Both optic fundi were normal. Non-contrast CT brain revealed bilateral frontal lobe hyperdense areas with mild cerebral oedema with minimal midline shift, suggestive of intra-cranial hemorrhages. His clotting parameters were within the normal limits. He was transfused with platelets to keep the platelet count more than 50×10^6/L and managed conservatively with adequate intravenous fluids, intravenous antibiotics and antiepileptic drugs. He was started on intravenous phenytoin sodium and later converted to oral phenytoin. Cerebral oedema was managed with intravenous dexamethasone and intravenous mannitol. He was administered with intravenous tranexamic acid to retard further bleeding. Critical phase was uneventful. His headache and drowsiness improved over the next 5 days and discharged with oral antiepileptics.

Case 4: (DEN 1 causing myocarditis and DHF together)
A-17-year-old previously healthy female presented to THP with a history of fever for 2 days associated with body aches and nausea. She didn't have any abdominal pain, bleeding manifestations or postural symptoms. On examination, she was flushed and febrile but was not pale or icteric. She was mildly dehydrated. Blood pressure was 100/70 mmHg, pulse rate 100 beats/min and capillary refilling time (CRFT) was less than 2 s. On abdominal examination, there was no free fluid. Lung fields were clear on respiratory system examination. Other systems examination was normal.

Her NS1 antigen was positive and serotype was identified as DEN1. She was managed as dengue fever with continuous monitoring. On the 3rd day of fever, she complained of retrosternal chest pain and undue tiredness. At that time her cardiovascular system examination was normal and electrocardiogram (ECG) showed acute T wave inversion in V2-V5 leads. Troponin I was negative and 2D echo showed global left ventricular hypokinesia and mild impairment of LV function. Ejection fraction was 40–45%. She was treated as having dengue fever complicated by myocarditis. Intravenous hydrocortisone 200 mg 8 hourly was administered for 2 days to reduce myocardial inflammation. On the 4rd day following admission, she complained of abdominal pain and ultrasound scanning revealed free fluid in hepato-renal pouch. Blood pressure was 100/70 mmHg, pulse rate 70 bpm, and CRFT was less than 2 s. She was taken to High Dependency Unit (HDU) and was managed as having DHF complicated with myocarditis with continuous monitoring and with careful administration of fluid to avoid fluid overload. She was discharged on day 7 of illness after recovering from critical phase of dengue fever. She was advised on limiting physical activities. During the follow up on day 14 of the illness, ECG showed reversal of T inversions. Echocardiogram showed improvement of left ventricular function with an ejection fraction of 55%.

Case 5: (acute GI bleeding and hepatitis in DF)
A-22-year old previously healthy male admitted to THP with a history of on and off fever for 10 days associated with 3 bouts of hematemesis and melaena. On examination, his pulse rate was 88 beats/m, blood pressure was 90/60 mmHg and CRFT was less than 2 s and lungs were normal. Abdomen was soft and there was no detectable free fluid. Rest of the examination was unremakable. Serology for dengue IgM and IgG were positive on admission. His liver enzymes were high on admission (AST 840 U/L and ALT 560 U/L) with a high INR value of 2.1. His complete blood count showed 11.5 g/dl of haemoglobin and platelet count of 144×10^9/l. Ultrasound examination of abdomen did not show any evidence of leaking thus, DHF was excluded. Hence, the patient was managed as in primary dengue fever with bleeding manifestations. Intravenous fluids were given along with tranexamic acid and vitamin K to reduce bleeding. Intravenous infusion of omeprazole was continued for 24 h and converted to twice day intravenous boluses. He was started in intravenous N acetyl cysteine infusion as liver transaminases were high. His symptoms resolved within the next few days, with symptomatic management.

Case 6: (DEN 2 primary infection and bleeding into GIT and GUT)
A-12-year old previously well female child was transferred to THP from a private hospital due to fever for 5 days associated with melena, haematemesis and haematuria with passage of blood clots. She did not have abdominal pain or any other warning signs of dengue on admission.

On examination, she was ill looking, adequately hydrated and GCS was 15/15. Blood pressure was 125/75 mmHg, pulse rate was 90 beats per minute and capillary refilling time was less than 2 s. On respiratory examination lungs were clear and on abdominal examination the abdomen was soft and non tender. Rest of the clinical examination was normal. Both NS1 and IgM were positive and dengue PCR revealed serotype of DEN 2. Ultrasound examination of abdomen did not show any evidence of plasma leaking. She was managed as having primary dengue fever with bleeding manifestations. Her liver enzymes were only mildly elevated (AST 87 u/L and ALT 56 u/L) with a normal clotting profile. Complete blood count revealed hemoglobin of 7 g/dl and platelet count of $17 \times 10^9/\mu L$. Due to low haemoglobin, she was transfused with 1 pint of blood and 4 units of platelets. Her symptoms resolved within the next few days.

Case 7: (DEN 2, severe diarrhoea, DHF, profound shock, sepsis and occult bleeding, need of massive transfusion)
A 14-year-old boy presented to THP with a history of fever for 2 days along with headache, arthralgia and myalgia. He did not complain of abdominal pain and did not have bleeding manifestations or any other warning symptoms. On examination, blood pressure was 110/70 mmHg and pulse rate was 100 beat per minute and capillary refilling time was less than 2 s. The abdomen was

soft and non-tender and there was no free fluid. Lung fields were clear on respiratory system examination. Rest of the examination was normal. His NS-1 was positive and the PCR appeared as DEN 2 serotype. The patient was managed as having dengue fever. He continued to have fever spikes for 4 days following admission. On the 5th day following admission, he developed postural dizziness, vomiting and heavy diarrhoea. On examination, he was febrile, dehydrated, flushed and had warm peripheries. Blood pressure was 90/60 mmHg, pulse rate was 130 beats per minute and a capillary refilling time of 2 s. Ultrasound examination of abdomen revealed free fluid in the hepato-renal pouch with increased gall bladder wall thickness. He was clinically diagnosed as having DHF complicated with septic shock and gastroenteritis. He was taken to HDU and critical phase monitoring commenced. His c-reactive protein was high 112 mg/dl. Broad-spectrum intravenous antibiotics (ceftriaxone and metronidazole) were started cover the sepsis after taking blood and urine cultures. Within about 1 h, the patient deteriorated significantly and continued to have vomiting and diarrhoea. Blood pressure dropped to 60/30 mmHg and the pulse rate increased to 120 beats/min. Several fluid boluses were given including normal saline and IV Dextran 40. The haematocrit value dropped from 36 to 30 and patient went into decompensated shock with no urine output. He needed continuous transfusion of whole blood amounting to 9 pints over 20 h to maintain blood pressure and urine output. However, there were no obvious bleeding sites. Further, intravenous noradrenaline infusion supported the blood pressure. Gradually patient improved with fluid, blood, antibiotics and vasopressors. He was given intravenous antibiotics for total of 7 days. Vasopressor was gradually weaned off. He was plethoric during convalescence due to over transfusion and was discharged on day 8 of admission.

Case 8 (presenting as dysentery and in compensated shock in DHF)

A previously well 36-year-old Buddhist monk presented to THP with a history of a febrile illness with generalized malaise for 4 days duration. His main complaint was vomiting and diarrhea of same duration. He did not have any postural symptoms, bleeding manifestations or abdominal pain at presentation. On examination, he was febrile and was not pale or icteric. Blood pressure was 120/100 mmHg with a pulse rate of 110 beats per minute and capillary refilling time of 2 s. On respiratory system examination, there was bilateral plural effusion and on examination of the abdomen there was shifting dullness. Other systems examination was normal. Ultrasound examination of abdomen revealed moderate amount of free fluid in the abdomen. Blood and urine were taken for investigations. His NS 1 antigen was positive, and serotype was identified as DEN 2. The patient was immediately taken to HDU and was managed as compensated shock of dengue hemorrhagic fever. Initial investigations revealed a platelet count of 15×10^9/l, and haematocrit of 57%. With meticulous fluid management he recovered. Thus, this patient had clinical picture of dysentery associated with DHF presenting at the peak of critical phase.

Case 9: (occult leaking of plasma leading to undetected decompensated shock)

A 51-one-year-old previously healthy female admitted with a history a febrile illness with arthralgia and myalgia for 4 days. Her NS1 antigen was positive on admission. She was ill and complained of postural dizziness and abdominal pain. On examination, she was ill looking, dehydrated and had bluish cold peripheries. She had central cyanosis and collapsed superficial veins. Her supine blood pressure was recorded as 90/80 mmHg and standing blood pressure was unable to measure due to severe postural symptoms. Capillary refilling time was prolonged, and her respiratory rate was 24 breaths per minute. Lungs were clear and clinically there was no evidence of free fluid in abdomen and pleura. She did not pass urine for 12 h. She was clinically diagnosed to have dengue haemorrhagic fever with decompensated shock. Then she was admitted to the HDU and critical phase management was started. Ultrasound scan of the abdomen did not show free fluid in peritoneal cavity despite patient was possibly in the peak of plasma leaking. However, 12 h after admission, repeat ultrasound scan showed thin rim of free fluid in the hepatorenal pouch. She was resuscitated with boluses of crystalloids and colloids., She became hemodynamically stable gradually and took about 8 h to gain warm peripheries. Fluid management and monitoring was continued, and her symptoms improved within the next 2 days. Although she went in to decompensated shock due to DHF, she had minimum detectable amount free fluid in the abdomen in the later phase of leaking.

Case 10: (DF complicating severe septic shock)

A 34-year-old female presented with a febrile illness with arthralgia and myalgia for 2 days duration. Her Dengue NS1 was positive. Her hemodynamic parameters were stable on admission. She was having continuous fever on day 6 of illness. There was no evidence of hemoconcentration or plasma leak and managed as uncomplicated dengue fever. She was kept on intravenous saline infusion at a slower rate. On 6th day of fever she developed cough and shortness of breath. Auscultation of lungs heard crepitations in bases. Over next 6 h she was not improving despite continuous infusion of normal saline and commencing antibiotics. Later, she became agitated and restless and was confused. She had warm peripheries despite blood pressure of 80/40 mmHg which further dropped to 60/30 mmHg. She had pulse rate of 108 beats/ min. There were widespread coarse crackles in the both lung fields involving all 3 zones. Her oxygen saturation dropped to 85% on room air. Her haematocrit remained within normal range. To counter the shock, she was given more intravenous normal saline, Dextran 40 and 2 units of blood transfusion. Then, she developed pulmonary oedema and required CPAP in the intensive care unit with high flow oxygen and intravenous frusemide. Patient was treated with intravenous meropenum 1 g 8 hourly and metronidazole. She had very high CRP and procalcitonin levels suggestive of severe sepsis. After 6 h of resuscitation her blood pressure got stabilized and she recovered completely over next 5 days. She was diagnosed as dengue fever complicated by septic shock probably originating from lungs even though, dengue shock syndrome (DSS) was contemplated at the outset.

Discussion and conclusion

Our case series compiles summaries of 10 confirmed dengue cases with wide array of unusual manifestation which are potentially fatal, in a single centre (THP) in the central hills of Sri Lanka. All these patients presented during mid-year outbreak of dengue in 2016 when serotype transition occurring from DEN 1 to DEN 2 that finally led to a massive outbreak of DEN 2 in 2017 in Sri Lanka. In these cases, females (n,6) out number males (n,4) and 7 patient had DHF. Out of 3 patients who had DF, 2 developed severe GI bleeding while other one developed severe septic shock that was mistaken for dengue shock syndrome (DSS) initially. Other unusual manifestations highlighted are hepatic dysfunction, myocarditis, erratic plama leak, ICH, occult blood loss, decompensated shock etc. Early detection of these manifestation and taking appropriate clinical decisions such as blood transfusions, antibiotics, and other empirical treatments saved all lives.

Most such manifestations of dengue infection are underreported, under recognized or not casually linked to dengue fever. Therefore, vigilance and anticipation are needed in managing dengue beyond the most common stable type of plasma leak in DHF.

Common life threatening complications related to DF and DHF include hepatic dysfunction leading to acute fulminant hepatic failure [3], musculoskeletal complications such as myositis and rhabdomyolysis [4], acute renal failure [5], cardiac complications such as myocarditis [6], life threatening bleeding such as gastrointestinal and intracranial bleeding [7], endocrine complications such as precipitating diabetic ketoacidosis [8] and neurological complications such as Guillain Barre syndrome and encephalopathy [9]. Early identification and early approach for appropriate management strategies are important to reduce morbidity and mortality of such cases. Better understanding of the disease dynamics has improved the outcome over time but still timely diagnosis and management is a challenge.

This case series comprises primary dengue infection, dengue fever (DF) and dengue hemorrhagic fever (DHF) all associated with unusual manifestaions. Importantly some life-threatening complications were observed in both primary dengue infection and DF without leaking. Patients in cases 1,2,3,4,7,8 and 9 developed DHF whereas patients in cases 5, 6 and 10 had DF. Some presented with bleeding manifestations while the others developed complications mentioned above.

Dengue can present with a diverse clinical spectrum ranging from asymptomatic infection or simple undifferentiated fever to DHF with multiorgan failure. Pathological hallmark of dengue hemorrhagic fever is increased capillary permeability with extravasation of fluids during the critical phase of dengue fever [3, 10]. The onset of critical phase is determined by clinically or radiologically demonstrable pleura effusion or ascites and/or evidence of hemoconcentration as shown by increased haematocrit in serial measurements [3, 11]. The critical phase lasts for a period of 24–48 h in which rate of plasma leak gradually peaks and comes down to the baseline. But this typical pattern is not appreciated all the time. Case 1 describes a young erratic leaker. His plasma leak peaked within 1st 12 h of critical phase evidenced by rapidly rising haematocrit and rapidly developing pleural effusions and ascites necessitating use of more than 60% of fluid quota within first 12 h. This type erratic leaker needs to be identified early with frequent monitoring of clinical parameters and haematocrit and fluid need to be titrated accordingly. The same patient had obvious fluid leak into peritoneal cavity and pleural spaces with hypoalbunaemia and took time for reabsorption. Case 9 describes a female who presented with decompensated shock. She had evidence of hemoconcentration with a high haematocrit. But on presentation clinically and ultrasonically she had no objective evidence of plasma leak into serous cavities. This highlights that although plasma leak is describes as selective to pleural, pericardial and peritoneal cavities, there can be substantial amount of fluid leaking in to 3rd space of unknown sites. Absence of objective fluid leak should not delay the treating physician making a diagnosis of DHF in the presence of evidence of intravascular volume depletion and hemoconcentration. However, frequent use of ultrasound examination has enhanced early detection of plasma leak. In THP, ultrasound scanners are available in the wards where dengue patients are treated to do bedside scaning without mobilizing patients to scanning rooms.

Liver dysfunction is a well-recognized feature in both dengue fever and DHF. Patients with dengue fever complaining of abdominal pain, nausea, vomiting and anorexia should alert the physician of the possibility of liver involvement [12]. Aetio-pathogenesis in liver dysfunction in dengue fever is yet to be elucidated. Direct effects of the virus or host immune response on liver cells, circulatory compromise, metabolic acidosis and/or hypoxia caused by hypotension or localized vascular leakage inside the liver are possible mechanisms postulated to explain the liver dysfunction [13, 14]. Case 2 describes patient with DHF developing acute liver failure and case 5 describes a patient with DF without leaking developing liver dysfunction, coagulopathy and gastrointestinal bleeding. Both cases were successfully managed with adequately maintaining the hydration status and intravenous N acetyl cysteine. NAC scavenges free radicals, improves antioxidant defense and acts as a vasodilator to improve oxygen delivery and consumption [15]. However, efficacy of NAC needs to be validated with further studies.

Bleeding manifestations are seen both in dengue fever and dengue hemorrhagic fever. Despite the name, cardinal feature that differentiate dengue fever from DHF is not hemorrhage but leaking. The underlying mechanisms responsible for bleeding in dengue infections remain poorly understood. Thrombocytopenia is universal in DHF and most of the patients with DF [16]. Platelet functions is abnormal in acute dengue fever mainly due to impaired ADP mediated platelet aggregation [17].Isarangkura et al. reported that platelet survival is less in acute dengue fever [18]. Mild prolongation of prothrombin time and activated partial thromboplastin times with reduction in fibrinogen levels were reported in some studies in patients without liver involvement [19, 20]. Patients with prolonged shock with multi-organ dysfunction and those with acute liver failure had major gastrointestinal bleeds contributed by deranged clotting and gut ischemia. Case 5 describes a patient with DF without leaking who had normal platelets with severe liver involvement leading to coagulopathy and gastrointestinal bleeding. In contrast in case 6, a primary DF patient developed severe gastrointestinal bleeding needing blood and platelet transfusions. Her liver enzymes were marginally elevated and had a normal clotting profile. Her main risk factor for a gastrointestinal bleed, haematuria was low platelet count.

Intracranial hemorrhage in dengue fever is a rare but a grave complication. Mechanism of intracranial bleeding is still not clearly described, it is postulated that it could be due to the interplay between coagulopathy, platelet dysfunction, thrombocytopenia, and vasculopathy [21, 22]. In our patient described in case 3 presented in the peak of leaking with postural symptoms. On admission, his platelet count was16 $\times 10^9/\mu l$. He had history of a fall with head impact and soon after admission patient sustained a generalized tonic clonic fit. Later he was found to have bilateral frontal lobe hemorrhages. This could be either traumatic following the fall or could be spontaneous which might have caused the fall. Management of an ICH in a dengue patient is controversial as the causative factors such as vasculopathy and platelet dysfunction are usually still present and irreversible while surgery is undertaken. No studies have been performed on place for surgery for ICH in dengue fever. Low platelets are the main risk factor for an ICH in dengue fever. There is no consensus on when to transfuse platelets and place for primary prophylaxis. Some studies have recommended prophylaxis platelet transfusions when the platelet count is very low [23, 24]. In 2011, Kurukularatne et al. strongly concluded that prophylactic platelet transfusion is associated with hazards and wastage without any hematological benefit and therefore, should not be adopted as a routine clinical practice [25]. Our patient received platelet transfusion as a secondary prophylactic measure as the platelet count was very low.

Dengue fever and DHF are associated with a wide spectrum cardiac complication. Kularatne et al. showed that 62.5% of 120 adults with dengue fever had an abnormal electrocardiogram [26]. Most cardiac complications are clinically mild and self-limiting, therefore, they are under diagnosed [27]. Myocardial involvement in dengue is yet to be fully described, but it can be due to direct viral invasion of the myocardium or cytokine mediated immune injury [28]. In case 4, young patient had evidence of myocarditis in ECG and left ventricular global hypokinesia in the 2D Echo. She was managed conservatively with meticulous fluid management and with a short course of steroids. Theoretically, steroids help to reduce inflammation of myocardium, thus improving contractility. Her follow up Echo in 2 weeks showed normalization of left ventricular systolic function.

Clinically considerable proportion of dengue patients who presented to the hospital can have bacterial co-infection [29]. Bacterial co-infection can be easily overlooked in the dengue epidemic setting. Delay in diagnosis and delay in anti-microbial therapy will have adverse outcome. Bacteremia in dengue fever is mainly Gram negative. It is probably caused by the breakdown of the intestinal mucosal barrier in severe dengue infection. In Case 7, the patient had DHF complicated with septic shock. The focus of sepsis is probably the gut, as he had diarrhoea and sepsis developed during leaking phase and gut ischemia probable led to breach in mucosal defense and gram-negative sepsis. Low blood pressure in tachycardia could have been easily overlooked attributing to dengue shock syndrome, but the disproportionately high pulse rate and warm peripheries in the background of shock alerted the treating physician of the possible underlying sepsis. Prompt use of antibiotics and judicious use of vasopressors were lifesaving. It is intriguing that he needed massive transfusions to maintain his blood pressure and save the life. This case provide empirical evidence for blood transfusion sever dengue infection Moreover, Case 10 describes a patient developed dengue fever and septic shock probably originating from the lung. Patient was treated with blood transfusion and intravenous crystalloids and colloids to overcome the shock which resulted in pulmonary edema. Judicious use of vasopressors is important in such instance to prevent volume overload. Supportive respiratory care over many hours maintained the oxygenation. The Case 8 describe presentation of dengue predominantly with diarrhea that might mislead the clinician as bacillary dysentery.

Lessons learnt from managing difficult cases of dengue as we presented here need sharing. Similar cases or situations may be happening at any given time in the globe as dengue is mostly seen everywhere. These clinical observations needs explanation on pathophysiological basis, but the knowledge about pathology and pathophysiology in dengue needs further improvement. Better treatment options are needed to improve the outcome of dengue.

Abbreviations

ADP: Adenine di-Phosphate; ALT: Alanine transaminase; AST: Aspartate transaminase; CPAP: Continuous Positive Airway Pressure; CRFT: Capillary Refilling Time; DEN1: Dengue virus serotype 1; DHF: Dengue Haemorrhagic Fever; FBC: Full Blood Count; HDU: High Dependency Unit; ICH: Intra Cranial Haemorrhage; NAC: N-Acetyl Cysteine; PCR: Polymerase chain reaction; PCV: Packed Cell Volume; THP: Teaching Hospital Peradeniya

Acknowledgements

We all express our gratitude to the patients, who kindly gave consent for the cases to be presented in this paper.

Funding

Not applicable.

Authors' contributions

SAMK, UR, PK and CD managed the patients. JJ and SR collected the data. All authors did intellectual contribution and participated in drafting the manuscript. All authors read and approved the final manuscript.

Consent for publication

Written informed consent was obtained from the patients and/or relatives for publication of this case report and any accompanying images. A copy of the written consent is available for review by the Editor-in-Chief of this journal.

Competing interests

The authors declare that they have no competing interests.

Author details

[1]Department of Medicine, Faculty of Medicine, University of Peradeniya, Peradeniya, Sri Lanka. [2]Teaching Hospital Peradeniya, Peradeniya, Sri Lanka.

References

1. Halstead SB. Dengue. CurrOpin Infect Dis. 2002;15(5):471–6.
2. Wilder-Smith A, Schwartz E. Dengue in travelers. N Engl J Med. 2005;353:924–32.
3. Kularatne SAM. Dengue fever. BMJ. 2015;351:h4661. https://doi.org/10.1136/BMJ.h4661.
4. Dalugama C, Ralapanawa U, Jayalath T. Dengue myositis and review of literature. Clin Case Rep Res Trials. 2017;2:16–8.
5. Lizarraga KJ, Nayer A. Dengue-associated kidney disease. J Nephropathol. 2014;3(2):57–62 http://doi.org/10.12860/jnp.2014.13.
6. Wali JP, Biswas A, Chandra S, Malhotra A, Aggarwal P, Handa R, Wig N, Bahl VK. Cardiac involvement in dengue haemorrhagic fever. Int J Cardiol. 1998;64(1):31–6.
7. Kumar R, Prakash O, Sharma BS. Intracranial hemorrhage in dengue fever: management and outcome: a series of 5 cases and review of literature. Surg Neurol. 2009;72(4):429–33.
8. Dalugama C, Gawarammana IB. Dengue hemorrhagic fever complicated with transient diabetic ketoacidosis: a case report. J Med Case Rep. 2017;11(1):302.
9. Ralapanawa DM, Kularatne SA, Jayalath WA. Guillain-Barre syndrome following dengue fever and literature review. BMC Res Notes. 2015;8:729. https://doi.org/10.1186/s13104-015-1672-0.
10. Stephenson JR. Understanding dengue pathogenesis: implications for vaccine design. Bull World Health Organ. 2005;83:308–14.
11. Guidelines on Management of Dengue Fever and Hemorrhagic Fever in adults: Epidemiology Unit, Ministry of Health; 2012. http://www.epid.gov.lk/web/images/pdf/Publication/guidelines_for_the_management_of_df_and_dhf_in_adults.pdf
12. Karoli R, Fatima J, Siddiqi Z, Kazmi KI, Sultania AR. Clinical profile of dengue infection at a teaching Hospital in North India. J Infect Dev Ctries. 2012;6:551–4.
13. Itha S, Kashyap R, Krishnani N, Saraswat VA, Choudhuri G, Aggarwal R. Profile of liver involvement in dengue virus infection. Natl Med J India. 2005;18:127–30.
14. Kularatne SAM, Imbulpitiya IVB, Abeysekera RA, Waduge R, Rajapakse RPVJ, Weerakoon KGAD. Extensive haemorrhagic necrosis of liver is an unpredictable fatal complication in dengue infection: a postmortem study. BMC Infect Dis. 2014;14:141.
15. Sklar GE, Subramaniam M. Acetylcysteine treatment for non-acetaminopheninduced acute liver failure. Ann Pharmacother. 2004;498–500(23):38.
16. World Health Organization. Dengue haemorrhagic fever: diagnosis, treatment, prevention and control. 2nd edi ed. Geneva: WHO; 1997. http://www.who.int/csr/resources/publications/dengue/Denguepublication/en/
17. Srichaikul TA, Nimmannitya SU, Sripaisarn T, Kamolsilpa MA, Pulgate CH. Platelet function during the acute phase of dengue hemorrhagic fever. Southeast Asian J Trop Med Public Health. 1989;20(1):19–25.
18. Isarangkura P, Tuchinda S. The behavior of transfused platelets in dengue hemorrhagic fever. Southeast Asian J Trop Med Public Health. 1993;24:222–4.
19. Mitrakul C, Poshyachinda M, Futrakul P, Sangkawibha N, Ahandrik S. Hemostatic and platelet kinetic studies in dengue hemorrhagic fever. Am J Trop Med Hyg. 1977;26(5):975–84.
20. Funahara Y, Shirahata A, Setiabudy-dharma RA. DHF characterized by acute type DIC with increased vascular permeability. Southeast Asian J Trop Med Public Health. 1987;18(3):346–50.
21. Cam BV, Fonsmark L, Hue NB, Phuong NT, Poulsen A, Heegaard ED. Prospective case-control study of encephalopathy in children with dengue hemorrhagic fever. Am J Trop Med Hyg. 2001;65:848–51.
22. Puccioni-Sohler M, Soares CN, Papaiz-Alvarenga R, Castro MJ, Faria LC, Peralta JM. Neurologic dengue manifestations associated with intrathecal specific immune response. Neurology. 2009;73:1413–7.
23. Makroo RN, Raina V, Kumar P, Kanth RK. Role of platelet transfusion in the management of dengue patients in a tertiary care hospital. Asian J Transfus Sci. 2007;1:4–7.

24. Dutta AK, Biswas A, Baruah K, Dhariwal AC. National guidelines for diagnosis and management of dengue fever/dengue haemorrhagic fever and dengue shock syndrome. J Indian Med Assoc. 2011;109:30–5.
25. Kurukularatne C, Dimatatac F, Teo DL, Lye DC, Leo YS. When less is more: can we abandon prophylactic platelet transfusion in dengue fever? Ann Acad Med Singap. 2011;40:539–45.
26. Kularatne SAM, Pathirage MMK, Kumarasiri PVR, Gunasena S, Mahindawanse SI. Cardiac complications of a dengue fever outbreak in Sri Lanka, 2005. Trans R Soc Trop Med Hyg. 2007;101(8):804–8.
27. Satarasinghe RL, Arultnithy K, Amerasena NL, Bulugahapitiya U, Sahayam DV. Asymptomatic myocardial involvement in acute dengue virus infection in a cohort of adult Sri Lankans admitted to a tertiary referral Centre. Br J Cardiol. 2007;14:171–3.
28. Hober D, Poli L, Roblin B, Gestas P, Chungue E, Granic G, Imbert P, Pecarere JL, Vergez-Pascal R, Watter P, Maniez-Montreuil M. Serum levels of tumor necrosis factor-alpha (TNF-alpha), interleukin-6 (IL-6), and interleukin-1 beta (IL-1 beta) in dengue-infected patients. Am J Trop Med Hyg. 1993;48(3):324–31.
29. See KC, Phua J, Yip HS, Yeo LL, Lim TK. Identification of concurrent bacterial infection in adult patients with Dengue. Am J Trop Med Hyg. 2013;89(4): 804–10 http://doi.org/10.4269/ajtmh.13-0197.

24

A case report of dengue haemorrhagic fever during the peripartum period: challenges in management and a case of vertical dengue transmission

B. V. K. M. Bopeththa[1*], Sardha Hemapriya[2], K. K. Gayan Niranga[2] and Danushka S. K. Kotigala[2]

Abstract

Background: Incidence of Dengue infection is on the increase in Sri Lanka with it being associated with significant maternal and neonatal morbidity in pregnancy.

Case presentation: A 33-year-old pregnant woman at 38 weeks of gestation, presented with acute onset of fever, was later diagnosed with Dengue illness. Due to the emergence of warning symptoms and signs and rapidly dropping platelet count, the baby was delivered by urgent caesarian section. She went into the critical phase during the postoperative period and due to concealed bleeding, required blood transfusion. On the 5th day of life, the neonate was also diagnosed with possible dengue by vertical transmission and required blood and PLT transfusions for recovery.

Conclusions: This case report illustrates how a high index of suspicion, early diagnosis, close monitoring, timely intervention and critical consideration of physiological changes of pregnancy when interpreting clinical situation, led to achieving a successful outcome.

Keywords: Dengue, Pregnancy, Vertical transmission, Physiological changes in pregnancy

Background

Dengue fever is an *Aedes* mosquito-borne flavivirus infection. It is becoming endemic in Sri Lanka, mainly due to changes in the rainfall patterns that increase the incidence. Dengue has become a major public health issue in Sri Lanka causing 215 deaths up to now, from 2017 [1]. Dengue is commonly defined as an acute febrile illness, associated with two or more of the following signs or symptoms: an intense headache, retro-orbital pain, myalgia, arthralgia, skin rash, leucopenia and hemorrhagic manifestations [2]. Although management of dengue in pregnancy is similar to non-pregnant dengue patient management, due to various physiological changes occurring in pregnancy, it may cause significant diagnostic and management issues in practical clinical situations.

Dengue infection is associated with a number of maternal and neonatal complications including maternal death, a most severe form of miscarriages, preterm deliveries, fetal anomalies and neonatal deaths respectively [3, 4]. Although increasing number of vertical transmission of dengue fever cases have been reported, details of vertical transmission is lacking [5]. Here, we report a case of dengue hemorrhagic fever during peripartum period that includes a possible case of vertical transmission.

Case presentation

A 33-year-old previously healthy mother in her 2nd pregnancy, was admitted at 38 weeks of gestation with a one-day history of high fever with chills, myalgia, arthralgia, and headache. Her first pregnancy ended up as lower segment caesarian section (LSCS) due to the unfavorable cervix. On admission, she was febrile (102 °F). Her pulse rate (PR) and blood pressure (BP) were 88 beats per minute and 94/60 mmHg respectively. Rest of the

* Correspondence: kameerabvkm@gmail.com
[1]Registrar in Emergency Medicine, Teaching Hospital Kandy, Kandy, Sri Lanka
Full list of author information is available at the end of the article

cardiac and respiratory examination was unremarkable. Abdominal examination revealed a soft abdomen with a single live fetus and symphysiofundal height was compatible with gestational age. Vaginal examination revealed an unfavorable cervix. Laboratory investigation results were as follows: total white cell count (WBC) 7100/mm^3, platelet count (PLT) 112,000/mm^3, haemoglobin (Hb) 11.5 g/dl, packed cell volume (PCV) 30%, C reactive protein (CRP) 31 mg/l and positive NS 1 antigen. Liver function and renal function tests were normal. Cardiotocograph (CTG) was normal and the fetal biophysical profile was compatible with the period of gestation (POG). There was no ultrasound evidence of free fluid in the abdomen or pelvis. The diagnosis was made of uncomplicated dengue and managed according to current national dengue management guidelines.

On the 2nd day, she developed two episodes of vomiting and had mild intermittent abdominal pain. Her PR was 98 beats per minute and blood pressure was 90/64 mmHg. There was mild right hypochondriac tenderness. Complete blood count (CBC) showed WBC 6900/mm^3, PLT 72000mm^3 and PCV 32%. Ultrasonically, there was no free in abdomen or chest. A multidisciplinary meeting was convened and a decision made to deliver her baby by urgent LSCS. Blood, fresh frozen plasma, and platelets were preserved and LSCS was performed under spinal anaesthesia. A healthy male baby weighing 3.0 kg was delivered with an uneventful intraoperative period. Although there was no significant bleeding as a prophylactic measure B lynch sutures were applied and an abdominal drain was also inserted. She was then transferred to intensive care unit (ICU) for further management.

On the 3rd day, fever was persisting and she continued to complain of right hypochondriac pain. She became tachycardic with PR of 105 beats per minute. BP was 92/66 mmHg. CBC revealed WBC of 5300/mm^3 with PLT of 63,000/mm^3 and PCV of 35%. Ultrasound (USS) examination showed pericholecystic oedema with a thin layer of free fluid in the hepatorenal pouch. The diagnosis of dengue hemorrhagic fever was made and observations conducted according to the observation chart for management of dengue in adult patients with fluid leakage. A 3 hourly PCV monitoring, hourly capillary refill time (CRFT), PR, supine BP and urine output was conducted. CBCs were performed twice daily with daily alanine transaminase (ALT) and aspartate transaminase (AST). Serum albumin was found to be low and 2D ECHO was normal. To cover unexpected nosocomial infections, IV of 4.5 g Piperazillin tazobactam, 8 hourly, was started. The summary of investigations is shown below (Table 1).

During the first 12 h of the critical phase (CP), vital parameters were stable and a flat rate of fluid administration was continued. Towards the peak of the leaking phase, her PR started to rise with a narrowing of pulse pressure. As there was a sudden drop in PCV, possible intra abdominal bleeding was suspected and 500 ml of packed cells was transfused. Although the abdominal draining was absent, USS confirmed the high possibility of the presence of blood in the peritoneal cavity. Haemodynamic parameters were improved following transfusion. At the same time, intravenous (IV) tranexamic acid 1 g was also given. Although there was a further drop in platelets, clotting studies were well within the normal range. At the beginning of the second half of the critical phase, she had developed pedal edema, mild ascites with right-sided mild pleural effusion without respiratory compromise. Around the 36th hour of CP, urine output dropped to less than 0.5 ml/kg/hour. Due to the high possibility of fluid overload, IV dextran 350 ml was given. Thereafter she had an uneventful recovery from rest of CP. She was then transferred to the high dependency unit and later to the postnatal ward, for further care. During the recovery phase, she became fever free and went into polyuric phase. Her CBC showed WBC 10000/mm^3, PLT 238000/mm^3 and Hb 9.8 g/dl. IV antibiotics were stopped after completion of the one week course following the negative urine and blood culture reports. Throughout the illness, her clotting studies and renal functions were normal. Later, she was discharged and underwent an uneventful recovery.

During her ICU stay, the baby was kept in the special baby unit (SBU) for the continuation of feeding and observation. He was never taken out of SBU and had no history of mosquito bites. The neonate was well until the 5th day of life but suddenly developed a high fever with jaundice. Sepsis or congenital dengue infection was suspected. Laboratory investigation results were as follows: WBC 5800/mm^3, Hb 13.8 g/dl, PLT 126000/mm^3, positive dengue NS 1 Antigen, AST 87 U/L, ALT 23 U/

Table 1 Summary of investigations performed during critical phase

	Hours of critical phase	WBC (cells/mm^3)	PLT (cells/mm^3)	Hb (g/dl)	PCV (%)	AST (U/L)	ALT (U/L)	Blood sugar (Mg/dl)	Corrected Serum calcium (mmol/l)	Arterial PH
Day 01	1–12	10.5	27,000	11.2	34	17	08	104		7.43
	13–24	11.98	26,000	10.9	36	55	6	138		
Day 02	25–36	20.9	18,000	8.9	26	141	62	118	2.26	7.46
	37–48	17.6	36,000	10.2	32	122	34	142		

L, CRP 5.8 mg/l with normal liver and renal functions with the exception of an elevated indirect bilirubin of 35 micro mol/L. Diagnosis of dengue fever was made and managed according to current guidelines. Later, on the 7th day of life, his PLT count dropped from 86,000/mm^3 to 43,000/mm^3 and he developed malena. However, bedside USS revealed no evidence of fluid leakage or intracranial bleed. Haemodynamic parameters were within normal ranges except tachycardia of 170 bpm during the period of malena. 30 ml of PLT and 45 ml of packed red cell transfusion were done. With close monitoring and judicious fluid balance, the baby improved and was discharged from the SBU with PLT of 146,000/mm^3 and Hb of 12 g/dl on the 11th day of life. However, his body weight had dropped to 2.580 kg upon discharge. On the 25th day of life, clinic review revealed weight gain up to 2.780 kg with age-appropriate milestone levels.

Discussion and conclusions

Currently, dengue is the most significant mosquito-borne disease in Sri Lanka. It is transmitted by the bite of an *Aedes* mosquito infected with any one of the four dengue viruses. Laboratory results have found that Dengue virus serotype 2 (DENV-2) to be the circulating strain in this outbreak [1]. Due to heavy monsoon rains and improper waste disposal leading to stagnation of rainwater, is attributed to the increasing number of dengue cases.

The clinical assessment, diagnosis, treatment, and monitoring of dengue fever or dengue hemorrhagic fever during pregnancy can be very difficult due to various physiological changes occurring in pregnancy and other obstetric complications mimicking a clinical presentation of dengue infection. Fever with low PLT count, elevated liver enzymes, and right hypochondriac pain could be a part of HELLP syndrome or dengue illness. Labor pain can be misinterpreted as right upper quadrant pain. Therefore diagnosis of dengue can be misled by the presentation of other obstetric complications. Hence, clinicians should have a high index of suspicion for the diagnosis [3].

Having higher baseline heart rate and a fall in systolic and diastolic blood pressure induced by a reduction in systemic vascular resistance, may cause difficulty in early detection of entering the dengue critical phase, dengue shock syndrome and assessing response to fluid boluses as in this case.

Plasma volume expansion accompanied by a lesser increase in red cell volume causes a modest reduction in hematocrit [6]. Therefore it is very important to determine the baseline PCV during the early part of dengue illness, as non-pregnant PCV values cannot be applied to pregnant patients. Without a baseline PCV, it is difficult to recognize the objective evidence of plasma leakage or concealed bleeding. In our patient, concealed bleeding was recognized by the sudden drop of PCV. However, a 20% rise of baseline PCV at the entrance into critical phase was not evident in this case, probably due to satisfactory hydration matching the rate of leaking. Over hydration in dengue can cause edema, pleural effusion, ascites and respiratory distress. Pregnancy itself can cause edema and mild respiratory discomfort due to gravid uterus. Clinical judgment alone may not be sufficient in such situations as in this case.

Pregnancy is associated with leukocytosis, primarily related to the increased circulation of neutrophils. In addition, the platelet count also begins to rise soon after delivery. Dengue infection causes leucopenia, thrombocytopenia, and a degree of thrombocytopenia is associated with the severity of dengue fever. Therefore, the interpretation of CBC and its correlation with the particular stage of dengue fever may not be accurate in pregnancy.

Still, there are no recommendations on mode and time of delivery for mothers with dengue infection. It was only due to this mother falling critically ill, was a multidisciplinary team approach considered. As fetal maturity was satisfactory but cervix not favorable, a CS was planned under spinal anaesthesia. It was carried out as urgent procedure due to several reasons. There was a high possibility of the patient entering the critical phase within the following few hours and if it did, the persistence of severe thrombocytopenia would last for next 2–3 days, with a high risk of bleeding during that period. Therefore immediate delivery was carried out.

Miscarriages, preterm labour, fetal abnormalities, increased risk of bleeding, low birth weight and maternal death in extreme cases, have been reported as adverse effects of dengue in pregnancy [4]. There are reported cases of vertical transmission of dengue infection and they have been confirmed by identification of dengue virus in cord blood samples [5]. Although dengue virus identification in cord blood was not performed in this case, development of fever on the 5th day of life and positive NS 1 antigen without a history of mosquito bites, supported the diagnosis of vertical transmission. The onset of fever following the 4–10 days of the normal incubation period of dengue is also favors the diagnosis [7]. All reported cases of vertical transmission have occurred around the delivery, probably due to lack of sufficient time to confer the passive immunity to the fetus [5]. Duration between the onset of maternal fever and delivery affects the time of onset of dengue fever in the neonate [8]. Only a few case reports of vertical transmission of dengue are currently available and according to this limited literature, the time of onset of fever in neonates, ranged from 16 h to 11 days after birth and lasted from 2 to 6 days [8].

In conclusion, it seems that, dengue infection during pregnancy can have various adverse effects on the mother as well as on the neonate. A high index of suspicion, early diagnosis, close monitoring, timely intervention and critical consideration of physiological changes of pregnancy when interpreting clinical situation, would have led us to achieve the successful outcome of this case.

Abbreviations

2DECHO: Two-dimensional echocardiogram; ALT: Alanine transaminase; AST: Aspartate transaminase; BP: Blood pressure; CBC: Complete blood count; CP: Critical phase; CRFT: Capillary refill time; CRP: C reactive protein; Hb: Hemoglobin; IV: Intravenous; LSCS: Lower segment caesarian section; NS-1: Non-structural protein 1; PCV: Packed cell volume; PLT: Platelet count; POG: Period of gestation; PR: Pulse rate; SBU: Special baby unit; USS: Ultrasound scan; WBC: White blood cell count

Acknowledgements

We would like to appreciate the neonatal intensive care team for their immense help received during the management of the neonate.

Authors' contributions

SH, BVKMB, KKGN and DSKK made equal contribution to the identification of the patient, conception of the work, diagnosis and treatment, data collection and analysis, drafting the manuscript, writing references, revising it critically for important intellectual content, final development of case report and all gave final approval of the version to be submitted.

Consent for publication

Written informed consent was obtained from the patient for publication of this case report. A copy of the written consent is available for review by the Editor-in-Chief of this journal.

Competing interests

The authors declare that they have no competing interests.

Author details

[1]Registrar in Emergency Medicine, Teaching Hospital Kandy, Kandy, Sri Lanka. [2]Consultant Obstetrician and Gynaecologist, Teaching Hospital Kandy, Kandy, Sri Lanka.

References

1. World Health Organization. Dengue fever – Sri Lanka. Geneva: World Health Organization; 2017. http://www.who.int/csr/don/19-july-2017-dengue-sri-lanka/en. Accessed 10 Oct 2017
2. Clinical Description for Case Definitions. Dengue | CDC. Cdc.gov. 2017. https://www.cdc.gov/dengue/clinicallab/casedef.html. Accessed 11 Oct 2017.
3. Phupong V. Dengue fever in pregnancy: a case report. BMC Pregnancy Childbirth. 2001;1:7.
4. Friedman EE, Dallah F, Harville EW, Myers L, Buekens P, Breart G, et al. Symptomatic dengue infection during pregnancy and infant outcomes: a retrospective cohort study. PLoS Negl Trop Dis. 2014;8:e3226.
5. Yin X, Zhong X, Pan S. Vertical transmission of dengue infection: the first putative case reported in China. Rev Inst Med Trop Sao Paulo. 2016;58:90.
6. Soma-Pillay P, Catherine NP, Tolppanen H, Mebazaa A, Tolppanen H, Mebazaa A. Physiological changes in pregnancy. Cardiovasc J Afr. 2016;27:89–94.
7. World Health Organization. Dengue and severe dengue. 2018. [online] Available at: http://www.who.int/en/news-room/fact-sheets/detail/dengue-and-severe-dengue. Accessed 23 Aug 2018.
8. Witayathawornwong P. Parturient and perinatal dengue hemorrhagic fever. Southeast Asian J Trop Med Public Health. 2004;34:797–9.

Heart and liver are infected in fatal cases of dengue: three PCR based case studies

S. A. M. Kularatne[1], M. M. Rajapakse[1], Udaya Ralapanawa[1*], R. Waduge[2], L. P. M. M. K. Pathirage[1] and R. P. V. J. Rajapakse[3]

Abstract

Background: Dengue is a global problem mainly in the tropics. Meticulous clinical management of cases has reduced the death rate significantly, but large numbers of people still succumb to severe complications of the infection. Presence of myocarditis is often overlooked leading to a poor outcome. Clinical management guidelines of dengue do not stress the importance of myocarditis as a manifestation in dengue infection. Severe hepatic dysfunction also needs emphasis.

Case presentation: We present three patients who had come to hospital on the 3rd day of fever. Two of them (case 1 and 3) were in shock on admission and case 2, who was stable on the3rd day, went into the critical phase and developed shock while in the hospital on the 4thday. All three had tachycardia on admission that got worse with time. The clinical course was unstable with fluctuations in urine output and deterioration of organ function. Despite frequent monitoring and life support they survived only 2–3 days in hospital. All three patients had myocarditis during the critical phase. In the first case, myocarditis was confirmed by troponin estimation and echocardiogram. In the second and third cases, histopathology confirmed myocarditis. Haemorrhagic necrosis of the liver was found in case 2 and 3 with exponential rise of transaminases. In all three cases, viral RNA was detected in both heart and liver tissues by PCR amplification.

Conclusions: We stress that detection of myocarditis and liver involvement in any dengue patient is important from the onset of the illness where treatment should be tailored to prevent development of hypotension. Our findings are novel as PCR and histology are rarely done on tissues of deceased dengue patients in the world. Studies are needed to find therapeutic interventions to reverse cardiac and hepatic dysfunction in dengue infection.

Keywords: Dengue, Myocarditis, Liver failure, Expanded dengue syndrome, RT-PCR, Sri Lanka

Background

Dengue is a global problem, mainly in the tropics, and travelers visiting endemic regions are at risk of contracting the infection [1–3]. Meticulous clinical management of cases has reduced the death rate significantly, but large numbers of people succumb to severe complications of the infection [4]. Sri Lanka experienced the worst dengue epidemic in mid-2017 with a total case load of the year amounting to 185,000 cases, with more than 400 deaths [5]. At institution level and centrally at the Ministry of Health, these unfortunate deaths are being reviewed in order to improve case management and to understand the contributory factors responsible for death. However, despite improvement of necessary infrastructure and guideline-based management, dengue infection still causes deaths [6]. The main pathology of dengue haemorrhagic fever is plasma leak from capillaries, where all kinds of cytokines are involved,but is amenable to meticulous fluid management [4, 6]. Moreover, WHO recognizes the expanded dengue syndrome to explain uncommon complications of the infection [7]. The majority of patients recover from the infection, if plasma leak is the sole pathology. Such a notion in the clinician's mind tends to overlook the concomitant vital organ dysfunction that is present in some cases of dengue. In these three case studies, we aim to demonstrate the presence of virus in the organ

* Correspondence: udayapralapanawa@yahoo.com
[1]Department of Medicine, Faculty of Medicine, University of Peradeniya, Peradeniya, Sri Lanka
Full list of author information is available at the end of the article

tissue at necropsy examination and to collate those findings with the clinical and laboratory manifestations prior to death to show evidence of dengue infection in the heart and lungs.

Case presentation

Case 1

A 34-year-old male presented to the THP on 11th May 2017 with a 3-day history of fever, arthralgia, backache, headache and skin flush. He had no cough, abdominal pain or diarrhoea. On admission, he was ill looking and had postural giddiness and cold peripheries. Blood pressure was 80/50 mmHg and pulse rate was 98 beats/min. Resuscitation was attempted with rapid infusion of 500 ml of normal saline followed by continuation normal saline infusion. His blood pressure (BP) picked up to 100/70 mmHg, but he remained oliguric over the next 12 h. Dextran 40 colloid 500 ml bolus infusion was given to raise the BP and to produce more urine. Twelve hours later, he developed generalized convulsions and needed immediate intubation and assisted ventilation in the Intensive Care Unit (ICU). Chest radiograph showed bilateral lung shadows suggestive of pulmonary oedema. Other investigations are shown in Table 1. In the ICU, at 3 PM, BP was 130/80 mmHg and pulse rate was 130 beats/min. However, at 3.30 PM, pulse rate was 160 beats /min, and BP dropped to 97/53 mmHg. The patient had central cyanosis, cold peripheries, feeble peripheral pulses and the haematocrit (HCT) rose to 55% requiring more Dextran 40 infusion.

On morning of the fifth day at 5 AM, HCT and haemoglobin dropped to 28% and 9 g/dl respectively without any obvious bleeding. With transfusion of one unit of blood, BP rose to 130/95 mmHg. With further transfusion HCT and urine output improved. Two dimensional echocardiogram showed global left ventricular hypokinesia with an ejection fraction of 40%. Cardiac troponintitre was high. From noon, the BP was falling - 80/50 mmHg and tachycardia persisted that needed continuous inotrope infusion. Despite meticulous management, the patient developed cardiac arrest and resuscitation failed.

Case 2

A 36-year-old male suffering from type 2 diabetes for 3 years was transferred to the Teaching Hospital, Kandy on the 15th July, 2017 with a 3-day history of fever and arthralgia.On admission he was febrile and BP was 130/80 and pulse rate was 90 beats per min. Lungs were clear and abdomen was soft with no hepatomegaly. Initial investigations revealed WBC of 3×10^9/l, platelets of 63×10^9/l and HCT of 45%. On day 1 of admission, his basic clinical parameters were normal and urine output was adequate throughout the day. On the next day, ultrasound scan examination of abdomen showed evidence of early plasma leaking, thus initiating critical phase monitoring from 9 am on 16th July. At this point his BP was 100/70 mmHg and HCT was 45%. His WBC was 3.7×10^9/l, platelet count was 34×10^9/l. His alanine transaminase (ALT) and aspartate transaminase (AST) were 383 U/l and 463 U/l respectively.

From the onset of the critical phase, the patient had tachycardia which persisted. He had satisfactory urine output initially, but his HCT continued to increase. At about 7 pm, a Dextran-40 colloid 500 ml bolus was given, but at midnight the urine output started dropping to a level of 35 ml/h. Thus, another bolus of 250 ml of dextran-40 was given. Meanwhile, the patient developed melaena, and 500 ml of whole blood was transfused. As the patient developed lactic acidosis, sodium bicarbonate infusion was given.

The patient was transferred to the ICU, Teaching hospital, Peradeniya (THP) at 3 am of 17th July while managing the critical phase into the 18th hour. On admission, blood pressure was 125/91 mmHg which rapidly dropped to 100/80 mmHg and the peripheries were cold to touch. The patient was conscious and rational. The urine output dropped to 20 ml/h. Pulse rate remained at 140 beats/min. Auscultation of the lungs revealed reduced breath sounds with fine crepitations in both lungs. Melaena was present on rectal examination. Arterial blood gasses showed lactic acidosis. Ultrasound examination of abdomen showed a significant amount of ascites. The patient was given two 250 ml boluses of dextran-40. The investigations are shown in Table 1. By about 7 AM, the patient became anuric with BP of 99/65 mmHg and HCT was 50%. The patient was transfused with 3 units of blood within the next 2 h but he remained anuric. By 9 AM, the patient was confused and disoriented and had cold peripheries with sluggish capillary refilling. He was intubated and ventilated electively. At 1.20 pm the patient developed bradycardia followed by cardiac arrest and resuscitation was unsuccessful.

Case 3

A 40-year-old female with a history of bronchial asthma for 17 years, presented to the THP with fever of 3 days duration associated with vomiting and postural giddiness on 22nd July 2017. On admission, pulse rate was 108 beats /min and blood pressure was unrecordable. Ultrasound scan of the abdomen showed evidence of fluid leaking. The onset of critical phase was calculated 8 h backward and prompt resuscitation was attempted. Despite fluid resuscitation tachycardia persisted with reduced urine output. On admission her ALT was 1365 U/l and AST was 2999 U/l. Serum albumin was 30.8 mg/dl and serum creatinine was 84 µmol/l. Her INR was 1.38. Serum amylase was 37 U/L.

On the evening of the same day she complained of abdominal pain with tenderness of the right hypochondrium.

Table 1 Summary of important clinical and laboratory data of 3 fatal cases of dengue with the list of complications

Description of case		Clinical status on admission and subsequently	Investigations		Complications	Duration of illness from onset to death
No	Age/Gender		Test	Results		
1	34 / M	Fever 3 days	WBC	3.5 × 10^9/l	Persistent hypotension	5 days
		Postural giddiness	Platelets	28 × 10^9/l	Fluid overload	
		Cold peripheries	Creatinine	193 μmol/l	Pulmonary oedema	
		BP: 80/50 mmHg	CRP	320 mg/l	Left ventricular-	
		Pulse rate 98/min	ALT	73 U/L	hypokinesia	
		Convulsions	AST	98 U/L	Hypoxaemia	
		Assisted ventilation	Troponin I	0.29 ng/ml	Sepsis	
			PH	7.1	Lactic acidosis	
			Pco2	44 mmHg	Bleeding	
			PaO2	61 mmHg	Renal failure	
2	36/M	Type 2 diabetes	WBC	3.7 × 10^9/l	Erratic critical phase	6 days
		Fever 3 days	Platelets	34 × 10^9/l	Undue tachycardia	
		BP 130/80 mmHg	Creatinine	82.5 μmol/l	Hypotension	
		Pulse rate 90/min	Blood sugar	233 mg/dl	Fulminant hepatic	
		Critical phase on	ALT (day- 3)	383 U/L	failure	
		4th day with pleural effusion, tachycardia and low BP 100 mmHg Melaena, Reduced urine out put	(day-4)	4905 U/L	GI- bleeding	
			AST (day-3)	463 U/L	Acute kidney injury	
			(day-4)	9371 U/L	Lactic acidosis	
			INR (day-5)	> 5		
			PH (day-5)	7.32		
3	40/F	Bronchial asthma	WBC	8.2 × 10^9/l	Profound shock on	6 days
		Fever 4 days	Platelet	28 × 10^9/l	admission	
		Vomiting, shock	HCt	37	Pleural effusions	
		Cold peripheries	Creatinine	84 μmol/l	Fulminant hepatic	
		BP – un-recordable	Albumin	30.8 g/l	failure	
		Pulse-108/ min	ALT(day-4)	1365 U/L	Encephalopathy	
		US-Ab: fluid leak	(day-7)	2590 U/L		
		Abdominal pain	AST (day-4)	2999 U/L		
		Melaena Confusion	(day-5)	6812 U/L		

She passed melaena stools. She had tachypnoea and blood gasses revealed acidosis. A small right sided pleural effusion was also present. She was transfused with one unit of whole blood. By the next morning her abdominal pain and postural symptoms increased and she developed mild icterus. She had tachycardia, but the blood pressure was maintained and urine output was satisfactory. She then developed ascites and bilateral pleural effusions. The next AST was 3661 U/l and ALT was 1579 U/l. By the evening her oxygen saturation dropped despite administering 100% oxygen. Subsequent AST and ALT were 8543 U/l and 2981 U/l respectively. The serum amylase was 48 U/l and serum creatinine was 105 μmol/l.

Towards the latter part of the critical phase the HCT started falling and the urine output declined to 25 ml/h. Several units of blood, FFP, and human albumin were infused to maintain the HCT. The patient rapidly developed difficulty in breathing with bilateral moderate pleural effusions. However, her AST and ALT levels reduced to 3661 U/l and 2685 U/l. On 24th July, the critical phase monitoring was over, but the patient gradually became confused and disoriented. She had high fever and oral bleeding but her other vital parameters and urine output were satisfactory. There were crepitations all over the lung fields and she needed assisted ventilation in the ICU. She died on the 2nd day in the ICU.

Discussion and conclusions

All three patients entered hospital on the 3rd day of fever.Two of them,cases 1 and 3, were in shock on admission and case 2, who was stable on admission on the 3rd day of fever,went into critical phase and shock while in the hospital on the 4th day. All three had tachycardia on admission that increased with time. The clinical course was unstable with fluctuations in urine output and deterioration of organ function. With very close monitoring and intense life support they lived only 2–3 days in the hospital. All three patients had myocarditis complicating the critical phase. In the first case, myocarditis was confirmed by cardiac troponin estimation and echocardiogram. In the second and third cases, post mortem histopathology confirmed myocarditis (Table 2, Fig. 1).PCR amplification was used to demonstrate the presence of dengue viral RNA in the myocardium in all three cases. The liver involvement is more marked in case 3 as evident by very high levels of hepatic transaminases. Case 2 and 3 had extensive haemorrhagic necrosis of the liver (Table 2, Fig. 2). In all three cases, viral RNA was detected by PCR in the liver. Moreover, viral RNA was detected in many tissues of these patients.

Postmortem studies are seldom reported in the world despite many dengue deaths. Further, histology and PCR studies of tissues of deceased victims are hardly happening despite availability of technology. Therefore, organ involvement in dengue infection has not been fully understood. This study shows extent of organ involvement in dengue and how it collates with the clinical manifestations in severe cases of dengue. There is a possibility that dengue virus infected blood cells entrapped in the organs would have given positive PCR results. However, taking clinical evidence of organ dysfunction, biochemical derangements and histology together, it is most likely that dengue virus could infect the organs.

Literature to support the existence of myocarditis in dengue infection has been available for more than a decade [8–15]. However, clinical management guidelines have given only little importance to myocarditis as a manifestation in dengue infection [6, 15]. In 2005, clinical experience in managing a large series of dengue cases with myocarditis in Sri Lanka was published where the causative serotype was DEN 3 [9, 13, 14]. Histopathological evidence of myocarditis was also found in 2009 [13]. A traveler returning from the Dominican Republic developing myocarditis has been published in 2014 [8]. Even though, there have been many deaths due to dengue, the literature available on necropsy studies dealing with detection of virus in tissues and related histopathology is scarce [16–21]. This deficit has curtailed critical analysis and identification of the true contributory causes for deaths. Clinicians are trapped in a straitjacket of orthodox thinking of clinical management of dengue where some patients die due to irreversible shock. It has been observed that fluid overload has contributed to most dengue deaths, like in case 1 in this series. In pure fluid leaking DHF, fluid overload does not occur if the cardiac status is normal. However, if myocarditis is present, the heart naturally fails when fluid is given in excess. The presence of tachycardia and development of shock early in the disease should sound the alarm of myocarditis. To prevent deaths, early detection

Table 2 Detection of Dengue virus RNA in different tissue samples obtained at necropsy examination and respective gross and microscopic changes in tissues of fatal cases of dengue

Tissue	Case 1		Case 2		Case 3	
	PCR	Macroscopy	PCR	Histology	PCR	Histology
Brain	–		+	Normal	–	Normal
Lungs	+	Congested, Haemorrhagic	*	Congested capillaries	+	Pulmonary oedema, capillary congestion in interstitium
Heart	+	Petechial haemorrages	+	Interstitial oedema with infiltration of neutrophils and lymphocytes	+	Marked interstitial oedema, lymphocytic infiltration in endomyseum
Liver	+	Congested	+	Extensive haemorrhagic necrosis	+	Submassive necrosis, haemorrhagic necrosis
Kidney	+		+	Acute tubular necrosis	–	Acute tubular necrosis
Spleen	–		–	Expansion of red pulp, extravasations of red cells	–	Expansion of red pulp with haemorrhage
Adrenal gland	*		*		+	Early autolysis
Pancreas	*		*		+	Early autolysis
Intestines	+		*			
Muscles	*		+	Occasional fibre necrosis, inflammation	+	
Skin	+		*		*	
Blood	+		*		*	

(+) detection of dengue (DEN 2) RNA in tissues, (––) Dengue RNA not detected, (*) Not tested as tissues samples were not available. In Case 1, histology of tissues were not done

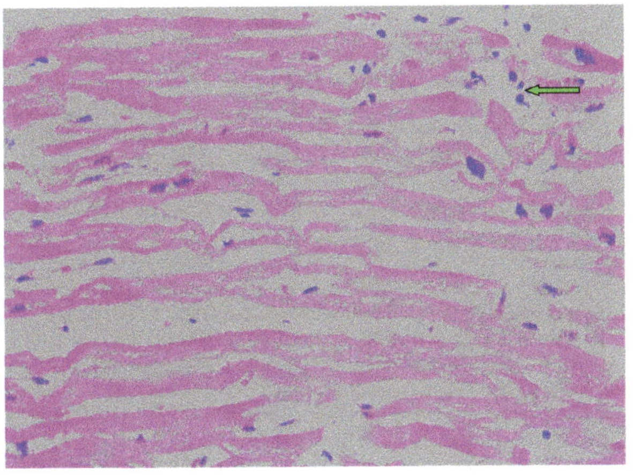

Fig. 1 Heart muscle × 400 inflammatory cell infiltration shown in arrow

of myocarditis is essential to institute extra precautions needed in management [9, 13, 14].

Hepatic involvement in dengue has been addressed in guidelines and literature [6, 7, 22, 23]. However, hepatic involvement has been ascertained by rising transaminases and in extreme cases development of fulminant hepatic failure. Very often, the pathophysiology that leads to hepatic dysfunction remains unknown. Speculation of ischemic hepatic damage during the critical phase is often entertained. In 2014, we demonstrated extensive haemorrhagic necrosis of liver in a necropsy study along with detection of viral RNA in liver tissue [23]. In the present case series, we found similar findings. In general, all cases of dengue infection have elevated transaminases at different levels [7, 24–26]. In some cases, elevation of transaminases is very high [24]. This suggests that the dengue virus infects the liver in virtually all cases, rarely causing severe hepatitis. Minimizing liver damage in dengue is a problem that needs resolving: some clinicians use N acetyl cystine infusions on a regular basis when hepatic transaminases are high [27, 28]. Studying these three cases suggests that the dengue virus could infect any tissue in the body even skin, muscles and intestine (Table 2). This is usually reflected in the clinical manifestations of dengue e.g. muscle pain, skin rashes, abdominal pain, diarrhoea etc. It is of interest that in this study viral RNA was not detected in the spleen. Clinically, these three cases demonstrate multiple organ dysfunction, metabolic abnormalities, sepsis and bleeding along with persistent hypotension contributing to death. Once the balance of critical parameters tilts towards deterioration, it becomes irreversible and death becomes inevitable despite giving the best of care and life support. We can extrapolate our findings to explain most of the fatalities in dengue in Sri Lanka and even the world over. Therefore, we stress that detection of myocarditis and liver involvement in any dengue patient is important from the onset of the illness where treatment should be tailored to prevent development of hypotension. Studies are needed to find therapeutic interventions to revert cardiac and hepatic dysfunction in dengue infections.

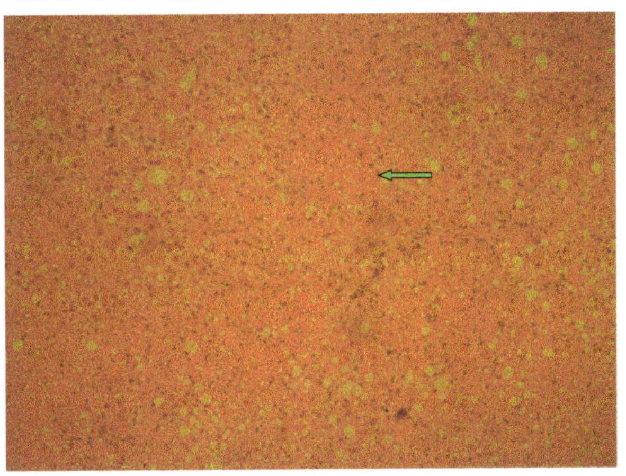

Fig. 2 Liver × 100 bringing necrosis shown in arrow

Abbreviations

ALT: Alanine transaminase; AST: Aspartate transaminase; CRP: Creactive protein; HCT: Haematocrit; ICU: Intensive Care Unit; PCR: Polymerase chain reaction; WBC: White blood cells

Acknowledgements

We wish to express our sincere thanks to Dr. Malik Fernando for copy-editing the manuscript.

Funding

Not applicable

Authors' contributions

SAMK, UR and LPMMKP managed patients. RW and RPVJR did histology and PCR respectively. MMR collected the data and coordinated the study. All authors did intellectual contribution and participated in drafting the manuscript. All authors read and approved the final manuscript.

Consent for publication

Postmortem examinationsin all three cases were performed as a legal requirement and the tissues were harvested for histology and viral studies with the consent of the next-of-kin in each case. We confirm that all procedures carried out on patients' tissues and blood samples including PCR were part of the routine postmortem examination. Written informed consent was obtained from the patients' relatives for publication of these case reports and any accompanying images. A copy of the written consent is available for review by the Editor-in-Chief of this journal.

Competing interests

The authors declare that they have no competing interests.

Author details
[1]Department of Medicine, Faculty of Medicine, University of Peradeniya, Peradeniya, Sri Lanka. [2]Department of Pathology, Faculty of Medicine, University of Peradeniya, Peradeniya, Sri Lanka. [3]Department of Veterinary Pathobiology, Faculty of Veterinary Medicine and Animal Science, University of Peradeniya, Peradeniya, Sri Lanka.

References

1. Bhatt S, Gething PW, Brady OJ, Messina JP, Farlow AW, Moyes CL, Drake JM, Brownstein JS, Hoen AG, Sankoh O, Myers MF, George DB, Jaenisch T, Wint GR, Simmons CP, Scott TW, Farrar JJ, Hay SI. The global distribution and burden of dengue. Nature. 2013;496(7446):504–7. https://doi.org/10.1038/nature12060 Epub 2013 Apr 7.
2. Dengue.WHO. http://www.who.int/ith/diseases/dengue/en/. Accessed 15 Apr 2018.
3. Wilder-Smith A. Dengue infections in travellers. Paediatr Int Child Health. 2012;32(s1):28–32. https://doi.org/10.1179/2F2046904712Z.00000000050.
4. Kularatne SAM. Dengue fever. BMJ. 2015;351:h4661.
5. Weekly epidemiological Report, Epidemiology Unit, Ministry of Health, Sri Lanka. 2018;45:2. http://www.epid.gov.lk/web/images/pdf/wer/2018/vol_45_no_02-english.pdf. Accessed 15 Apr 2018.
6. Ministry of Health - Sri Lanka, National Guidelines on Management of Dengue Fever & Dengue Haemorrhagic Fever In Adults, Revised and expanded edition November 2012. http://www.epid.gov.lk/web/images/pdf/Publication/guidelines_for_the_management_of_df_and_dhf_in_adults.pdf. Accessed 15 Apr 2018.
7. Ralapanawa DMPUK, Kularatne SAM. Current Management of Dengue in adults: a review. Int Med J Malays. 2015;14(1):29–42.
8. Zea D, Foley K, Case Report CJ. Myocarditis in a traveler returning from the Dominican Republic:an unusual presentation of dengue fever. Am J Trop Med Hygine. 2014;91(1):156–8. https://doi.org/10.4269/ajtmh.13-0637.
9. Kularatne S, Pathirage MMK, Medagama UAB, Gunasena S, Gunasekera MB. Myocarditis in three patients with dengue virus type DEN 3 infection. Ceylon Med J. 2009;51(2):75–6. https://doi.org/10.4038/cmj.v51i2.1362.
10. Sane S, Saulova A, McLaren R, White H. A fatal case of primary dengue infection with myocarditis and cerebral oedema. AMJ. 2015;8(9):299–303. https://doi.org/10.4066/AMJ.2015.2489.
11. Ku Y-H, Yu W-L. Case Report-Fatal dengue myocarditis despite the use of Extracoporal membrane oxygenation. Case Rep Infect Dis. 2016. https://doi.org/10.1155/2016/5627217.
12. Torres AF, Braga DN, Muniz F, Mendonca C, Olivera DN, de Souza ET, Bruke A, Tavora F. Lymphocytic myocarditis at autopsy in patients with dengue fever. Braz J Infect Dis. 2013;17(5):619–21. https://doi.org/10.1016/j.bjid.2013.03.009.
13. Weerakoon GAD, Kularatne SAM, Edussuriya DH, Kodikara KAS, Gunathilake PGL, Pinto VG, Seneviratne GS. Histopathological diagnosis of myocarditis in a dengue outbreak in Sri Lanka, 2009. BMC Res Notes. 2011;4:268. https://doi.org/10.1186/1756-0500-4-268.
14. Kularatne SAM, Pathitage MMK, Kumarasiri PVR, Gunasena S, Mahindawansa SI. Cardiac complications of a dengue fever outbreak in Sri Lanka, 2005. Trans R Soc Tro Med Hyg. 2007;101:804–8. https://doi.org/10.1016/j.trstmh.2007.02.021.
15. Lim SMS, Hoo FK, WAW S. A case of dengue haemorrhagic fever with myocarditis and complete heart block. Rawal Medical Journal. 2014;39(1):104–6.
16. Bhamarapravati N, Tuchinda P, Boonyapaknavik V. Pathology of Thailand haemorrhagic fever: a study of 100 autopsy cases. Ann Trop Med Parasitol. 1967;61(4):500–10.
17. Fresh JW, Reyes V, Clarke EJ, Uylangco CV. Philippine hemorrhagic fever: a clinical, laboratory, and necropsy study. J Lab Clin Med. 1969;73(3):451–8.
18. Couvelard A, Marianneau P, Bedel C, Drouet MT, Vachon F, Hénin D, Deubel V. Report of a fatal case of dengue infection with hepatitis: demonstration of dengue antigens in hepatocytes and liver apoptosis. Hum Pathol. 1999; 30(9):1106–10.
19. Rosen L, Drouet MT, Deubel V. Detection of dengue virus RNA by reverse transcription-polymerase chain reaction in the liver and lymphoid organs but not in the brain in fatal human infection. Am J Trop Med Hyg. 1999; 61(5):720–4.
20. Rathi KR, Arora MM, Sahai K, Tripathi S, Singh SP, Raman DK, Anand KB. Autopsy findings in fatal dengue haemorrhagic fever - 06 cases. Med J Armed Forces India. 2013;69(3):254–9. https://doi.org/10.1016/j.mjafi.2012.08.021.
21. Aye KS, Charngkaew K, Win N, Wai KZ, Moe K, Punyadee N, Thiemmeca S, Suttitheptumrong A, Sukpanichnant S, Prida M, Halstead SB. Pathologic highlights of dengue hemorrhagic fever in 13 autopsy cases from Myanmar. Hum Pathol. 2014;45(6):1221–33. https://doi.org/10.1016/j.humpath.2014.01.022.
22. World Health Organization. Dengue Guidelines For Diagnosis, Treatment, Prevention And Control, New edition 2009. http://www.who.int/tdr/publications/documents/dengue-diagnosis.pdf.
23. Kularatne SA, Imbulpitiya IV, Abeysekera RA, Waduge RN, Rajapakse RP, Weerakoon KG. Extensivehaemorrhagic necrosis of liver is an unpredictable fatal complication in dengue infection: a postmortem study. BMC Infect Dis. 2014;14:141. https://doi.org/10.1186/1471-2334-14-141.
24. Ageep A. Degree of liver injury in dengue virus infection. J Gen Mol Virol. 2012;4(October):1–5. https://doi.org/10.5897/JGMV11.023.
25. Samanta J. Dengue and its effects on liver. World J Clin Cases. 2015;3:125. https://doi.org/10.12998/wjcc.v3.i2.125.
26. Fernando S, Wijewickrama A, Gomes L, Punchihewa CT, Madusanka SDP, Dissanayake H, Jeewandara C, Peiris H, Ogg GS, Malavige GN. Patterns and causes of liver involvement in acute dengue infection. BMC Infect Dis. 2016; 16:319. https://doi.org/10.1186/s12879-016-1656-2.
27. Habaragamuwa BWP, Dissanayaka P. N-acetylcystein in dengue associated severe hepatitis. Indian J Crit Care Med. 2014;18(3):181–2. https://doi.org/10.4103/0972-5229.128712.
28. Kumarasena RS, Senanayake SM, Sivaraman K, de Silva AP, Dassanayake AS, Premaratna R, Wijesiriwardena B, de Silva HJ. Intravenous *N*-acetylcysteine in dengue-associated acute liver failure. Hepatol Int. 2010;4(2):533–4. https://doi.org/10.1007/s12072-010-9176-4 Published online 2010 May 28.

Accuracy and reliability of an NS1 rapid immunochromatographic test for DENV-1 diagnosis at point of care and in the laboratory

Verónica Elizabeth Mata[1*], Sonia Regina Lambert Passos[1], Yara Hahr Marques Hökerberg[1], Guilherme Miguéis Berardinelli[1], Maria Angelica Borges dos Santos[2], Levy Vilas Boas Fukuoka[1], Anna Carolina Fontoura Seixas Rangel Maciel[1], Cintia Damasceno dos Santos Rodrigues[3], Aline da Silva Santos[3] and Raquel de Vasconcellos Carvalhaes de Oliveira[1]

Abstract

Background: Rapid immunochromatographic tests (ICT) for dengue non-structural protein 1 (NS1) have shown good performance for diagnosing acute-phase dengue in serum in laboratory settings, but rarely have been assessed in whole blood and at point of care (POC). This study compare the accuracy and inter- and intra-observer reliability of the NS1 Bioeasy™ ICT in whole blood at POC versus serum in the laboratory, during a DENV-1 epidemic.

Methods: Cross-sectional study involving 144 adults spontaneously demanding care in an emergency department within 4 days of onset of acute febrile illness. Accuracy of NS1 Bioeasy™ ICT was compared in whole blood and serum, both at 15 and 30 min, blinded to the reference RT-PCR or NS1 ELISA. Non-dengue patients were also tested for Zika virus with RT-PCR. Reliability of whole blood and serum readings by the same or different observers was measured by simple kappa (95% CI).

Results: At 15 min, sensitivity (Sn) of NS1 Bioeasy™ ICT in whole blood/POC was 76.7% (95% CI: 68.0–84.1) and specificity (Sp) was 87.0% (95% CI: 66.4–97.2). Sn in serum/laboratory was 82% (95% CI: 74.1–88.6) and Sp 100% (95% CI: 85.8–100). Positive likelihood ratio was 5.9 (95% CI: 2.0–17.0) for whole blood/POC and 19.8 (95% CI: 2.9–135.1) for serum/laboratory. Reliability of matched readings of whole blood/POC and serum/laboratory by the same observer ($k = 0.83$, 95% CI: 0.74–0.93) or different observers ($k = 0.81$, 95% CI: 0.72–0.92) was almost perfect, with higher discordant levels in the absence of dengue. Results did not differ statistically at 5%.

Conclusions: NS1 Bioeasy™ ICT in DENV-1 epidemics is a potentially confirmatory test. Invalid results at 15 min should be reread at 30 min. To optimize impact of implementing ICT in the management of false-negatives it should be incorporated into an algorithm according to setting and available specimen.

Keywords: Dengue, Sensitivity and specificity, Diagnosis, Point-of-care systems, NS1, Reproducibility of results

* Correspondence: veronica.mata@ini.fiocruz.br
[1]Av. Brasil 4036 sala 201 A, CEP 21040-361 Rio de Janeiro, RJ, Brasil
Full list of author information is available at the end of the article

Background

Dengue virus (DENV) is an international public health problem, especially serotype 1 (DENV-1), which shows the highest frequency in the world [1]. The continents with the highest incidence of dengue are America and Asia with 84% of the 390 million cases in the world per year [2]. A systematic analysis on the global burden of dengue suggested that, in 2013, disease costs worldwide may have reached U$ 8.9 billion [3].

Clinical suspicion of dengue is based on the signs and symptoms described in the World Health Organization (WHO) guidelines, i.e., nausea/vomiting, rash, aches and pains, leucopenia, any warning sign (abdominal pain or tenderness, persistent vomiting, clinical fluid accumulation, mucosal bleeding, lethargy/restlessness, liver enlargement, and hemoconcentration concurrent with rapid decrease in platelet count). However, this criterion shows low specificity due to the absence of confirmatory laboratory tests [4].

A study conducted in the United States showed that laboratory diagnostic tests assist health decisions in 60–70% of cases [5]. The World Health Organization (WHO) recommends that ideal laboratory diagnostic tests should be affordable, sensitive, specific, user-friendly, robust, rapid (can be stored at room temperature and interpreted within 30 min), equipment-free, and deliverable to those who need them (ASSURED) [6].

Rapid immunochromatographic tests (ICT) for dengue with the detection of non-structural protein 1 (NS1) meet some of the characteristics of an ASSURED test: high specificity, ranging from 82.8% [7] to 100% [8–12], simple presentations, whether in cassette or strip format, and rapid interpretation of results (15 to 30 min) [13]. However, the sensitivity showed substantial discrepancy, ranging from 55.2% to 94.3% [10, 11].

In addition, the advantages of ICT in cassette format include the possibility of performing the test in whole blood specimens rather than serum and not requiring a specific infrastructure (equipment-free). This allows their deployment in sites with limited resources, for example at point of care (POC) [7, 12–15]. The tests offer rapid results – allowing the implementation of adequate therapy and care in time to avoid possible complications and even unnecessary costs [16]. Meanwhile, ICT in strip test format requires the use of a centrifuge, reagents, storage in a refrigerator, and test tubes to perform the reaction [7–12, 17].

Dengue NS1 ICTs in cassette or strip format have been evaluated in the last decade, mainly for serotypes 1, 2, and 3, with the best performance in the first 5 days of the illness. Still, these studies mostly used serum specimens, whether from biobanks [8, 10, 11] or processed in laboratory settings [8–12]. Lack of the test's evaluation in whole blood specimens hinders evaluation of ICT performance at POC and the recommendation of its deployment by health systems in epidemic situations [18].

The accuracy and reliability of ICTs for dengue NS1 are essential for guaranteeing quality tests. Still, few published studies on dengue have evaluated agreement between observers with different levels of training [19] or similar levels [14, 20], varying from moderate to almost perfect agreement. No studies were identified that evaluated the reliability of ICTs according to the types of specimens (whole blood versus serum) or settings.

A literature search detected only one study that evaluated duo ICT (NS1/IgM/IgG) and single NS1 using whole blood at POC, with sensitivities of 93.9% (95% CI: 88.8–96.8) and 81.6% (95% CI:74.6–87.1), and specificities of 92% (95% CI: 81.2–96.9) and 98% (95% CI: 89.5–99.7), respectively. Inter-observer reliability proved almost perfect (kappa = 1 95% 95% CI: 0.84–1) [21].

The current study thus aimed to compare the accuracy and reliability of NS1 Bioeasy™ ICT in whole blood at POC and in serum in the laboratory in adults during a DENV-1 epidemic in Rio de Janeiro State, Brazil.

Methods

This was a prospective diagnostic cross-sectional study that evaluated accuracy of the NS1 Bioeasy™ rapid immunochromatographic test and inter- and intra-observer reliability in whole blood specimens at point of care (POC) and serum specimens in the laboratory. The study was conducted according to the Standards for Reporting Studies of Diagnostic Accuracy (STARD) [22].

The study population consisted of patients over 18 years of age with up to 4 days of acute febrile syndrome without an established diagnosis, treated consecutively and by spontaneous demand at an emergency hospital of the Resende Municipal Health Secretariat, Rio de Janeiro State, Brazil, during a dengue epidemic in March 2015.

Data collection

The selected patients answered a questionnaire on clinical signs and symptoms associated with dengue according to WHO 2009 criteria for Dengue diagnosis [4, 23]. All of them signed the free and informed consent form.

Three blood specimens were drawn in vacuum tubes by a nurse and four medical students. Prior asepsis was performed with 70% alcohol, followed by brachial venipuncture with a 25 × 7 mm BD Vacutainer® needle. One tube with EDTA K2 was sent to the hospital laboratory for performing a complete blood count, another with heparin for ICT with whole blood at POC and the third with clotting activator and gel separator for obtaining serum. The latter was transported to the Flavivirus Laboratory, where it remained frozen at −70 °C for subsequent characterization of the specimen and ICT with serum.

The ICTs with whole blood were performed at point of care in the hospital by a nurse, and the ICTs with serum by a biologist and the same nurse (that performed ICT with blood at POC), in the Flavivirus Laboratory of the Oswaldo Cruz Institute, FIOCRUZ, the regional reference laboratory in Rio de Janeiro State. The observers were blinded to the reference test.

Diagnosis

Index test

The index test used was Dengue Eden Test NS1 ICT from the Bioeasy™ company. This is a rectangular cassette with an orifice to add whole blood, serum, or plasma, and which contains an immunochromatographic membrane coated with NS1 antigen on the test line (T) and a window to view the result. When only the control line (C) is visible, the test is considered negative; if lines C and T are visible, the result is positive; and when no line or only the T line is visible, the test result is invalid [13].

The tests were performed according to manufacturer's instructions and with readings at 15 and 30 min. Tests with invalid results at 15 min were reread at 30 min.

Reference test

All samples were tested using Reverse Transcription Polymerase Chain Reaction (RT-PCR) for dengue and Platelia™ Dengue NS1 Ag-ELISA (Bio-Rad™ Laboratories, France) as reference, performed according to the protocol described by Lanciotti et al. [24] and the manufacturer's specifications, respectively [25]. Dengue cases were defined by a positive result in at least one of them and non-dengue by negative results in both. Positive specimens according to the reference test were tested by Dengue Serion ELISA classic dengue virus IgM and IgG tests (Virion/Serion, Würzburg, Germany) [26], according to manufacturers' specifications for characterization of primary and secondary cases, respectively.

Non-dengue patients were also tested for Zika virus with RT-PCR [27] to investigate co-circulation of these viruses.

The reference tests were performed at the Flavivirus Laboratory by two biologists blinded to the index test.

Statistical analysis

The qualitative variables were described by simple frequencies and the quantitative variables by the median with interquartile range (IQR) or minimum and maximum. Shapiro-Wilk test showed rejection of normality for the quantitative variables, indicating the use of a non-parametric test. Verification of association in the dengue and non-dengue groups used the Mann-Whitney non-parametric test and Pearson's chi-square test for quantitative and qualitative variables, respectively.

To assess the performance of the index test, dengue NS1 ICT, in each setting using whole blood at point of care (POC) and serum in the laboratory in readings at 15′ and 30′, compared to the standard reference, the following measures of accuracy were considered: sensitivity (Sn), specificity (Sp), positive and negative predictive values (PPV, NPV), and positive and negative likelihood ratios (LR+) and (LR-) with the respective 95% confidence intervals (95% CI). Post-test probabilities were calculated for scenarios with prevalence rates of 30%, 50%, and 83.3%, using the Fagan nomogram [28].

The sensitivity and specificity of the index test in different settings were compared for using the χ^2 McNemar test [29].

Reliability was assessed by the variability of the ICT results in whole blood/POC and serum/laboratory with readings at 15 min. Inter-observer reliability was analyzed by the readings done by the two professionals (nurse and biologist) and intra-observer reliability by the same professional (nurse), in blinded fashion. The proportions of positive agreement (Ppos) and negative agreement (Pneg) were calculated, as well as simple and prevalence-adjusted bias-adjusted kappa (PABAK) coefficients with respective 95% CI [30]. Kappa values (k) were interpreted according to the classification by Landis & Koch [31]: poor ($k < 0.0$), slight ($0.0 < k < 0.2$), fair ($0.2 < k < 0.4$), moderate ($0.4 < k < 0.6$), substantial ($0.6 < k < 0.8$), almost perfect ($0.8 < k < 1.00$), and perfect agreement ($k = 1$).

Statistical significance was set at $p < 0.05$.

The software packages used were R Commander 3.2.1, WinPepi 11.50, and MedCalc 15.8 [32–34].

Results

Of 148 patients recruited, four were excluded due to five or more days of fever (Fig. 1). Of the 144 patients included, 52.8% were women. Patients' median age was 34.5 years, with higher ages in the dengue group (median: 36.1 years, ranging from 18 to 82.4) than in the non-dengue group (median: 27 years, ranging from 18.8 to 62.9), $p = 0.019$.

Patients presented a median of 1.4 days of fever (95% IQR: 1–2), and the most frequent symptoms were myalgia (91%), headache (89.6%), asthenia (83.3%), and arthralgia (73%). None of the patients evidenced clinical severity signs according to WHO 2009 criteria [4].

Prevalence of the disease was 83.3%. Of the 120 positive cases, 40.3% ($n = 58$) were primary infections. The dengue virus was characterized by RT-PCR in 105 samples and 15 exclusively by NS1 ELISA. Four samples that were negative for dengue by RT-PCR and NS1 ELISA

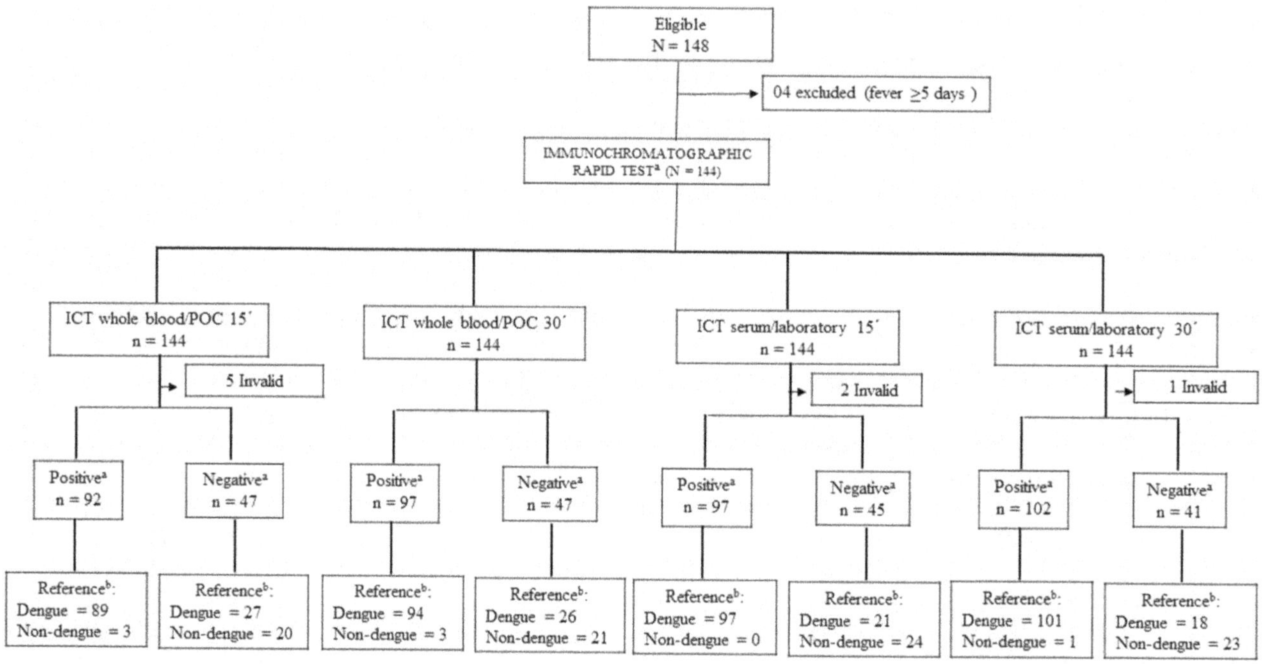

Fig. 1 Sample selection and laboratory analysis of 144 suspected dengue cases during a DENV-1 epidemic. a: rapid immunocromatographic test (index test), b: RT-PCR or ELISA NS1 positive (reference test)

were positive for Zika virus. One Zika Positive sample tested positive in IgM ELISA.

For all the five invalid cases on readings performed at 15 min in whole blood at POC, readings repeated at 30 min tested positive. For two serum samples at the laboratory showing invalid readings at 15 min, one turned positive at 30 min and the other remained invalid (Fig. 1).

ICT performance was similar in the two settings independently of reading times, both in the point estimate and 95% CI. Sensitivity of ICT with the 15-min reading varied from 76.7% in whole blood at point of care to 82.2% in serum in the laboratory. For the 30-min reading, sensitivity was 78.3% using whole blood at point of care and 84.9% in serum in the laboratory (Table 1). Specificity at 15-was 87% for whole blood at point of care and 100% for serum at the laboratory. For 30-min readings, specificity was 87.5% for whole blood at point of care and 95.8% for serum in the laboratory.

Positive predictive value was high (Table 1) in the prevalence observed in the study (83.3%). In scenarios with prevalence rates of 30% (72.4% CI: 49.3–87.7) or 50% (86%, 95% CI: 69.3–94.3), the PPV remains high. The negative predictive value would increase to 78.9% (95% CI: 72.3–84.3) with a decrease in prevalence in a scenario with 50% prevalence and to 89.7% (95% CI: 85.9–92.6) in a scenario with 30% prevalence.

The reliability between whole blood/POC and serum/laboratory was almost perfect, when evaluated both by the same observer (k = 0.83 CI: 0.74–0.93) and by different observers (k = 0.81 CI: 0.72–0.92), and remained almost perfect even when adjusted by prevalence bias. However, considering the lower limit of Kappa 95% Confidence Interval, reliability interpretation decreased from almost perfect to substantial both for inter-observer (0.73) and for intra-observer 0.75) (Table 2).

Discussion

This study assessed the Bioeasy™ rapid immunochromatographic test for DENV-1 NS1 antigen in a high-prevalence setting with adults in Rio de Janeiro State, Brazil, and found similar performance when testing was compared in whole blood/POC and serum/laboratory.

This was the first study to date comparing the performance of NS1 Bioeasy™ ICT in two scenarios, one in a laboratory setting with professionals trained to perform diagnostic tests and the other in a real-world setting (point of care). The evaluation at POC was conducted in the spontaneous treatment flow in an emergency care unit during an epidemic period, with whole blood samples drawn by different professionals. The accuracy of NS1 Bioeasy™ ICT in whole blood/POC showed sensitivity of 76.7% and specificity of 87% at the 15-minuute reading, similar to that found by Gan et al. [21] for Bioline™ ICT SD with whole blood/POC in a predominantly DENV-2 sample, i.e., Sn = 81.6%, 95% CI: 74.6–87.1 and Sp = 98%, 95% CI: 89.5–99.7.

Table 1 Accuracy of Bioeasy™ rapid immunochromatographic test at point of care and in the laboratory

	Readings at 15′		Readings at 30′	
	Whole blood/POC[a]	Serum/Laboratory[b]	Whole blood/POC[a]	Serum/Laboratory[b]
Sensitivity	76.7%[c]	82.2%[c]	78.3%[c]	84.9%[c]
(95%CI)	(68.0–84.1)	(74.1–88.6)	(69.9–85.3)	(77.2–90.8)
Specificity	87.0%[d]	100.0%[d]	87.5%[d]	95.8%[d]
(95% CI)	(66.4–97.2)	(85.8–100.0)	(67.6–97.3)	(78.9–99.9)
PPV	96.7%	100.0%	96.9%	99.0%
(95%CI)	(90.8–99.3)	(96.3% - 100.0)	(91.2–99.4)	(95.4–99.8)
NPV	42.6%	53.3%	44.7%	56.1%
(95%CI)	(28.3–57.8)	(37.9–68.3)	(30.2–59.9)	(39.8–71.5)
LR+	5.9	19.8[e]	6.27	20.4
(95%CI)	(2.0–17.0)	(2.9–135.1)	(2.2–18.1)	(3.0–139.0)
LR-	0.27	0.18	0.25	0.16
(95%CI)	(0.19–0.39)	(0.12–0.26)	(0.17–0.36)	(0.10–0.24)

POC point of care, *95% CI* 95% confidence interval, *PPV* positive predictive value, *NPV* negative predictive value, *LR+* positive likelihood ratio, *LR-* negative likelihood ratio

[a]Performed with whole blood

[b]Performed with serum

[c]P-value <0.01

[d]P-value >0.05 of χ^2 McNemar test

[e]LR+ calculated using 97.9% specificity

DENV-1 ICT in serum in the laboratory showed a slight increase in accuracy, i.e., Sn = 82.2% and Sp = 100%. The literature reports variability in sensitivity according to serotype, with better performance in serotypes 1, 2, and 3, varying from 69% [7] to 81.8% [8] in DENV-1, from 62% [7] to 81.8% in DENV-2, and from 61.3% to 81.2% [8] in DENV-3, as compared to variation from 44.5% [23] to 84.8% [8] in DENV-4, so that the tests need to be improved in order to perform independently of serotype.

NS1 ICT manufacturers recommend readings at 15 or 20 min [13, 35]. However, in the current study five cases of whole blood specimens at point of care that were invalid at 15 min turned positive at 30 min, and one of the two invalid results at 15 min with serum in the laboratory turned positive at 30 min. Dussart et al. [8] and Osorio et al. [14] used ICT with serum in the laboratory and also reported improved accuracy at the 30-min reading.

Table 2 Reliability at 15′ of rapid immunochromatographic test comparing whole blood/POC and serum/laboratory

	Kappa	Ppos	Pneg	PABAK
Inter-observer[a] (*n* = 135)	0.81	94%	86.7%	0.83
(95% CI)	(0.73–0.88)	(90.6–97.3)	(79.6–93.8)	
Intra-observer[b] (*n* = 137)	0.82	94.2%	87.6%	0.84
(95% CI)	(0.75–0.89)	(90.9–97.5)	(80.8–94.5)	

Kappa simple kappa, *Ppos* positive proportion, *Pneg* negative proportion, *PABAK* prevalence-adjusted bias-adjusted kappa, *95% CI* confidence interval, *n* absolute number

[a]inter-observer: nurse (blood/POC) and biologist (serum/laboratory)

[b]intra-observer: nurse (blood/POC and serum/laboratory)

The high number of false-negatives suggests that this ICT should not be used to screen for cases, as recommended even by the manufacturer [13] and Andries et al. [15]. The low number of false-positives and the high likelihood of post-testing in this study suggest that the test could be used for diagnostic confirmation. Robustness of this result is strengthened by the use of composite reference test, comprising PCR Dengue [24] and ELISA Dengue NS1 Platelia. The latter has shown very high specificity (100%) in DENV-1 in a previous study [36].

Inter and intra-observer reliability was almost perfect in this study independently of the type of specimen examined (whole blood or serum), the setting (POC or laboratory), and the level of training of the professionals that performed the test. This result corroborates Gan et al. [21].

Evidence for Zika and Dengue cross reactivity has, so far, been identified for IgM ELISA dengue but not for ELISA NS1 dengue tests [27, 37]. In our study, one of four Zika positive samples showed cross-reactivity with IgM Dengue ELISA, but none cross-react with NS1 ELISA Dengue. Increasingly acute febrile syndromes will demand investigation for several flaviviruses.

A possible limitation to the study was the high prevalence of dengue, but the post-test likelihoods were provided for different prevalence scenarios. The evaluation of a single serotype, DENV-1, may have been a limitation, but it resulted from a consecutive patient sample in an epidemic period. The comparison of whole blood/POC and serum/laboratory precludes other comparisons such as serum/POC and whole blood/laboratory, but it represents the possible routine use in emergency care departments without the necessary infrastructure for processing serum specimens during epidemics.

Considering NS1 Bioeasy™ ICT an ASSURED test [6], these recommendations may be particularly useful at sites without laboratory infrastructure or in hyperendemic scenarios, since they would offer faster turnaround of test results, thus favoring diagnosis in emergencies or remote sites [16].

In health services with some laboratory infrastructure, we recommend the use of NS1 ICT with serum in the laboratory, since it is approximately three times more positive in individuals with dengue than without (LR + = 19.8) when compared to whole blood specimens at point of care (LR + = 5.9). However, in services without laboratory infrastructure or during DEN-V 1 epidemics, we recommend screening according to WHO criteria [4] based on clinical signs followed by NS1 Bioeasy™ ICT in whole blood/POC and reading at 15 min and rereading of invalid results at 30 min.

In addition, investment to improve the performance of these tests in whole blood would allow better diagnostic confirmation, potentially optimizing the flow and efficiency of care and treatment. Training strategies for different levels of health professionals involved in performing and reading the NS1 ICT in whole blood at point of care can guarantee the reliability and adequate implementation in the clinical management of suspected cases.

Conclusions

Bioeasy™ NS1 antigen rapid immunochromatographic test showed a good accuracy during the epidemic of DENV-1, particularly for confirmatory diagnosis. It may be useful at the point of care, with no more than a drop of whole blood, since it is rapid and simple to do by minimal trained health personnel. In this context, Bioeasy™ is relevant for the early diagnosis of dengue, particularly at sites without laboratorial infrastructure and in epidemic or hyperendemic scenarios.

Abbreviations

ASSURED: Affordable, sensitive, specific, user-friendly, robust, rapid, equipment-free, and deliverable to those who need them; C: Control line; CI: Confidence interval; DALYs: Disability-adjusted life years; DENV: Dengue virus; DENV-1: Dengue virus serotype 1; DENV-2: Dengue virus serotype 2; DENV-3: Dengue virus serotype 3; DENV-4: Dengue virus serotype 4; EDTA: Ethylenediaminetetraacetic acid; ELISA: Enzyme-linked immunosorbent assay; ICR: Immunochromatographic rapid test; IgG: Immunoglobulin G; IgM: Immunoglobulin M; Kappa: Simple Kappa; LR–: Negative likelihood ratio; LR+: Positive likelihood ratio; NPV: Negative predictive value; NS1: Nonstructural protein-1; PABAK: Prevalence and bias adjusted kappa; POC: Point of care; PPV: Positive predictive value; RT-PCR: Reverse-transcription polymerase chain reaction; S: Sensitivity; Sp: Specificity; STARD: Standards for Reporting of Diagnostic Accuracy Study; T: Test line; WHO: World Health Organization

Acknowledgements

The authors wish to thank for field work, Rogério Ferrari, Ana Victória Palagi Viganó, Indiara Firmino Brito and Letícia Borges dos Santos.

Funding

This study was supported by the National Council for Scientific and Technological Development (CNPq) [grant numbers 401,366/2013–8] - Brazilian Network for Technological and Health Assessment (REBRATS), Excellence Program in Clinical Research of the Oswaldo Cruz Foundation (PROEP/PCLIN) [grant numbers N° 402,068/2012–2] and the Foundation for Research Support in the State of Rio de Janeiro (FAPERJ) [grant numbers E-25/110.188/2014]. Fellowship grant from CNPq [grant numbers 311,414/2013–3] and UNESA - Productivity Research to [SRLP] and scholarship from FAPERJ [grant numbers 221,354 E_01/2016] to [VEM].

Authors' contributions

VEM conceived of the study, participated in its design, data collection, recording, carried out rapid immunochromatographic test and coordination and helped to draft the manuscript. SRLP conceived of the study, participated in its design and coordination and helped to draft the manuscript. YHMH and MABS participated in the study design, data analysis and interpretation and helped to draft the manuscript. GMB, LVBF and ACFSRM participated in its design, data collection and recording. CDSR and ASS carried out the immunoassays, viral characterization and writing the manuscript. RVCO participated in the design of the study and performed the statistical analysis. All authors read and approved the final manuscript.

Consent for publication

Not applicable.

Competing interests

The authors declare that they have no competing interests.

Author details

[1]Av. Brasil 4036 sala 201 A, CEP 21040-361 Rio de Janeiro, RJ, Brasil. [2]Rua Leopoldo Bulhões 1480 sala 601, Rio de Janeiro, RJ CEP 21040-361, Brazil. [3]Av. Brasil 4365, CEP 21040-360 Rio de Janeiro, RJ, Brasil.

References

1. Guzman MG, Halstead SB, Artsob H, Buchy P, Farrar J, Gubler DJ, et al. Dengue: a continuing global threat. Nat Rev Microbiol. 2010;8(12 Suppl):S7–16.
2. Constenla D, Armien B, Arredondo J, Carabali M, Carrasquilla G, Castro R, et al. Costing dengue fever cases and outbreaks: recommendations from a costing dengue working group in the Americas. Value Health Reg Issues. 2015;8C:80–91.
3. Shepard DS, Undurradga EA, Halasa YA, Stanaway JD. The global economic burden of dengue: a systematic analysis. Lancet Infect Dis. 2016;16(8):935–41.
4. World Health Organization. Dengue – Guidelines for diagnosis, treatment, prevention and control. Geneva: WHO; 2009. p. 11. http://www.who.int/tdr/publications/documents/dengue-diagnosis.pdf. Accessed 09 Apr 2016.

5. Goodman C, Faulkner E, Gould C, Karnes E, Smith A, Aguiar C, et al. The Value of Diagnostics Innovation, Adoption and Diffusion into Health Care. The Lewin Group, Inc. AdvaMed. 2005. https://dx.advamed.org/sites/dx.advamed.org/files/resource/Lewin%20Value%20of%20Diagnostics%20Report.pdf. Accessed 15 Dec 2016.
6. Peeling RW, Mabey D. Point-of-care tests for diagnosing infections in the developing world. Clin Microbiol Infect. 2010;16(8):1062–9.
7. Fry SR, Meyer M, Semple MG, Simmons CP, Sekaran SD, Huang JX, et al. The diagnostic sensitivity of dengue rapid test assays is significantly enhanced by using a combined antigen and antibody testing approach. PLoS Negl Trop Dis. 2011;5(6):e1199.
8. Dussart P, Petit L, Labeau B, Bremand L, Leduc A, Moua D, et al. Evaluation of two new commercial tests for the diagnosis of acute dengue virus infection using NS1 antigen detection in human serum. PLoS Negl Trop Dis. 2008;2(8):e280.
9. Pok KY, Lai YL, Sng J, Ng LC. Evaluation of nonstructural 1 antigen assays for the diagnosis and surveillance of dengue in Singapore. Vector-Borne and Zoonotic Dis. 2010;10(10):1009–16.
10. Tricou V, Vu HTT, Quynh NVN, Nguyen CW, Tran CT, Farrar J, et al. Comparison of two dengue NS1 rapid tests for sensitivity, specificity and relationship to viraemia and antibody responses. BMC Infect Dis. 2010;10:142.
11. Lima MdRQ, Nogueira RMR, Schatzmayr HG, Santos FBd. Comparison of three commercially available dengue NS1 antigen capture assays for acute diagnosis of dengue in Brazil. PLoS Negl Trop Dis. 2010;4(7):e738.
12. Ferraz FO, Bomfim MRQ, Totola AH, Ávila TV, Cisalpino D, Pessanha JEM, et al. Evaluation of laboratory tests for dengue diagnosis in clinical specimens from consecutive patients with suspected dengue in Belo Horizonte, Brazil. J Clin Virol. 2013;58:41–6.
13. Dengue Eden Test Bioeasy®. Korea: Bioeasy Diagnóstica Ltda. 2015. http://www.masterdiagnostica.com.br/public/files/produtos/1394214631139421463132631 16009.pdf. Accessed 6 May 2017.
14. Osorio L, Ramirez M, Bonelo A, Villar LA, Parra B. Comparison of the diagnostic accuracy of commercial NS1-based diagnostic tests for early dengue infection. Virol J. 2010;7:361.
15. Andries AC, Duong V, Ngan C, Ong S, Huy R, Sroin KK, et al. Field evaluation and impact on clinical management of a rapid diagnostic kit that detects dengue NS1, IgM and IgG. PLoS Negl Trop Dis. 2012;6(12):e1993.
16. Pai NP, Vadnais C, Denkinger C, Engel N, Pai M. Point-of-care testing for infectious diseases: diversity, complexity, and barriers in low- and middle-income countries. PLoS Med. 2012;9(9):e1001306.
17. Ty Hang V, Minh Nguyet N, The Trung D, Tricou V, Yoksan S, Dung NM, et al. Diagnostic accuracy of NS1 ELISA and lateral flow rapid tests for dengue sensitivity, specificity and relationship to viraemia and antibody responses. PLoS Negl Trop Dis. 2009;3(1):e360.
18. Palamountain KM, Baker J, Cowan LP, Essajee S, Mazzola LT, Metzler M, et al. Perspectives on introduction and implementation of new point-of-care diagnostic tests. J Infect Dis. 2012;205(Suppl 2):S181–90.
19. Martínez-Veja RA, Díaz-Quijano FA, Coronel-Ruiz C, Gómez SY, Villar-Centeno LA. Evaluación de la utilidad de la prueba rápida de casete por imunocromatografía para el diagnóstico de dengue en una región endémica colombiana. Biomedica. 2009;29:616–24.
20. Hunsperger EA, Yoksan S, Buchy P, Nguyem VC, Sekaran SD, Enria DA, et al. Evaluation of commercially available diagnostic tests for the detection of dengue virus NS1 antigen and anti-dengue virus IgM antibody. PLoS Negl Trop Dis. 2014;8(10):e3171.
21. Gan VC, Tan L-K, Lye DC, Pok K-Y, Mok S-Q, Chua RC-R, et al. Diagnosing dengue at the point-of-care: utility of a rapid combined diagnostic kit in Singapore. PLoS ONE. 2014;9(3):e90037.
22. Korevaar DA, Wang J, van Enst WA, Leeflang MM, Hooft L, Smidt N, et al. Reporting diagnostic accuracy studies: some improvements after 10 years of STARD. Radiology. 2015;274:781–9.
23. Buonora SN, Passos SRL, do Carmo CN, Quintela FM, de Oliveira DNR, dos Santos FB, et al. Accuracy of clinical criteria and an immunochromatographic strip test for dengue diagnosis in a DENV-4 epidemic. BMC Infect Dis. 2016;16:37.
24. Lanciotti RS, Calisher CH, Gubler DJ, Chang GJ, Vorndam AV. Rapid detection and typing of dengue viruses from clinical samples by using reverse transcriptase-polymerase chain reaction. J Clin Microbiol. 1992;30(3): 545–51.
25. Platelia™ Dengue NS1 AG®. France: Bio-Rad Laboratories, Inc.. 2008. http://www.biorad.com/webroot/web/pdf/inserts/CDG/en/72830_881149_EN.pdf. Accessed 6 May 2017.
26. Lanciotti RS, Kosoy OL, Laven JJ, Velez JO, Lambert AJ, Johnson AJ, et al. Genetic and serologic properties of Zika virus associated with an epidemic, Yap State, Micronesia, 2007. Emerg Infect Dis. 2008;14(8):1232–9.
27. Serion Elisa Classic Dengue Virus IgG/IgM Virion\Serion®. Germany: Institut Virion\Serion GmbH. 2012. http://www.virionserion. de/download/flyer/Flyer_ELISA_classic_Dengue_Virus_EN.pdf. Accessed 6 May 2017.
28. Fagan TJ. Nomogram for Bayes theorem [letter]. N Engl J Med. 1975;293(5):257.
29. Trajman A, Luiz RR. McNemar $\chi 2$ test revisited: comparing sensitivity and specificity of diagnostic examinations. Scand J Clin Lab Invest. 2007;68(1):77–80.
30. Byrt T, Bishop J, Carlin JB. Bias, prevalence and kappa. J Clin Epidemiol. 1993; 46(5):423–9.
31. Landis JR, Koch GG. The measurement of observer agreement for categorical data. Biometrics. 1977;33:159–74.
32. R Core Team. R: A language and environment for statistical computing. Vienna: R Foundation for Statistical Computing; 2015. https://www.R-project.org/.
33. Abramson JH. WINPEPI updated: computer programs for epidemiologists, and their teaching potential. Epidemiol Perspect Innov. 2011;8:1.
34. MedCalc Statistical Software version 12.7.8. Ostend: MedCalc Software bvba; 2014. https://www.medcalc.org.
35. IVB Dengue Ag NS1 OrangeLife®. Brazil: Orangelife comércio e indústria Ltda. 2016. http://www.dmed.com.br/manuais/denguens1orangelife.pdf. Accessed 07 Jan 2016.
36. Pal S, Dauner AL, Mitra I, Forshey BM, Garcia P, Morrison AC, Halsey ES, Kochel TJ, Wu SJ. Evaluation of dengue NS1 antigen rapid tests and Elisa kits using clinical samples. PLoS One. 2014;9(11):e113411.
37. Matheus S, Boukhari R, Labeau B, Ernault V, Bremand L, Kazanji M, Rousset D. Specificity of Dengue NS1 antigen in differential diagnosis of dengue and Zika virus infection. Emerg Infect Dis. 2016;22(9):1691–2.

27

Genetic variants of *MICB* and *PLCE1* and associations with the laboratory features of dengue

James Whitehorn[1,2*], Duong Thi Hue Kien[2], Nguyen Than Ha Quyen[2], Bridget Wills[2,3], Nguyen Van Vinh Chau[4], Dong Thi Hoai Tam[4], Nguyen Minh Tuan[5], Thomas Jaenisch[6], Martin Hibberd[1,7], Chiea Chuen Khor[8,9,10] and Cameron P. Simmons[11]

Abstract

Background: A previous genome-wide association study identified 2 susceptibility loci for severe dengue at *MICB* rs3132468 and *PLCE1* rs3740360 and further work showed these mutations to be also associated with less severe clinical presentations. The aim of this study was to determine if these specific loci were associated with laboratory features of dengue that correlate with clinical severity with the aim of elucidating the functional basis of these genetic variants.

Methods: This was a case-only analysis of laboratory-confirmed dengue patients obtained from 2 prospective cohort studies and 1 randomised clinical trial in Vietnam (Trial registration: ISRCTN ISRCTN03147572. Registered 24th July 2012). 2742 dengue cases were successfully genotyped at *MICB* rs3132468 and *PLCE1* rs3740360. Laboratory variables were compared between genotypes and stratified by DENV serotype.

Results: The analysis showed no association between *MICB* and *PLCE1* genotype and early viraemia level, platelet nadir, white cell count nadir, or maximum haematocrit in both overall analysis and in analysis stratified by serotype.

Discussion: The lack of an association between genotype and viremia level may reflect the sampling procedures within the included studies. The study findings mean that the functional basis of these mutations remains unclear.

Background

Dengue viruses (DENV) cause a spectrum of clinical manifestations ranging from asymptomatic infection through to life-threatening shock and haemorrhage [1, 2]. Single nucleotide polymorphisms (SNPs) at two genomic loci are associated with DSS in Vietnamese children [3]. These SNPs were in the major histocompatibility complex class I polypeptide-related sequence B gene (*MICB*) on chromosome 6 (rs3132468) and in the phospholipase C epsilon 1 (*PLCE 1*) gene on chromosome 10 (rs3740360). Further work demonstrated that these variations are also significantly associated with less severe but medically attended dengue cases dengue [4, 5]. The *MICB* gene encodes a surface protein that contributes to natural killer (NK) cell activation. The observed association with a SNP in the *MICB* gene and dengue shock syndrome (DSS) may reflect dysfunctional NK and CD8 cell activity in severe disease, suggesting a key role for these cells in disease control and pathogenesis. Mutations in *PLCE1* are associated with nephrotic syndrome, a condition characterised by proteinuria, reduced vascular oncotic pressure and subsequent oedema [6]. The association with mutations in *PLCE1* and dengue raises the possibility of a role for this gene in the maintenance of normal endothelial integrity. Despite these speculations, the functional basis for the association of these mutations with DSS remains unclear.

The aim of this study was to measure if an association existed between the aforementioned *MICB* and *PLCE1* specific mutations and virological and hematological features of dengue that have been shown to have correlation with the clinical outcome of infection. For example, the level of

* Correspondence: james.whitehorn@lshtm.ac.uk
[1]Department of Clinical Research, London School of Hygiene and Tropical Medicine, London, UK
[2]Oxford University Clinical Research Unit, Hospital for Tropical Diseases, 764 Vo Van Kiet, District 5, Ho Chi Minh City, Viet Nam
Full list of author information is available at the end of the article

viremia in the first days of illness is positively associated with the severity of the disease phenotype [7]. Similarly, the degrees of lymphopenia and thrombocytopenia are associated with development of DSS [8, 9]. Thus this study tested the hypothesis that the *MICB* (rs3132468) and *PLCE1* (rs3740360) variants were associated with clinically important laboratory features of dengue.

Methods

The specific aims of this analysis were to measure the association between individuals with different *MICB* rs3132468 and *PLCE1* rs3740360 genotypes (wild-type, heterozygous carriers, and homozygous variant) and various laboratory features. The laboratory features that were compared between the groups were (1) early plasma viremia level, (2) platelet nadir, (3) white cell count nadir, and (4) maximum haematocrit.

Samples were obtained from participants who gave written informed consent to participate in the previously reported prospective studies detailed in Table 1 [10–12]. Parents or guardians of the children involved in the studies gave written informed consent on their behalf. All these studies took place in southern Vietnam. The protocols of these studies were reviewed and approved by the Institutional Review Boards of each study site (Hospital for Tropical Diseases Ho Chi Minh City (HCMC), Children's Hospital 1 and 2 HCMC, and Tien Giang Hospital) and by the Oxford University Tropical Research Ethics Committee. The inclusion criteria for 13DX were (1) fever or history of fever for less than 72 h, (2) clinical suspicion of dengue, (3) 1–15 years of age, (4) written informed consent, and (5) accompanying family member has a mobile phone. The exclusion criteria were (1) deemed unlikely to attend follow-up, and (2) in whom an alternative diagnosis was thought more likely. The inclusion criteria for 22DX were (1) fever or history of fever for less than 72 h, (2) clinical suspicion of dengue, (3) aged 5 years or over, (4) written informed consent. The exclusion criteria were (1) localising features suggesting an alternative diagnosis, and (2) inability to attend daily follow-up. The inclusion criteria for 26DX were (1) age 18 or over, (2) presenting within 72 h of fever onset with an illness consistent with dengue, (3) positive rapid test for dengue non-structural protein 1 (NS1 (NS1 Ag-STRIP, Bio-Rad). The exclusion criteria were (1) alanine transaminase (ALT) level > 150 U/L, (2) creatine kinase (CK) level > 1000 U/L, (3) platelet count <50 × 10^9/L, (4) pregnancy or lactation, and (5) a history of cirrhosis or myopathy.

This was a case-only analysis of laboratory-confirmed dengue patients obtained from two prospective cohort studies and one randomised clinical trial in Vietnam. The cohort studies were conducted in both adults and children and aimed to create diagnostic and prognostic algorithms to improve the clinical management of dengue in this setting. The randomised clinical trial was an investigation of lovastatin therapy in adult patients with dengue.

DNA extractions were performed using a MagNA Pure 96 DNA and Viral NA Small Volume Kit (Roche, Germany) according to the manufacturer's instructions. Candidate SNPs were genotyped using a TaqMan genotyping assay to amplify and detect the specific alleles in the DNA samples as per the manufacturer instructions. Samples failing picogreen QC (<5 ng/uL in concentration) were excluded from further analysis. Similarly, during the genotyping process, samples, which fail to show adequate allelic discrimination on the Taqman RT-PCR melt-curve, were also excluded from analysis. Each SNP has been shown previously to show good call rate exceeding >95%.

Statistical analysis was performed in Stata 13 (Stata Statistical Software: Release 13. College Station, TX. StataCorp LP). Laboratory variables were compared between genotypes and stratified by DENV serotype using the binary chi-squared test, the Kruskal-Wallis nonparametric test and the analysis of variance test. A sample size calculation was not performed, as a priori, the variance of the viremia measurements was not known.

Results

Two thousand seven hundred forty two dengue cases were successfully genotyped at *MICB* rs3132468 and *PLCE1* rs3740360. 573 cases were in adults (age ≥ 15) and 2180 were in children. There were 109 cases of severe dengue across the cohorts (6 in adults and 103 in children). The baseline characteristics of the study participants are summarised in Table 2.

Association between MICB rs3132468 and enrolment viremia

The mean viremia was compared between patients with the spectrum of *MICB* genotypes. The mean viremia in patients carrying the C/C allele was 7.16 (95% CI: 6.84–7.47) $\log_{10}$-copies/mL. In those with the C/T allele it was 7.05 (95% CI: 6.92–7.18) $\log_{10}$-copies/mL, and in those with the T/T allele it was 7.08 (95% CI: 7.01–7.15) $\log_{10}$-

Table 1 Details of studies included in analysis

Study	Setting	Study type	Age criteria (years)	Number (% male)	Laboratory sampling procedure	Median age (range 5th–95th centile)
13DX	Outpatient	Prospective cohort	1–15	1951 (57)	Enrolment only	9 (3–14)
22DX	Outpatient	Prospective cohort	5 or over	749 (60)	Multiple time points	18 (6–39)
26DX	Inpatient	Randomised clinical trial	18 or over	42 (57)	Multiple time points	24 (18–51)

Table 2 Collated study population characteristics (n = 2730)

	DENV1 (n = 1042)	DENV2 (n = 593)	DENV3 (n = 263)	DENV4 (n = 832)	All (n = 2730)
Age (median, IQR), years	10(7–13)	10(7–14)	9(6–13)	11(8–15)	10(7–14)
Sex (n,%)					
Male	596(57.2)	357(60.2)	147(55.9)	474(57.0)	1574(57.7)
Female	446(42.8)	236(39.8)	116(44.1)	358(43.0)	1156(42.3)
Days of illness at enrolment (n,%)					
0	9(0.86)	1(0.17)	0(0)	3(0.36)	13(0.48)
1	323(31.0)	174(29.3)	85(32.3)	195(23.4)	777(28.5)
2	437(41.9)	271(45.7)	113(43.0)	354(42.5)	1175(43.0)
3	269(25.8)	146(24.6)	64(24.3)	279(33.5)	758(27.8)
4	2(0.19)	1(0.17)	1(0.4)	0(0)	4(0.15)
Viremia (mean, 95% CI), log10 copies/mL	7.39(7.29–7.50)	6.89(6.77–7.01)	7.14(6.94–7.33)	6.80(6.71–6.88)	7.08(7.02–7.14)
Clinical classification (n,%)					
Dengue	950(91.2)	553(93.3)	257(97.7)	780(93.8)	2540(93.0)
Severe dengue	39(3.74)	32(5.4)	6(2.3)	32(3.85)	109(3.99)

copies/mL. The difference between these values was not statistically significant. The comparison in viremia levels between *MICB* genotypes was repeated with data stratified by DENV serotype. Again, no significant differences were demonstrated. These data are summarised in Table 3. Collectively, these data indicate some variation in the viremia between the serotypes but no significant difference between the *MICB* genotypes.

Association between PLCE1 rs3740360 and enrolment viraemia

The mean viremia was compared between the *PLCE1* genotypes. The mean viremia in patients carrying the A/A allele was 7.08 (95% CI: 7.00–7.15) $\log_{10}$-copies/mL. In those carrying the A/C allele it was 7.09 (95% CI: 6.99–7.19) $\log_{10}$-copies/mL, and in those with the C/C allele it was 7.02 (95% CI: 6.78–7.26) $\log_{10}$-copies/mL. The difference between these values was not statistically significant. The comparison in viremia levels between *PLCE1* genotypes was repeated with data stratified by DENV serotype. Again, no significant differences were demonstrated. These data are summarised in Table 3. As above, these data indicate some variation in the viremia level between the serotypes but no significant difference between the *PLCE1* genotypes.

Association between MICB rs3132468 and other laboratory variables

After excluding data from 13DX, which only included enrolment results, the platelet nadir, the maximum haematocrit and the minimum white cell count were

Table 3 Viremia by *MICB* and *PLCE* genotype by dengue serotype and overall (mean (IQR) (N))

MICB				
Serotype	C/C	C/T	T/T	*P*-value
DENV1	7.32 (6.7–7.95) (n = 24)	7.28 (7.03–7.53) (n = 211)	7.43 (7.31–7.55) (n = 761)	0.238
DENV2	7.04 (6.32–7.76) (n = 18)	7.03 (6.77–7.29) (n = 125)	6.84 (6.7–6.98) (n = 450)	0.833
DENV3	6.99 (5.24–8.75) (n = 7)	7.15 (6.7–7.6) (n = 50)	7.14 (6.91–7.36) (n = 206)	0.836
DENV4	7.13 (6.67–7.59) (n = 28)	6.75 (6.56–6.93) (n = 184)	6.8 (6.7–6.9) (n = 620)	0.86
Overall	7.16 (6.84–7.47) (n = 78)	7.05 (6.92–7.18) (n = 583)	7.08 (7.01–7.15) (n = 2081)	0.315
PLCE				
Serotype	A/A	A/C	C/C	*P*-value
DENV1	7.38 (7.24–7.53) (n = 578)	7.39 (7.22–7.56) (n = 397)	7.47 (7.03–7.91) (n = 67)	0.972
DENV2	6.83 (6.67–7) (n = 334)	6.99 (6.79–7.19) (n = 215)	6.83 (6.38–7.29) (n = 44)	0.938
DENV3	7.08 (6.82–7.34) (n = 157)	7.19 (6.87–7.5) (n = 87)	7.32 (6.35–8.29) (n = 19)	0.198
DENV4	6.87 (6.75–6.98) (n = 472)	6.74 (6.99–7.19) (n = 306)	6.51 (6.18–6.83) (n = 54)	0.867
Overall	7.08 (7–7.15) (n = 1546)	7.09 (6.99–7.19) (n = 1012)	7.02 (6.78–7.26) (n = 184)	0.7

compared between the *MICB* genotypes in both an overall analysis and then stratified by serotype. The median platelet nadir in patients with the C/C allele was 82.5 (IQR: 47–101) × 10^9/L, in those with the C/T allele was 80 (IQR: 48–115) × 10^9/L, and in those with the T/T allele was 70 (41–113) × 10^9/L. These differences were not statistically significant. The minimum white cell count in those with the C/C allele was 2.6 (IQR: 2.3–3.1) × 10^9/L, in those with the C/T allele was 2.9 (IQR: 2.3–3.8) × 10^9/L and in those with the T/T allele was 2.7 (IQR: 2.1–3.4) × 10^9/L. These differences were not statistically significant. The median maximum haematocrit in patients with the C/C allele was 45.4% (IQR: 44–49.2%), in those with the C/T allele was 45% (IQR: 42–48.3%), and in those with the T/T allele was 44.7% (IQR: 41.8–48.4%). These differences were not statistically significant. When these data were stratified by DENV serotype again no significant differences were demonstrated. These data suggest no measurable association between *MICB* genotype and the laboratory variables explored in this analysis.

These data are summarised in Table 4.

Association between PLCE1 rs3740360 and other laboratory variables

The platelet nadir, the maximum haematocrit and the minimum white cell count were compared between the *PLCE1* genotypes in both an overall analysis and then stratified by serotype. The median platelet nadir in patients with the A/A allele was 71 (IQR: 41–109) × 10^9/L, in those with the A/C allele was 76.5 (IQR: 45–118) × 10^9/L, and in those with the C/C allele was 66 (37–114) × 10^9/L. These differences were not statistically significant. The minimum white cell count in those with the A/A allele was 2.7 (IQR: 2.1–3.4) × 10^9/L, in those with the A/C allele was 2.8 (IQR: 2.2–3.6) × 10^9/L and in those with the C/C allele was 2.9 (IQR: 2.2–3.6) × 10^9/L. These differences were not statistically significant. The median maximum haematocrit in patients with the A/A allele was 44.6% (IQR: 41.9–48.1%), in those with the A/C allele was 45.1% (IQR: 42–48.3%), and in those with the C/C allele was 45% (IQR: 42.4–50.3%). These differences were not statistically significant. When these data were stratified by DENV, serotype again no significant differences were demonstrated. These data suggest no measurable association between *PLCE1* genotype and the laboratory variables explored in this analysis.

These data are summarised in Table 4.

Discussion

This study did not find an association between *MICB* and *PLCE* genotype and early viremia level, platelet nadir, white cell count nadir or maximum haematocrit in both overall analysis and in analysis stratified by serotype. Given the possibility that *MICB* may have an important role in the establishment of antiviral effector function we proposed that mutations in this gene might be associated with higher dengue viraemia. Our analysis in 2742 adults and children with dengue showed no difference in the enrolment viraemia levels between the different *MICB* and *PLCE1* genotypes in both an overall analysis and analysis stratified by DENV serotype. The enrolment viremia was taken in the vast majority of patients in the first 72 h of clinical illness (Table 2). While our understanding of DENV kinetics suggests that this is likely to correspond near to the peak viraemia level it only gives a snapshot of the in vivo viral dynamics. It is possible that the viral clearance patterns varied across genotypes. In addition, measuring plasma viremia only provides a surrogate of what is happening in other tissues – obviously, however, invasive assessments of this would not be appropriate in large prospective studies. However, an interesting finding was the range of early viraemia levels across the DENV serotypes and between the different *MICB* and *PLCE* genotypes. While the observed variation was not statistically significant, it does suggest that there are factors that influence the early viremia level. This may be a combination of intrinsic genetic susceptibility, host immune status and various viral factors [13]. Determining the factors that influence the DENV "set point" would be intriguing and would advance our understanding of dengue pathogenesis.

Table 4 Laboratory features by *MICB* and *PLCE* genotype

MICB				
Laboratory/clinical feature	C/C (n = 18)	C/T (n = 150)	T/T (n = 554)	*P*-value
Platelet nadir (median(IQR))	82.5 (47–101)	80 (48–115)	70 (41–113)	0.494
Minimum white cell count (median(IQR))	2.6 (2.3–3.1)	2.9 (2.3–3.8)	2.7 (2.1–3.4)	0.214
Maximum haematocrit (median(IQR))	45.4 (44–49.2)	45 (42–48.3)	44.7 (41.8–48.4)	0.244
PLCE				
Laboratory/clinical feature	A/A (n = 409)	A/C (n = 266)	C/C (n = 47)	*P*-value
Platelet nadir (median(IQR))	71 (41–109)	76.5 (45–118)	66 (37–114)	0.675
Minimum white cell count (median(IQR))	2.7 (2.1–3.4)	2.8 (2.2–3.6)	2.9 (2.2–3.6)	0.268
Maximum haematocrit (median(IQR))	44.6 (41.9–48.1)	45.1 (42–48.3)	45 (42.4–50.3)	0.336

As no associations between viremia and genotype were shown, it is perhaps not surprising that no associations were demonstrated between genotype and the pre-selected routine haematological laboratory variables both in overall analysis and in analysis stratified by DENV serotype. These variables were chosen because they have been previously shown to have some correlation with dengue severity [8, 9]. However, differences in the study designs, particularly the frequency of laboratory investigations, across the cohorts described meant that the largest study in terms of patient numbers (13DX) was excluded from this component of the analysis.

While previous work has demonstrated an association between genetic variants of *MICB* and *PLCE1* and both severe and non-severe dengue, the functional basis of these associations is not clear [3, 4]. *MICB* encodes an activating ligand for natural killer cells, and possibly CD8+ T cells, raising the possibility that mutations in this gene may result in altered antiviral effector functions and an associated increased viral burden, a recognised risk factor for the development of severe dengue [7]. It is possible that the associations reflect an aspect of dengue pathogenesis unrelated to control of early viral replication. The association of *PLCE1* and dengue is harder to explain. It is interesting to note that mutations in this gene have been associated with nephrotic syndrome, regulation of blood pressure and oesophageal malignancy [6, 14, 15]. While it is plausible that the relationship between mutations in *PLCE1* and both severe dengue and nephrotic syndrome suggests some role in the maintenance of endothelial integrity, it is more difficult to relate this potential function to oesophageal malignancy. The role of *PLCE1* in control of blood pressure warrants further exploration as it raises the possibility of some overlap in function in dengue given hypotension is seen in severe dengue. While the hypotension in dengue shock is mediated largely by plasma leak, it is possible that variants in *PLCE1* play a contributory role. This relationship with diverse conditions suggests an important, but as yet unclear, role for *PLCE1* in human health and disease.

Our study has limitations. The number of patients with the "risk" alleles for *MICB* and *PLCE1* was relatively small, reflecting the low frequency of these allelic variants. The small number of cases may mean that the analysis lacked the power to detect a true association. This is especially true as the dose effect of a given SNP is likely to be small. Further work with a larger sample size may allow further exploration of a potential dose effect of a homozygous allelic variant on initial viremia. In addition, the study methodology varied between the studies included in the analysis meaning that it was only possible to explore the relationship between genotype and laboratory variable in a smaller group of patients. The functional basis of these observed associations remains unclear but it is possible that pooled data from prospective intervention studies will provide clearer insights. The potential offered by this study approach reflects the more frequent sampling that typically occurs in this type of study. It would be intriguing to explore whether these associations have an effect on cytokine levels – this could be explored within the context of prospective studies. Greater insights into dengue host susceptibility have the potential to expand our knowledge of disease pathogenesis and, in the longer term, assist the development of vaccines and therapeutics.

Conclusions

This study aimed to explore the functional basis of specific mutations in the *MICB* and *PLCE1* genes previously shown to be associated with severe dengue. We assessed whether these specific loci were associated with laboratory features of dengue that correlate with clinical severity. Our analysis showed no association between *MICB* and *PLCE1* genotype and early viraemia level, platelet nadir, white cell count nadir, or maximum haematocrit in both overall analysis and in analysis stratified by serotype. These results mean that the functional basis of these mutations remains unclear. It is possible that greater insights into dengue susceptibility and pathogenesis will be gained from careful analysis conducted within prospective studies.

Abbreviations

DENV: Dengue virus; DSS: Dengue shock syndrome; HCMC: Ho Chi Minh City; MICB: Major histocompatibility complex class I polypeptide-related sequence B gene; NK: Natural killer cells; PLCE1: Phospholipase C epsilon 1 gene; SNP: Single nucleotide polymorphism

Acknowledgements

Not applicable

Authors' contributions

Conception and design of study: JW, BW, NVVC, MH, TJ, DTHT, CCK, CPS. Patient recruitment and laboratory work: JW, DTHK, NTHQ, NVVC, DTHT, NMT, CCK. Analysis: JW, CCK, CPS. Writing: JW, BW, CCK, CPS with input from all authors. All authors read and approved the final manuscript.

Funding

This work was funded by the Wellcome Trust (grant numbers 097430/Z/11/Z and 084368/Z/07/Z and Genome Institute of Singapore intramural funding.

Competing interests

JW receives consulting fees from Janssen Pharmaceuticals related to their work on dengue antiviral development. CPS. is an occasional paid consultant to GlaxoSmithKline, Tibotec, and Unither Virology on the development of antiviral drugs for dengue. BW receives consulting fees for serving on the data monitoring committee for the Takeda Dengue Vaccine Trials program.

Consent for publication

Not applicable

Ethics approval and consent to participate

Samples were obtained from participants who gave written informed consent to participate in three previously reported prospective studies

13DX, 22DX and 22DX). These studies were conducted according to the principles of the Declaration of Helsinki. The protocols of these studies were reviewed and approved by the Institutional Review Boards of each study site (Hospital for Tropical Diseases Ho Chi Minh City (HCMC), Children's Hospital 1 and 2 HCMC, and Tien Giang Hospital) and by the Oxford University Tropical Research Ethics Committee. The ethics approval codes for 13DX were CS/ND/10/10 and OxTREC 35-10. The ethics approval codes for 22DX were CS/ND/11/08 and OxTREC 40-11. The ethics approval codes for 26DX were CS/ND/12/09 and OxTREC 40-11

Author details

[1]Department of Clinical Research, London School of Hygiene and Tropical Medicine, London, UK. [2]Oxford University Clinical Research Unit, Hospital for Tropical Diseases, 764 Vo Van Kiet, District 5, Ho Chi Minh City, Viet Nam. [3]Centre for Tropical Medicine, Nuffield Department of Medicine, University of Oxford, Oxford, UK. [4]Hospital for Tropical Diseases, 764 Vo Van Kiet, District 5, Ho Chi Minh City, Viet Nam. [5]Children Hospital Number 1, Ho Chi Minh City, Viet Nam. [6]Department of Infectious Diseases, Heidelberg University Hospital, Heidelberg, Germany. [7]Genome Institute of Singapore, Biopolis Way, Singapore, Singapore. [8]School of Public Health, National University of Singapore, Singapore, Singapore. [9]Department of Paediatrics, National University of Singapore, Singapore, Singapore. [10]Department of Ophthalmology, National University of Singapore, Singapore, Singapore. [11]Department of Microbiology and Immunology, University of Melbourne, at the Peter Doherty Institute, Melbourne, VIC 3010, Australia.

References

1. Simmons CP, Farrar JJ, Nguyen VV, Wills B. Dengue. N Engl J Med. 2012;366: 1423–32.
2. WHO. Dengue: guidelines for diagnosis, treatment, prevention and control. New ed. Geneva: World Health Organisation; 2009.
3. Khor CC, Chau TN, Pang J, Davila S, Long HT, et al. Genome-wide association study identifies susceptibility loci for dengue shock syndrome at MICB and PLCE1. Nat Genet. 2011;43:1139–41.
4. Whitehorn J, Chau TN, Nguyet NM, Kien DT, Quyen NT, et al. Genetic variants of MICB and PLCE1 and associations with non-severe dengue. PLoS One. 2013;8:e59067.
5. Dang TN, Naka I, Sa-Ngasang A, Anantapreecha S, Chanama S, et al. A replication study confirms the association of GWAS-identified SNPs at MICB and PLCE1 in Thai patients with dengue shock syndrome. BMC Med Genet. 2014;15:58.
6. Hinkes B, Wiggins RC, Gbadegesin R, Vlangos CN, Seelow D, et al. Positional cloning uncovers mutations in PLCE1 responsible for a nephrotic syndrome variant that may be reversible. Nat Genet. 2006;38:1397–405.
7. Libraty DH, Young PR, Pickering D, Endy TP, Kalayanarooj S, et al. High circulating levels of the dengue virus nonstructural protein NS1 early in dengue illness correlate with the development of dengue hemorrhagic fever. J Infect Dis. 2002;186:1165–8.
8. Kalayanarooj S, Vaughn DW, Nimmannitya S, Green S, Suntayakorn S, et al. Early clinical and laboratory indicators of acute dengue illness. J Infect Dis. 1997;176:313–21.
9. Noisakran S, Chokephaibulkit K, Songprakhon P, Onlamoon N, Hsiao HM, et al. A re-evaluation of the mechanisms leading to dengue hemorrhagic fever. Ann N Y Acad Sci. 2009;1171(Suppl 1):E24–35.
10. Whitehorn J, Nguyen CV, Khanh LP, Kien DT, Quyen NT, et al. Lovastatin for the treatment of adult patients with dengue: a randomized, double-blind, placebo-controlled trial. Clin Infect Dis. 2016;62:468–76.
11. Tuan NM, Nhan HT, Chau NV, Hung NT, Tuan HM, et al. Sensitivity and specificity of a novel classifier for the early diagnosis of dengue. PLoS Negl Trop Dis. 2015;9:e0003638.
12. Jaenisch T, Tam DT, Kieu NT, Van Ngoc T, Nam NT, et al. Clinical evaluation of dengue and identification of risk factors for severe disease: protocol for a multicentre study in 8 countries. BMC Infect Dis. 2016;16:120.
13. Chan KR, Wang X, Saron WA, Gan ES, Tan HC, et al. Cross-reactive antibodies enhance live attenuated virus infection for increased immunogenicity. Nat Microbiol. 2016;1:16164.
14. Ehret GB, Munroe PB, Rice KM, Bochud M, Johnson AD, et al. Genetic variants in novel pathways influence blood pressure and cardiovascular disease risk. Nature. 2011;478:103–9.
15. Abnet CC, Freedman ND, Hu N, Wang Z, Yu K, et al. A shared susceptibility locus in PLCE1 at 10q23 for gastric adenocarcinoma and esophageal squamous cell carcinoma. Nat Genet. 2010;42:764–7.

Permissions

All chapters in this book were first published in ID, by BioMed Central; hereby published with permission under the Creative Commons Attribution License or equivalent. Every chapter published in this book has been scrutinized by our experts. Their significance has been extensively debated. The topics covered herein carry significant findings which will fuel the growth of the discipline. They may even be implemented as practical applications or may be referred to as a beginning point for another development.

The contributors of this book come from diverse backgrounds, making this book a truly international effort. This book will bring forth new frontiers with its revolutionizing research information and detailed analysis of the nascent developments around the world.

We would like to thank all the contributing authors for lending their expertise to make the book truly unique. They have played a crucial role in the development of this book. Without their invaluable contributions this book wouldn't have been possible. They have made vital efforts to compile up to date information on the varied aspects of this subject to make this book a valuable addition to the collection of many professionals and students.

This book was conceptualized with the vision of imparting up-to-date information and advanced data in this field. To ensure the same, a matchless editorial board was set up. Every individual on the board went through rigorous rounds of assessment to prove their worth. After which they invested a large part of their time researching and compiling the most relevant data for our readers.

The editorial board has been involved in producing this book since its inception. They have spent rigorous hours researching and exploring the diverse topics which have resulted in the successful publishing of this book. They have passed on their knowledge of decades through this book. To expedite this challenging task, the publisher supported the team at every step. A small team of assistant editors was also appointed to further simplify the editing procedure and attain best results for the readers.

Apart from the editorial board, the designing team has also invested a significant amount of their time in understanding the subject and creating the most relevant covers. They scrutinized every image to scout for the most suitable representation of the subject and create an appropriate cover for the book.

The publishing team has been an ardent support to the editorial, designing and production team. Their endless efforts to recruit the best for this project, has resulted in the accomplishment of this book. They are a veteran in the field of academics and their pool of knowledge is as vast as their experience in printing. Their expertise and guidance has proved useful at every step. Their uncompromising quality standards have made this book an exceptional effort. Their encouragement from time to time has been an inspiration for everyone.

The publisher and the editorial board hope that this book will prove to be a valuable piece of knowledge for researchers, students, practitioners and scholars across the globe.

List of Contributors

Sibelle Nogueira Buonora, Sonia Regina Lambert Passos, Fernanda Moisés Quintela, Diana Neves Rodrigues de Oliveira and Yara Hahr Marques Hökerberg
Laboratory of Clinical Epidemiology, Evandro Chagas National Institute of Infectious Diseases, Oswaldo Cruz Foundation, Rio de Janeiro, Brazil

Cleber Nascimento do Carmo
National School of Public Health, Oswaldo Cruz Foundation, Rio de Janeiro, Brazil

Regina Paiva Daumas
Germano Sinval Faria Teaching Primary Care Center, National School of Public Health, Oswaldo Cruz Foundation, Rio de Janeiro, Brazil

Flavia Barreto dos Santos and Rita Maria Ribeiro Nogueira
Flavivirus Laboratory, Oswaldo Cruz Institute, Oswaldo Cruz Foundation, Rio de Janeiro, Brazil

Felipe Maia de Toledo Piza, Thiago Domingos Corrêa, Alexandre Rodrigues Marra, João Carlos Campos Guerra, Andrea Aparecida Rocco Villarinho, Valdir Fernandes de Aranda, Sandra Christina Pereira Lima Shiramizo and Maria Roza de Jesus de Lima
Department of Intensive Care Medicine, Hospital Israelita Albert Einstein, Av. Albert Einstein, 627/701, 5° andar, São Paulo CEP: 05651-901, Brazil

Roseny dos Reis Rodrigues
Department of Intensive Care Medicine, Hospital Israelita Albert Einstein, Av. Albert Einstein, 627/701, 5° andar, São Paulo CEP: 05651-901, Brazil
Hospital das Clinicas da Faculdade de Medicina da Universidade de São Paulo, São Paulo, Brazil

Esper Georges Kallas and Alexandre Biasi Cavalcanti
Hospital das Clinicas da Faculdade de Medicina da Universidade de São Paulo, São Paulo, Brazil

Ai Li Quake
Infectious Diseases Programme, Saw Swee Hock School of Public Health, National University of Singapore, Singapore, Singapore

Arnaud Tarantola and Anne Rachline
Epidemiology Unit, Institut Pasteur du Cambodge, Phnom Penh, Cambodia

Yee Sin Leo
Infectious Diseases Programme, Saw Swee Hock School of Public Health, National University of Singapore, Singapore, Singapore
Institute of Infectious Disease and Epidemiology, Tan Tock Seng Hospital, Singapore, Singapore

Moniboth Duch and Yuvatha Kdan
National Paediatric Hospital, Phnom Penh, Cambodia

Rekol Huy
National Dengue Control Program (NDCP), National Center for Parasitological, Entomology and Malaria Control, Ministry of Health, Phnom Penh, Cambodia

Veasna Duong
Virology Unit, Institut Pasteur in Cambodia, Phnom Penh, Cambodia

Jeremy L. Brett
Medical Affairs Department, Sanofi Pasteur, Singapore, Singapore
Takeda Vaccines Pte Ltd., Singapore, Singapore

Philippe Cavailler
Infectious Diseases Programme, Saw Swee Hock School of Public Health, National University of Singapore, Singapore, Singapore
Agence de Médecine Préventive, 13 Chemin du Levant, Ferney-Voltaire 01210, France

Andrew A. Lover
Infectious Diseases Programme, Saw Swee Hock School of Public Health, National University of Singapore, Singapore, Singapore
Global Health Group, University of California, San Francisco, USA

Philippe Buchy
Virology Unit, Institut Pasteur in Cambodia, Phnom Penh, Cambodia
GlaxoSmithKline vaccines, 150 Beach road, Singapore, Singapore

Nathália Barbosa Furlan and Caroline Tukasan
Faculdade de Medicina, União das Faculdades dos Grandes Lagos, São José do Rio Preto, São Paulo, Brazil

Cássia Fernanda Estofolete
Faculdade de Medicina, União das Faculdades dos Grandes Lagos, São José do Rio Preto, São Paulo, Brazil
Laboratório de Pesquisas em Virologia, Faculdade de Medicina de São José do Rio Preto, São Paulo, Brazil

Maurício Lacerda Nogueira
Laboratório de Pesquisas em Virologia, Faculdade de Medicina de São José do Rio Preto, São Paulo, Brazil

Natal Santos da Silva
Faculdade de Medicina, União das Faculdades dos Grandes Lagos, São José do Rio Preto, São Paulo, Brazil
Laboratório de Pesquisas em Virologia, Faculdade de Medicina de São José do Rio Preto, São Paulo, Brazil
Laboratório de Modelagens Matemática e Estatística em Medicina, União das Faculdades dos Grandes Lagos, São José do Rio Preto, São Paulo, Brazil
Laboratório de Modelagens Matemática e Estatística em Medicina, Faculdade de Medicina, União das Faculdades dos Grandes Lagos, Rua Dr. Eduardo Nielsem, 960 Jardim Novo Aeroporto, São Jose do Rio Preto, São Paulo CEP 15030-070, Brazil

Eduardo Fernández and Stephen D. Walter
Department of Clinical Epidemiology and Biostatistics, McMaster University, Hamilton, Ontario, Canada

Marek Smieja and Mark Loeb
Department of Clinical Epidemiology and Biostatistics, McMaster University, Hamilton, Ontario, Canada
Department of Pathology and Molecular Medicine, McMaster University, Hamilton, Ontario, Canada
Institute for Infectious Diseases Research, McMaster University, Hamilton, Ontario, Canada

Samitha Fernando, Laksiri Gomes, Chameera T. Punchihewa and S. D. P. Madusanka
Department of Microbiology, Centre for Dengue Research, Faculty of Medical Sciences, University of Sri Jayewardenepura, Nugegoda 10250, Sri Lanka

Gathsaurie Neelika Malavige
Department of Microbiology, Centre for Dengue Research, Faculty of Medical Sciences, University of Sri Jayewardenepura, Nugegoda 10250, Sri Lanka
MRC Human Immunology Unit, Weatherall Institute of Molecular Medicine, Oxford NIHR Biomedical Research Centre and University of Oxford, Oxford OX3 9DS, UK

Harsha Dissanayake
Department of Anatomy, Faculty of Medical Sciences, University of Sri Jayewardenepura, Nugegoda 10250, Sri Lanka

Chandima Jeewandara
Department of Family Medicine, Faculty of Medical Sciences, University of Sri Jayewardenepura, Nugegoda 10250, Sri Lanka

Hemantha Peiris
Department of Biochemistry, Faculty of Medical Sciences, University of Sri Jayewardenepura, Nugegoda 10250, Sri Lanka

Ananda Wijewickrama
Infectious Diseases Hospital, Angoda, Sri Lanka

Graham S. Ogg
MRC Human Immunology Unit, Weatherall Institute of Molecular Medicine, Oxford NIHR Biomedical Research Centre and University of Oxford, Oxford OX3 9DS, UK

Sibelle Nogueira Buonora and Sonia Regina Lambert Passos
National Institute of Infectious Diseases Evandro Chagas, Laboratory of Clinical Epidemiology, Oswaldo Cruz Foundation, Av. Brasil, 4036 sala 201 A - Manguinhos, Rio de Janeiro CEP: 21040-361, Brazil

Flavia Barreto dos Santos, Manoela Heringer da Silva, Monique Rocha de Lima and Rita Maria Ribeiro Nogueira
Oswaldo Cruz Institute, Instituto Oswaldo Cruz - Pavilhão Hélio e Peggy Pereira, Flavivirus Laboratory, Oswaldo Cruz Foundation, Avenida Brasil, 4365, Manguinhos, Rio de Janeiro CEP: 21040-900, Brazil

Regina Paiva Daumas
Germano Sinval Faria Teaching Primary Care Center, National School of Public Health, Oswaldo Cruz Foundation, Rua Leopoldo Bulhões, 1480 - Bonsucesso, Rio de Janeiro CEP: 21041-210, Brazil

Pui-Jen Tsai
Center for General Education, Aletheia University, New Taipei City 25103, Taiwan, ROC

Hwa-Jen Teng
Center for Diagnostics and Vaccine Development, Centers for Disease Control, Taipei, Taiwan, ROC

Hu Suk Lee and Hung Nguyen-Viet
International Livestock Research Institute, Regional Office for East and Southeast Asia, Room 301-302, B1 Building, Van Phuc Diplomatic Compound,298 Kim Ma Street, Ba Dinh District, Hanoi, Vietnam

Vu Sinh Nam
Vector Borne Diseases and Training, National Institute of Hygiene and Epidemiology, Hanoi, Vietnam

Mihye Lee
Medical microbiology Department, The Royal Bournemouth Hospital, Bournemouth, UK

Sungho Won
Graduate School of Public Health, Seoul National University, Seoul, Korea
Interdisciplinary Program of Bioinformatics, Seoul National University, Seoul, Korea
Institute of Health and Environment, Seoul National University, Seoul, Korea

Phuc Pham Duc
Center for Public Health and Ecosystem Research (CENPHER), Hanoi School of Public Health, Hanoi, Vietnam

Delia Grace
International Livestock Research Institute, Nairobi, Kenya

Lucimeire Antonelli da Silveira and Adriana Oliveira Guilarde
Institute of Tropical Pathology and Public Health of Federal University of Goiás, Rua 235, St Universitário, Goiânia 74.605-050, GO, Brazil

Celina Maria Turchi Martelli
Institute of Tropical Pathology and Public Health of Federal University of Goiás, Rua 235, St Universitário, Goiânia 74.605-050, GO, Brazil
Centro de Pesquisas Aggeu Magalhães da Fundação Oswaldo, Av. Prof. Moraes Rego, 1235, Cidade Universitária, 50.670-901 Recife, PE, Brazil

Angela Ferreira Lopes de Teive e Argolo
Institute of Tropical Pathology and Public Health of Federal University of Goiás, Rua 235, St Universitário, Goiânia 74.605-050, GO, Brazil
Public Health Laboratory of Secretaria Estadual de Saúde de Goiás (LACEN-GO), Av. Contorno, 3.556, Jd. Bela Vista, 74.853-120 Goiânia, GO, Brazil

Valéria Christina de Rezende Féres
Pharmacy College of Federal University of Goiás, Av. Universitaria, St. Universitario, 74.605-220 Goiânia, GO, Brazil

Marli Tenório Cordeiro and Wayner Vieira de Souza
Centro de Pesquisas Aggeu Magalhães da Fundação Oswaldo, Av. Prof. Moraes Rego, 1235, Cidade Universitária, 50.670-901 Recife, PE, Brazil

Ernesto Torres de Azevedo Marques Jr.
Centro de Pesquisas Aggeu Magalhães da Fundação Oswaldo, Av. Prof. Moraes Rego, 1235, Cidade Universitária, 50.670-901 Recife, PE, Brazil
Center for Vaccine Research, Department of Infectious Diseases and Microbiology, University of Pittsburgh, Pittsburgh, PA, USA

Yuan Chen and Zhong Min Liu
Department of Laboratory Medicine, The First Affiliated Hospital of Guangzhou Medical University, Guangdong, China

Yong Ping Lin
Department of Laboratory Medicine, The First Affiliated Hospital of Guangzhou Medical University, Guangdong, China
Research Centre of Translational Medicine, The First Affiliated Hospital of Guangzhou Medical University, Guangdong, China

Qiang Zhou and Xiao Han Yang
Department of Laboratory Medicine, The Second Affiliated Hospital of Guangzhou University of Chinese Medicine, Guangdong, China

Mart Matthias Lamers, Sumana Sanyal and Chris Ka Pun Mok
HKU-Pasteur Research Pole, School of Public Health, HKU Li Ka Shing Faculty of Medicine, The University of Hong Kong, Hong Kong, China

Yasha Luo
Department of Laboratory Medicine, The Second Affiliated Hospital of Guangzhou University of Chinese Medicine, Guangdong, China
Department of Laboratory Medicine, Guangdong Women and Children Hospital, Guangzhou, China

Tian Tang, Liu Zhang, Gang Chen, Jing Yu, Fu-Qiang Zhang and Quan-Shui Fan
Center for Disease Control and Prevention, Chengdu Military Region, 168 Daguan Road, Kunming 650032, People's Republic of China

Hai-Lin Zhang
Center for Disease Control and Prevention, Chengdu Military Region, 168 Daguan Road, Kunming 650032, People's Republic of China
Yunnan Institute of Endemic Diseases Control and Prevention, Dali, Yunnan, People's Republic of China

Yun Feng
Yunnan Institute of Endemic Diseases Control and Prevention, Dali, Yunnan, People's Republic of China

Jian-Hua Fan, Jin Zu, Hong-Bin Li and Yuan-Yuan Li
Xishuangbanna Center for Disease Control and Prevention, Jinghong, Yunnan, People's Republic of China

Yong-Hua Liu and Xiao-Xiong Yin
Ruili Center for Disease Control and Prevention, Ruili, Yunnan, People's Republic of China

Hua-Chang Li
Lincang Center for Disease Control and Prevention, Lincang, Yunnan, People's Republic of China

Ting-Song Hu
Center for Disease Control and Prevention, Chengdu Military Region, 168 Daguan Road, Kunming 650032, People's Republic of China
The Postdoctoral Programme of Kunming General Hospital, Chengdu Military Region, Kunming, People's Republic of China

Thaker A. A. Alyousefi
Department of Hematology, Faculty of Medical Sciences, Al-Razi University, Sana'a, Yemen

Samira M. A. Al-Eryani and Abdulsalam M. Al-Mekhlafi
Department of Parasitology, Faculty of Medicine and Health Sciences, Sana'a University, Sana'a, Yemen

Rashad Abdul-Ghani and Mohammed A. K. Mahdy
Department of Parasitology, Faculty of Medicine and Health Sciences, Sana'a University, Sana'a, Yemen
Tropical Disease Research Center, University of Science and Technology, Sana'a, Yemen

Yahia A. Raja
Faculty of Public Health and Informatics, Umm Al-Qura University, Mecca, Saudi Arabia

Shamusul Azhar Shah
Department of Community Health, Universiti Kebangsaan Malaysia Medical Centre, Kuala Lumpur, Malaysia

John C. Beier
Department of Public Health Sciences, University of Miami Miller School of Medicine, Miami, FL, USA

Chee Fu Yung
Infectious Disease Service, Department of Paediatrics, KK Women's and Children's Hospital, Singapore, Singapore
Communicable Disease Centre, Institute of Infectious Diseases and Epidemiology, Tan Tock Seng Hospital, Singapore, Singapore

Siew Pang Chan
Department of Medicine, Yong Loo Lin School of Medicine, National University of Singapore, Singapore, Singapore
Faculty of Science, Technology and Engineering, La Trobe University, Melbourne, Australia

Tun Linn Thein and Siaw Ching Chai
Communicable Disease Centre, Institute of Infectious Diseases and Epidemiology, Tan Tock Seng Hospital, Singapore, Singapore

Caroline Tukasan and Nathália Barbosa Furlan
Faculdade de Medicina, União das Faculdades dos Grandes Lagos, São José do Rio Preto, São Paulo, Brazil

Yee Sin Leo
Department of Medicine, Yong Loo Lin School of Medicine, National University of Singapore, Singapore, Singapore
Communicable Disease Centre, Institute of Infectious Diseases and Epidemiology, Tan Tock Seng Hospital, Singapore, Singapore
Lee Kong Chian School of Medicine, Nanyang Technological University Singapore, Singapore, Singapore
Saw Swee Hock School of Public Health, National University Singapore, Singapore, Singapore

Cássia Fernanda Estofolete and Maurício Lacerda Nogueira
Laboratório de Pesquisas em Virologia, Faculdade de Medicina de São José do Rio Preto, São José do Rio Preto, São Paulo, Brazil

Natal Santos da Silva
Faculdade de Medicina, União das Faculdades dos Grandes Lagos, São José do Rio Preto, São Paulo, Brazil
Laboratório de Pesquisas em Virologia, Faculdade de Medicina de São José do Rio Preto, São José do Rio Preto, São Paulo, Brazil
Laboratório de Modelagens Matemática e Estatística em Medicina, Faculdade de Medicina, União das Faculdades dos Grandes Lagos, São José do Rio Preto, São Paulo, Brazil

Kuan-Ting Liu
Graduate Institute of Clinical Medicine, College of Medicine, Kaohsiung Medical University, No.100, Shih-Chuan 1st Road, Kaohsiung 807, Taiwan
Department of Emergency Medicine, Kaohsiung Medical University Hospital, Kaohsiung Medical University, No.100, Tzyou 1st Road, Kaohsiung 807, Taiwan
School of Medicine, College of Medicine, Kaohsiung Medical University, Kaohsiung 807, Taiwan

Yao-Hua Liu and Meng-Chi Yen
Department of Emergency Medicine, Kaohsiung Medical University Hospital, Kaohsiung Medical University, No.100, Tzyou 1st Road, Kaohsiung 807, Taiwan

Chun-Yu Lin
School of Medicine, College of Medicine, Kaohsiung Medical University, Kaohsiung 807, Taiwan
Division of Infectious Diseases, Department of Internal Medicine, Kaohsiung Medical University Hospital, Kaohsiung Medical University, Kaohsiung 807, Taiwan

Ming-Ju Tsai
Division of Pulmonary and Critical Care Medicine, Kaohsiung Medical University Hospital, Kaohsiung Medical University, Kaohsiung 807, Taiwan

Ya-Ling Hsu
Graduate Institute of Medicine, College of Medicine, Kaohsiung Medical University, Kaohsiung 807, Taiwan

Po-Lin Kuo
Graduate Institute of Clinical Medicine, College of Medicine, Kaohsiung Medical University, No.100, Shih-Chuan 1st Road, Kaohsiung 807, Taiwan
Institute of Medical Science and Technology, National Sun Yat-Sen University, Kaohsiung 804, Taiwan

Manoela Heringer, Thiara Manuele A Souza, Monique da Rocha Q Lima, Priscila Conrado G Nunes, Nieli Rodrigues da C Faria, Fernanda de Bruycker-Nogueira, Thaís Chouin-Carneiro and Flavia Barreto dos Santos
Viral Immunology Laboratory, Oswaldo Cruz Institute/FIOCRUZ, Av Brasil 4365, Manguinhos, Rio de Janeiro, RJ 21045-360, Brazil

Rita Maria R Nogueira
Flavivirus Laboratory, Oswaldo Cruz Institute, Rio de Janeiro, Brazil

Getachew Ferede, Moges Tiruneh, Yitayih Wondimeneh and Belay Tessema
Department of Medical Microbiology, School of Biomedical and Laboratory Sciences, College of Medicine and Health Sciences, University of Gondar, Gondar, Ethiopia

Ebba Abate
Ethiopian Public Health Institute, Addis Ababa, Ethiopia

Endalamaw Gadisa, Rawleigh Howe and Abraham Aseffa
Armauer Hansen Research Institute, Addis Ababa, Ethiopia

Saiful Safuan Md Sani, Winn Hui Han, Hui Jen Ding and Kiah Loon Ng
Department of Medicine, Hospital Kuala Lumpur, Jalan Pahang, 50586 Kuala Lumpur, Malaysia

Mohamad Adam Bujang
Biostatistic Unit, National Clinical Research Centre, 1st Floor, MMA Building, 124 Jalan Pahang, 53000 Kuala Lumpur, Malaysia

Mohd Azizuddin Amir Shariffuddin
Clinical Research Centre, Hospital Kuala Lumpur, Jalan Pahang, 50586 Kuala Lumpur, Malaysia

Eduardo Fernández and Stephen D. Walter
Department of Clinical Epidemiology and Biostatistics, McMaster University, Hamilton, ON, Canada

Marek Smieja and Mark Loeb
Department of Clinical Epidemiology and Biostatistics, McMaster University, Hamilton, ON, Canada
Department of Pathology and Molecular Medicine, Institute for Infectious
Disease Research McMaster University, Hamilton, ON, Canada

Judith Kirstein
Advanced Clinical Research, West Jordan, UT, USA

William Douglas
Benchmark Research, Sacramento, CA, USA

Manoj Thakur and Mark Boaz
Sanofi Pasteur, Global Clinical Immunology, Discovery Drive, Swiftwater, PA 18370, USA

Thomas Papa, Anna Skipetrova and Eric Plennevaux
Sanofi Pasteur, Siège Social, 14 Espace Henry Vallée, 69007 Lyon, France

Tun Linn Thein and Jing Jin
Institute of Infectious Diseases and Epidemiology, Tan Tock Seng Hospital, 144 Moulmein Road, Singapore 308089, Singapore

Junxiong Pang
Institute of Infectious Diseases and Epidemiology, Tan Tock Seng Hospital, 144 Moulmein Road, Singapore 308089, Singapore
Saw Swee Hock School of Public Health, National University of Singapore, Singapore, Singapore

Zoe Jane-Lara Hildon
Saw Swee Hock School of Public Health, National University of Singapore, Singapore, Singapore
Johns Hopkins Center for Communication Programs, Johns Hopkins University, Baltimore, USA
Department of Global Health and Development, Faculty of Public Health & Policy, London School of Hygiene and Tropical Medicine, London, UK

Yee Sin Leo
Institute of Infectious Diseases and Epidemiology, Tan Tock Seng Hospital, 144 Moulmein Road, Singapore 308089, Singapore
Saw Swee Hock School of Public Health, National University of Singapore, Singapore, Singapore
Yong Loo Lin School of Medicine, National University of Singapore, Singapore, Singapore
Lee Kong Chian School of Medicine, Nanyang Technological University, Singapore, Singapore

S. A. M. Kularatne, Udaya Ralapanawa, Chamara Dalugama, Jayanika Jayasinghe, M. M Rajapakse, L. P. M. M. K. Pathirage and Sawandika Rupasinghe
Department of Medicine, Faculty of Medicine University of Peradeniya, Peradeniya, Sri Lanka

Prabashini Kumarihamy
Teaching Hospital Peradeniya, Peradeniya, Sri Lanka

B. V. K. M. Bopeththa
Registrar in Emergency Medicine, Teaching Hospital Kandy, Kandy, Sri Lanka

Sardha Hemapriya, K. K. Gayan Niranga and Danushka S. K. Kotigala
Consultant Obstetrician and Gynaecologist, Teaching Hospital Kandy, Kandy, Sri Lanka

R. Waduge
Department of Pathology, Faculty of Medicine, University of Peradeniya, Peradeniya, Sri Lanka

R. P. V. J. Rajapakse
Department of Veterinary Pathobiology, Faculty of Veterinary Medicine and Animal Science, University of Peradeniya, Peradeniya, Sri Lanka

Verónica Elizabeth Mata, Sonia Regina Lambert Passos, Yara Hahr Marques Hökerberg, Guilherme Miguéis Berardinelli, Levy Vilas Boas Fukuoka, Anna Carolina Fontoura Seixas Rangel Maciel and Raquel de Vasconcellos Carvalhaes de Oliveira
Av. Brasil 4036 sala 201 A, CEP 21040-361 Rio de Janeiro, RJ, Brasil

Maria Angelica Borges dos Santos
Rua Leopoldo Bulhões 1480 sala 601, Rio de Janeiro, RJ CEP 21040-361, Brazil

Cintia Damasceno dos Santos Rodrigues and Aline da Silva Santos
Av. Brasil 4365, CEP 21040-360 Rio de Janeiro, RJ, Brasil

James Whitehorn
Department of Clinical Research, London School of Hygiene and Tropical Medicine, London, UK
Oxford University Clinical Research Unit, Hospital for Tropical Diseases, 764 Vo Van Kiet, District 5, Ho Chi Minh City, Viet Nam

Duong Thi Hue Kien and Nguyen Than Ha Quyen
Oxford University Clinical Research Unit, Hospital for Tropical Diseases, 764 Vo Van Kiet, District 5, Ho Chi Minh City, Viet Nam

Bridget Wills
Oxford University Clinical Research Unit, Hospital for Tropical Diseases, 764 Vo Van Kiet, District 5, Ho Chi Minh City, Viet Nam
Centre for Tropical Medicine, Nuffield Department of Medicine, University of Oxford, Oxford, UK

Nguyen Van Vinh Chau and Dong Thi Hoai Tam
Hospital for Tropical Diseases, 764 Vo Van Kiet, District 5, Ho Chi Minh City, Viet Nam

Nguyen Minh Tuan
Children Hospital Number 1, Ho Chi Minh City, Viet Nam

Thomas Jaenisch
Department of Infectious Diseases, Heidelberg University Hospital, Heidelberg, Germany

Martin Hibberd
Department of Clinical Research, London School of Hygiene and Tropical Medicine, London, UK
Genome Institute of Singapore, Biopolis Way, Singapore, Singapore

Chiea Chuen Khor
School of Public Health, National University of Singapore, Singapore, Singapore
Department of Paediatrics, National University of Singapore, Singapore, Singapore
Department of Ophthalmology, National University of Singapore, Singapore, Singapore

Cameron P. Simmons
Department of Microbiology and Immunology, University of Melbourne, at the Peter Doherty Institute, Melbourne, VIC 3010, Australia

Index

www.ingramcontent.com/pod-product-compliance
Lightning Source LLC
LaVergne TN
LVHW080724210926
848485LV00003B/515